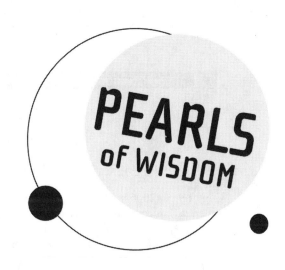

USMLE
Step 2 and Step 3
REVIEW

Second Edition

Scott H. Plantz
Gillian Emblad
Peter Emblad
Nicholas Lorenzo

McGraw-Hill
Medical Publishing Division

New York Chicago San Francisco Lisbon London
Madrid Mexico City Milan New Delhi
San Juan Seoul Singapore
Sydney Toronto

USMLE Step 2 and Step 3 Review, Second Edition

Copyright © 2006 by The McGraw-Hill Companies, Inc. All rights reserved. Printed in the United States of America. Except as permitted under the United States Copyright Act of 1976, no part of this publication may be reproduced or distributed in any form or by any means, or stored in a data base or retrieval system, without the prior written permission of the publisher.

1 2 3 4 5 6 7 8 9 0   CUS/CUS   0 9 8 7 6 5

ISBN 0-07-146455-7

The editors were Catherine A. Johnson and Marsha Loeb.
The production supervisor was Phil Galea.
The cover designer was Handel Low
Von Hoffmann Graphics was printer and binder.

This book is printed on acid-free paper.

Cataloging-in-Publication data for this title is on file at the Library of Congress.

INTERNATIONAL EDITION ISBN: 0-07-110895-5

DEDICATION

To my mother, Pauline Plantz, for all her love, kindness, and support.

Scott H. Plantz

To Peter, I am both honored and thrilled to spend the rest of my life with you. Watch out world, here we come!

Gillian Emblad

To Bermt amd Omga-Karin Emblad, my close friends and grandparents. Thank you for helping me achieve my dream, and inspiring me to keep on dreaming.

Peter Emblad

To my wife Anne, my son Adam, and to my two wonderful parents

Nicholas Lorenzo

EDITORS:

Scott H. Plantz, MD
Associate Professor
Chicago Medical School
Mt. Sinai Medical Center
Chicago, IL

Gillian Emblad, PA-C, MA
Physician Assistant
Summit Medical Center
Oakland, CA

Peter Emblad, MD
Kaiser Permanente
San Francisco, CA

Nicholas Lorenzo, MD
Founding Editor-in-Chief
eMedicine Neurology Online Reference
Founder, Neurological Consulting
of Nebraska, Kansas, and Minnesota

CONTRIBUTING AUTHORS:

Bobby Abrams, MD
Attending Physician
Macomb Hospital
Macomb, MI

Jonathan Adler, MD
Instructor of Medicine
Harvard Medical School
Boston, MA

David F. M. Brown, MD
Instructor in Medicine
Harvard Medical School
Massachusetts General Hospital
Boston, MA

Eduardo Castro, MD
Instructor in Medicine
Harvard Medical School
Massachusetts General Hospital
Boston, MA

C. James Corrall, MD, MPH
Clinical Associate Professor
University of Illinois College of Medicine
Peoria, IL

Leslie S. Carroll, MD
Assistant Professor
Chicago Medical School
Toxicology Director

Carl W. Decker, MD
Madigan Army Medical Center
Fort Lewis, WA

Craig Feied, MD
Clinical Associate Professor
George Washington University
Washington Hospital Center

William Gossman, MD
Chicago Medical School
Mt. Sinai Medical Center
Chicago, IL

James F. Holmes, MD
University of California, Davis
School of Medicine
Sacramento, CA

Eddie Hooker, MD
Assistant Professor
University of Louisville
Louisville, KY

Lance W. Kreplick, MD
Assistant Professor
University of Illinois
EHS Christ Hospital
Oak Lawn, IL

Bernard Lopez, MD
Assistant Professor
Thomas Jefferson Medical College
Thomas Jefferson University Hospital
Philadelphia, PA

Mary Nan S. Mallory, MD
Instructor
University of Louisville
Louisville, KY

David Morgan, MD
University of Texas
Southwestern Medical Center
Parkland Memorial Hospital
Dallas, TX

Edward A. Panacek, MD
Associate Professor
University of California, Davis
School of Medicine
Sacramento, CA

Karen Rhodes, MD
University of Chicago Medical Center
Chicago, IL

Carlo Rosen, MD
Instructor in Medicine
Harvard Medical School
Massachusetts General Hospital
Boston, MA

Dana Stearns, MD
Instructor in Medicine
Harvard Medical School
Massachusetts General Hospital
Boston, MA

Jack Stump, MD
Attending Physician
Rogue Valley Medical Center
Medford, OR

Joan Surdukowski, MD
Assistant Professor
Chicago Medical School
Mt. Sinai Hospital
Chicago, IL

Introduction

Congratulations! *USMLE Step 2 and Step 3 Review: Pearls of Wisdom* will help you learn some medicine. Originally designed as a study aid to improve performance on the USMLE Step 2 and Step 3, this book is full of useful information. A few words are appropriate discussing intent, format, limitations, and use.

Since *USMLE Step 2 and Step 3 Review* is primarily intended as a study aid, the text is written in rapid-fire question/answer format. This way, readers receive immediate gratification. Moreover, misleading or confusing "foils" are not provided. This eliminates the risk of erroneously assimilating an incorrect piece of information that makes a big impression. Questions themselves often contain a "pearl" intended to reinforce the answer. Additional "hooks" may be attached to the answer in various forms, including mnemonics, visual imagery, repetition, and humor. Additional information not requested in the question may be included in the answer. Emphasis has been placed on distilling trivia and key facts that are easily overlooked, that are quickly forgotten, and that somehow seem to be needed on board examinations.

Many questions have answers without explanations. This enhances ease of reading and rate of learning. Explanations often occur in a later question/answer. Upon reading an answer, the reader may think, "Hm, why is that?" or, "Are you sure?" If this happens to you, go check! Truly assimilating these disparate facts into a framework of knowledge absolutely requires further reading on the surrounding concepts. Information learned in response to seeking an answer to a particular question is retained much better than information that is passively observed. Take advantage of this! Use this book with your preferred source texts handy and open.

The first half of the text is presented in topic areas found on the *USMLE Steps 2 and 3* examinations. Information presented is mostly limited to straightforward, basic facts. The second section of the book, "Random Pearls," consists of questions grouped into small clusters by topic, presented in no particular order. This section repeats some of the factual information previously covered and builds on this foundation with emphasis on linking information and filling in gaps from the topical chapters.

USMLE Step 2 and Step 3 Review has limitations. We have found many conflicts between sources of information. We have tried to verify in several references the most accurate information. Some texts have internal discrepancies further confounding clarification.

USMLE Step 2 and Step 3 Review risks accuracy by aggressively pruning complex concepts down to the simplest kernel—the dynamic knowledge base and clinical practice of family medicine is not like that! Furthermore, new research and practice occasionally deviates from that which likely represents the right answer for test purposes. This text is designed to maximize your score on a test. Refer to your most current sources of information and mentors for direction for practice.

USMLE Step 2 and Step 3 Review is designed to be used, not just read. It is an interactive text. Use a 3 x 5 card and cover the answers; attempt all questions. A study method we recommend is oral group study, preferably over an extended meal or pitchers. The mechanics of this method are simple and no one ever appears stupid.
One person holds <u>Pearls</u>, with answers covered, and reads the question. Each person, including the reader, says "Check!" when he or she has an answer in mind. After everyone has "checked" in, someone states his/her answer. If this answer is correct, on to the next one; if not, another person says their answer or the answer can be read. Usually the person who "checks" in first receives the first shot at stating the answer. If this person is being a smarty-pants answer-hog, then others can take turns. Try it, it's almost fun!

USMLE Step 2 and Step 3 Review is also designed to be re-used several times to allow, dare we use the word, memorization. A hollow bullet is provided for any scheme of keeping track of questions answered correctly or incorrectly.

We welcome your comments, suggestions and criticism. Great effort has been made to verify these questions and answers. Some answers may not be the answer you would prefer. Most often this is attributable to variance between original sources. Please make us aware of any errors you find. We hope to make continuous improvements and would greatly appreciate any input with regard to format, organization, content, presentation, or about specific questions. We look forward to hearing from you!

Study hard and good luck!

S.H.P., G.E., P.E., & N.L.

TABLE OF CONTENTS

INTERNAL
MEDICINE
PEARLS

CARDIOVASCULAR

○ **Are aortic aneurysms more common in men or women?**

Men (10:1). Other risk factors include hypertension, atherosclerosis, diabetes, hyperlipidemia, smoking, syphilis, Marfan's disease, and Ehlers-Danlos disease.

○ **A patient presents with sudden-onset chest and back pain. Further workup reveals an ischemic right leg. What is your diagnosis?**

Suspect an acute aortic dissection when chest or back pain is associated with ischemic or neurologic deficits.

○ **What physical findings suggest an acute aortic dissection?**

Blood pressure differences between arms and/or legs, cardiac tamponade, and aortic insufficiency murmur.

○ **What CXR findings occur with a thoracic aortic aneurysm?**

Change in aortic appearance, mediastinal widening, hump in the aortic arch, pleural effusion (most commonly on the left), and extension of the aortic shadow.

○ **A 74-year-old male presents with acute-onset testicular pain. Ecchymosis is present in the groin and scrotal sac. What is the diagnosis?**

A ruptured aortic or iliac artery aneurysm.

○ **What x-ray study should be ordered for a patient with an abdominal mass and a suspected ruptured AAA?**

None. The patient should go to the OR immediately. About 60% of AAAs occur with calcification and appear on a lateral abdominal x-ray.

○ **What may an x-ray of a patient with an aortic dissection reveal?**

Widening of the superior mediastinum, a hazy or enlarged aortic knob, an irregular aortic contour, separation of the intimal calcification from the outer aortic contour that is greater than 5 mm, a displaced trachea to the right, and cardiomegaly.

○ **What is the most common symptom of aortic dissection?**

Interscapular back pain.

○ **Where do aortic dissections most often occur?**

Proximal ascending aorta (60%). Twenty percent of aortic dissections are found between the origin of the left subclavian and the ligamentum arteriosum in the descending aorta, and 10% are found in the aortic arch or the abdominal aorta. Dissection involves intimal tears propagated by hematoma formation.

○   **What aortic aneurysm diameter is generally considered to be an indication for surgery: a) in the thorax and b) in the abdomen?**

Those with non-dissecting thoracic aneurysm larger than 7 cm in diameter are candidates for surgery. However, surgery should be considered with smaller aneurysms for those with Marfan's syndrome, because of a higher incidence of rupture. Non-dissecting abdominal aortic aneurysms larger than 4 cm in diameter should be considered for surgical repair.

○   **Describe DeBakey's classification of aortic dissections.**

Type I: Dissection of the aortic root, arch, and descending aorta
Type II: Ascending aorta only
Type III: Distal aorta only

○   **Describe the Stanford classification of aortic dissections.**

Stanford Type A: Involve ascending aorta.
Stanford Type B: Do not involve ascending aorta.

○   **What dissections can be treated medically?**

Patients with Type B (and DeBakey's Type III) are eligible for medical, rather than, surgical treatment. Surgical treatment may be required for those with uncontrollable pain, aortic bleeding, hemodynamic instability, increasing hematoma size, or an impending rupture.

○   **What is the prognosis for an untreated aortic dissection?**

20% of afflicted individuals die within 24 hours, 60% within 2 weeks, and 90% within 3 months. With surgical treatment, the 10 year survival rate is 40%. Redissection occurs in 25% of these patients within 10 years of the original episode.

○   **What murmur is expected in patients with substantial aortic stenosis?**

A prolonged, harsh, loud (IV, V, or VI) systolic murmur.

○   **Where is the most common site of peripheral aneurysms that develop from arteriosclerosis?**

The popliteal artery. Other sites include the femoral, carotid, and subclavian arteries.

○   **How long can ST and T changes persist after an episode of pain in unstable angina?**

Several hours.

○   **Among those with Marfan's syndrome, at what age does aortic aneurysm become problematic?**

Thirties and forties.

○   **Matching:**

1) Quincke's pulse   a) Uvular pulsation during systole
2) Corrigan's pulse   b) Head bobbing
3) de Musset's sign   c) Visible pulsations in nail bed capillaries
4) Muller's sign   d) Femoral artery murmurs during systole if the artery is compressed
                                 proximally and during diastole if the artery is compressed distally
5) Duroziez's sign   e) Collapsing pulse
6) Pulsus paradoxus   f) Drop in the systolic blood pressure > 10 mm Hg with inspiration

Answers: (1) c, (2) e, (3) b, (4) a, (5) d, and (6) f. These are all signs pertaining to aortic insufficiency.

○   **What is the most common cause of aortic regurgitation in children?**

Aortic valve prolapse associated with a congenital ventricular septal defect.

○   **What is the most common cause of aortic regurgitation in adults?**

Mild aortic regurgitation frequently develops as a result of a bicuspid aortic valve. A severe aortic regurgitation is induced by rheumatic heart disease, syphilis, endocarditis, trauma, an idiopathic degeneration of the aortic valve, a spontaneous rupture of the valve leaflets, or aortic dissection.

○   **What are the signs and symptoms of acute aortic regurgitation?**

Dyspnea, tachycardia, tachypnea, and chest pain.

○   **What is the most common cause of aortic stenosis in patients under age 50? Over age 50?**

Under 50:   Calcification of congenital bicuspid aortic valves (1% of the population has congenital bicuspid valves).
Over 50:   Calcification of degenerating leaflets.

○   **What triad of symptoms characterizes aortic stenosis?**

Syncope, angina, and left heart failure. As the disease progresses, systolic BP decreases and pulse pressure narrows.

○   **What are the clinical findings in a patient with aortic stenosis?**

Angina, dyspnea on exertion, syncope, sustained apical impulse, narrow pulse pressure, parvus et tardus, systolic ejection crescendo-decrescendo murmur that radiates to the neck, systolic ejection click (not heard in severe cases when the valve is so stenosed that it is immobile), paradoxically split S1 and soft S2, and audible S4.

○   **How does a heart murmur reflect the severity of aortic stenosis?**

A longer duration associated with an increasing in intensity indicates severe aortic stenosis. The "loudness" of the murmur is not as important in assessing its severity.

○   **When should surgery be considered for patients with aortic stenosis?**

Only when symptoms are displayed. The risk of morbidity and mortality associated with the replacement of an aortic valve outweighs any benefit of operating on asymptomatic patients.

○   **What are the common causes of multifocal atrial tachycardia?**

COPD, CHF, sepsis, and methylxanthine toxicity. Treat the arrhythmia with magnesium, verapamil, or ß-blocking agents.

○   **How is atrial flutter treated?**

Initiate AV nodal blockade with ß-blockers, calcium channel blockers, or digoxin. If necessary, treat a stable patient with chemical cardioversion by using a class IA agent, such as procainamide or quinidine, fter digitalization. If this treatment fails or if the patient is unstable, electrocardiovert at 25 to 50 J.

O   **What are some causes of atrial fibrillation?**

Hypertension, rheumatic heart disease, pneumonia, thyrotoxicosis, ischemic heart, pericarditis, ethanol intoxication, PE, CHF and COPD.

O   **How is atrial fibrillation treated?**

Control rate with ß-blockade or calcium channel blocker, (such as verapamil or diltiazem) then convert with procainamide, quinidine, or verapamil. Digoxin may be considered, although its effect will be delayed. Synchronized cardioversion at 100 to 200 J should be performed on an unstable patient. In a stable patient with a-fib of unclear duration, anticoagulation should be considered for 2 to 3 weeks prior to chemical or electrical cardioversion. Watch for hypotension with the administration of negative inotropes.

O   **What are some causes of SVT?**

Digitalis toxicity, pericarditis, MI, COPD, pre-excitation syndromes, mitral valve prolapse, rheumatic heart disease, pneumonia, and ethanol.

O   **What mechanism most commonly produces SVTs?**

Reentry. Another common cause is abnormal automaticity. (i.e., ectopic foci).

O   **What is the treatment for SVT caused by digitalis toxicity?**

Stop the digitalis, treat the hypokalemia, and administer magnesium or phenytoin. Provide digoxin specific antibodies to the unstable patient. Avoid cardioversion.

O   **What is the treatment for stable SVT not caused by digitalis toxicity or WPW syndrome?**

Vagal maneuvers, adenosine, verapamil, or ß-blockers.

O   **Describe the key feature of Mobitz I (Wenckebach) second degree AV block.**

A progressive prolongation of the PR interval until the atrial impulse is no longer conducted. If symptomatic, atropine and transcutaneous/transvenous pacing is required.

O   **Describe the key feature of Mobitz II second degree AV block.**

A constant PR interval in which one or more beats fail to conduct.

O   **What is the treatment for Mobitz II second degree AV block?**

Atropine and transcutaneous/transvenous pacing, if symptomatic.

O   **Carotid massage or Valsalva maneuver is useful for slowing supraventricular rhythms. When is carotid massage contraindicated?**

With ventricular arrhythmias, dig toxicity, stroke, syncope, seizures, or in those with a carotid bruit.

O   **What are some common vagal maneuvers?**

Breath holding, valsalva (bearing down as if having a bowel movement,) stimulating of the gag reflex, squatting, pressure on the eyeballs, and immersing the face in cold water.

O   **Which is more common: premature atrial beats or ventricular beats?**

Premature atrial beats. Palpitations that occur because of premature atrial beats are generally benign and asymptomatic. Reassurance is the only treatment. Less frequent but more serious causes of atrial premature beats include pheochromocytoma and thyrotoxicosis. Random PVCs are also benign but common in the general population. Runs of PVCs or associated symptoms of dyspnea, angina, or syncope require investigation and are most likely related to an underlying heart disease.

❍   **What is the most common side effect of esmolol, labetalol, and bretylium?**

Hypotension.

❍   **What side effect can occur with a rapid infusion of procainamide?**

Hypotension. Other side effects include QRS/QT prolongation, ventricular fibrillation, and Torsade de pointes.

❍   **What are some adverse drug effects of lidocaine?**

Drowsiness, nausea, vertigo, confusion, ataxia, tinnitus, muscle twitching, respiratory depression, and psychosis.

❍   **Patients with abdominal aorta stenosis may complain of impotence. What causes this?**

Decreased blood flow through the hypogastric arteries. Stenosis is caused by luminal narrowing secondary to ulcerating atherosclerotic plaques, thrombi, emboli, or fibrointimal thickening. Stenosis of the abdominal aorta also results in claudication.

❍   **What artery is usually affected by arterial occlusive disease in diabetics?**

The popliteal artery. Because of diabetic neuropathy and the potential for the development of a necrotizing infection in a leg with compromised circulation, it is very important that patients with diabetes are knowledgeable about pedal hygiene.

❍   **What is the Budd-Chiari syndrome?**

Thrombosis in the hepatic vein resulting in abdominal pain, jaundice, and ascites.

❍   **A mother has rubella in the first trimester of her pregnancy and her baby is born with a congenital heart disease. The baby probably has which type of heart disease?**

Patent ductus arteriosus.

❍   **What is the cause of Prinzmetal's angina?**

Coronary artery vasospasm with or without fixed stenotic lesions. Prinzmetal's angina is more often associated with ST segment elevation than with depression. Calcium channel blockers are the drugs of choice to treat this condition. ß-Blockers are contraindicated in patients who have vasospasm without fixed stenotic lesions.

❍   **Eighty to ninety percent of patients who experience sudden non-traumatic cardiac arrest are in what rhythm?**

Ventricular fibrillation. Early defibrillation is the key. In an acute MI, the infarction zone becomes electrically unstable. Ventricular fibrillation is most common during original coronary occlusion or when the coronaries begin to reperfuse.

❍   **In CPR, what is the ventilation to compression ratio for one rescuer? For two rescuers?**

1 rescuer: 2 breaths to 15 compressions
2 rescuers: 1 breath to 5 compressions
(note: new BLS quidelines do not require any breaths, only compressions)

○   **Which is the most common type of cardiomyopathy?**

Dilated cardiomyopathy (all 4 chambers). This condition is induced by progression of myocarditis, alcohol, adriamycin, diabetes,, pheochromocytoma, thiamine deficiency, thyroid disease, and valve replacement. The other types of cardiomyopathies are hypertrophic and restrictive/obliterative pregnancy.

○   **Which is the most common type of cardiac failure: high or low output?**

Low output failure. Reduced stroke volume, lowered pulse pressure, and peripheral vasoconstriction are all signs of low output failure.

○   **What is the most common cause of low output heart failure in the world?**

Chagas' disease. In addition to heart failure, patients present with prolonged fever, hepatosplenomegaly, megaesophagus, megacolon, edema, and lymphadenopathy. This disease is most prevalent in Latin America.

○   **What is the most common cause of low output heart failure in the US?**

CAD. Other causes include congenital heart disease, cor pulmonale, dilated cardiomyopathy, hypertension, hypertrophic cardiomyopathy, infection, toxins, and valvular heart disease.

○   **Compare the mortality rate from CHF between the sexes.**

Women fare slightly better. The 5 year mortality rate for a female with CHF is 45%, as compared to 60% for males. The majority of deaths from CHF result from ventricular arrhythmias.

○   **Describe the 3 stages of CXR findings in CHF.**

Stage I: Pulmonary arterial wedge pressure (PAWP) of 12 to 18 mm Hg. Blood flow increases in the upper lung fields (cephalization of pulmonary vessels).

Stage II: PAWP of 18 to 25 mm Hg. Interstitial edema is evident with blurred edges of blood vessels and Kerley B lines.

Stage III: PAWP > 25 mm Hg. Fluid exudes into alveoli with the generation of the classic butterfly pattern of perihilar infiltrates.

○   **Which do nitrates affect: preload or afterload?**

Predominantly preload.

○   **Which does hydralazine affect: preload or afterload?**

Afterload.

○   **Do prazosin, captopril, and nifedipine affect afterload?**

Yes.

○   **When is dobutamine used in CHF?**

When heart failure is not accompanied with severe hypotension. Dobutamine is a potent inotrope with some vasodilation activity.

○ **When is dopamine selected in CHF?**

When a patient is in shock. Dopamine is a vasoconstrictor and a positive inotrope.

○ **What is the most common cause of right ventricular heart failure?**

Left ventricular heart failure.

○ **Match the sign or symptom with left (L) or right (R) sided heart failure.**

1) Hypotension
2) Hepatomegaly
3) Orthopnea
4) Cough
5) Dyspnea on exertion
6) Abdominal distention
7) Paroxysmal nocturnal dyspnea

8) Hemoptysis
9) S3 gallop
10) Early satiety
11) Jugular venous distention
12) Ascites
13) Rales

Answers : (1) L, (2) R, (3) L, (4) L, (5) L, (6) R, (7) L, (8) L, (9) L, (10) R, (11) R, (12) R, and (13) L.

○ **What is the rate of restenosis after percutaneous transluminal coronary angioplasty?**

20% to 30% restenose within 6 months, 40% restenose within the year. Successful dilation occurs in 90% of the cases but because of the high rate of restenosis, this option is less attractive than CABG.

○ **How are acute MI, angina pectoralis, and Prinzmetal's angina differentiated?**

The pain is similar but typically differs in radiation, duration, provocation, and palliation. Obtaining an accurate history is the most important tool for diagnosing chest pain!

Angina pectoralis is aggravated by exercise, cold, and excitement, but it is relieved by rest and nitro.

Prinzmetal's angina occurs at rest, during normal activity, and generally at night or in the early morning. It lasts longer than angina pectoralis.

Acute MIs produce pain with a greater radius of radiation that may last for hours.

○ **A patient presents to the hospital one month after placement of a mechanical prosthetic valve with fever, chills, and a leukocytosis. Endocarditis is suspected. Which bacterium is most common?**

Staphylococcus aureus or *Staphylococcus epidermidis*.

○ **Lovastatin (Mevacor) and niacin are used to treat hyperlipoproteinemia. Both of these drugs lower triglycerides and LDL. Which one raises HDL?**

Only niacin. Lovastatin has little affect on HDL. However, because niacin often produces significant side effects, such as gastritis, reactivation of peptic ulcers, gout, hyperglycemia, cutaneous flushing, and scaling skin, lovastatin remains the drug of choice.

○ **What hypertensive medications should be avoided in diabetics?**

Diuretics and ß-blockers. These drugs increase insulin resistance. ACE inhibitors are the drugs of choice for the treatment of hypertension in diabetics.

❍   **While taking your boards, why might you become severely annoyed if seated next to a person on ACE inhibitors?**

ACE inhibitors produce a cough in 15% of patients.

❍   **What are the most common side effects of ß-blockers?**

Fatigue will occur early in treatment, followed later by depression.

❍   **What percentage of hypertension is secondary?**

Five percent. Secondary hypertension should be suspected in patients under age 35, patients with a sudden-onset hypertension, and those without a family history for hypertension.

❍   **What is the most common cause of secondary hypertension?**

Renal parenchymal disease. In women, the most common cause is oral contraceptives. In patients over age 50, secondary hypertension can usually be attributed to renal artery stenosis. Other causes include pheochromocytoma, coarctation of the aorta, drugs (cocaine), hyperthyroidism, aldosteronism, and Cushing's syndrome.

❍   **What percentage of patients with aortic dissection are hypertensive?**

70 to 90%.

❍   **What percentage of hypertensive patients are afflicted with left ventricular hypertrophy?**

50%. This is the primary reason that hypertension is a major risk factor for MI, CHF, and sudden death.

❍   **What are the side effects of thiazide diuretics?**

Hyperglycemia, hyperlipidemia, hyperuricemia, hypokalemia, hypomagnesemia, and hyponatremia.

❍   **Which drugs should be administered to lower the BP in a patient with thoracic aortic dissection?**

Sodium nitroprusside. A ß-blocker should also be used to reduce the dp/dt (Propagation Speed).

❍   **A patient has a history of episodic blood pressure elevations. She complains of headache, diarrhea, and skin pallor. Probable diagnosis?**

Pheochromocytoma.

❍   **What is the most common complication of nitroprusside?**

Hypotension. Thiocyanate toxicity accompanied by blurred vision, tinnitus, change in mental status, muscle weakness, and seizures is more prevalent in patients with renal failure or prolonged infusions. Cyanide toxicity is uncommon. However, this type of toxicity may occur with hepatic dysfunction, after prolonged infusions, and in rates greater than 10 mg/kg per minute.

❍   **Define a hypertensive emergency.**

Elevated diastolic blood pressure > 115 mm Hg with associated end organ dysfunction or damage.

○   **How quickly should a patient's blood pressure be lowered in a hypertensive emergency?**

Gradually over 2 to 3 hours to 140 to 160 mm Hg systolic and 90 to 110 mm Hg diastolic. To prevent cerebral hypoperfusion, the blood pressure should not be decreased by more than 25% of the mean arterial pressure.

○   **What drug can be used for almost all hypertensive emergencies?**

Sodium nitroprusside. It assists in relaxing smooth muscle tissue through the production of cGMP. As a result, there is decreased preload and afterload, decreased oxygen demand, and a slightly increased heart rate with no change in myocardial blood flow, cardiac output, or renal blood flow. The duration of action is 1 to 2 minutes. Sometimes, ß-blockade is required to treat rebound tachycardia.

○   **Define a hypertensive urgency.**

Dangerously elevated diastolic blood pressure > 115 mm Hg without signs of end organ damage. Blood pressure should be gradually reduced over 24 to 48 hours.

○   **Define uncomplicated hypertension.**

Diastolic blood pressure < 115 mm Hg without symptoms of end organ damage. Uncomplicated hypertension does not require acute treatment.

○   **What lab findings confirm a hypertensive emergency?**

U/A: RBCs, red cell casts, and proteinuria.
BUN and CR: Elevated.
X-ray: Aortic dissection, pulmonary edema, or coarctation of the aorta.
ECG: LVH and cardiac ischemia.

○   **What are the signs and symptoms of hypertensive encephalopathy?**

Nausea, vomiting, headache, lethargy, coma, blindness, nerve palsies, hemiparesis, aphasia, retinal hemorrhage, cotton wool spots, exudates, sausage linking, and papilledema. Treat with labetalol or sodium nitroprusside and lower the mean arterial pressure to approximately 120 mm Hg.

○   **Cardiac hypertrophy will most likely displace the point of maximal impulse to where?**

The normal apical impulse at the medial to midclavicular line in the fourth or fifth intercostal space will be displaced downwards to the sixth intercostal space.

○   **What maneuvers will *increase* hypertrophic cardiomyopathy murmurs?**

Valsalva, standing, and amyl nitrate.

○   **What maneuvers will *decrease* hypertrophic cardiomyopathic murmurs?**

Handgrip, squatting, and leg elevation in the supine patient.

○   **Livedo reticularis commonly develops on what body parts?**

The legs. Livedo reticularis is a bluish red discoloration of the skin resulting from vasospasm of the arterioles. This condition is worsened by exposure to cold.

○   **What is the most common source of acute mesenteric ischemia?**

Arterial embolism (40 to 50%). The source is usually the heart, generally from a mural thrombus. The most common point of obstruction is the superior mesenteric artery.

O   **What lab results strongly suggest that a patient has mesenteric ischemia?**

Leukocytosis > 15,000, metabolic acidosis (sometimes with anion gap), hemoconcentration, and elevated phosphate and amylase.

O   **Which type of myocardial infarction is more often associated with thrombosis: transmural or subendocardial?**

Transmural. Thrombolytic therapy increases left ventricle ejection fraction post MI, reduces the development of post infarction CHF, and can reduce early MI mortality by 25%.

O   **How much aspirin should a post MI patient ingest daily to reduce the incidence of reinfarction?**

160 to 325 mg/day.

O   **What is the most common cause of death during the first few hours of a MI?**

Cardiac dysrhythmias, generally ventricular fibrillation.

O   **When treating early MIs, ß-blockers decrease the risk of reinfarction. Which patients should not receive ß-blockers?**

Patients with hypotension, diabetes, CHF, severe left ventricular dysfunction, AV block, bradycardia, asthma, or another bronchospastic disease.

O   **How common are PVCs in post MI patients?**

90% will have PVCs within the first few weeks. Concern arises if the PVCs are complex, which is the case in 20 to 40% of MI patients. Risk of sudden death in post MI patients with complex PVCs increases 2 to 5 times.

O   **What percentage of the LV myocardium must to be damaged to induce cardiogenic shock?**

40%. Twenty-five percent or more results in heart failure.

O   **What percentage of MIs are clinically unrecognized?**

5 to 10%.

O   **A non-Q wave infarction is usually associated with what?**

Subsequent angina or recurrent infarction. Non-Q wave infarctions also have lower in-hospital mortality rate compared to Q wave MIs.

O   **What ECG changes arise in a true posterior infarction?**

Large R wave and ST depression in V1 and V2.

O   **What conduction defects commonly occur in an anterior wall MI?**

The dangerous kind. Damage to the conducting system results in a Mobitz II second or third degree AV block.

○   **How should PSVT be treated during an AMI?**

Vagal maneuvers, adenosine, or cardioversion. Stable patients may be able to tolerate negative inotropes, such as verapamil or even ß-blockers.

○   **A patient presents one day after discharge for an AMI with a new, harsh systolic murmur along the left sternal border and pulmonary edema. What is the diagnosis?**

Ventricular septal rupture. Diagnosis is confirmed with Swan-Ganz catheterization or echo. The treatment regime includes nitroprusside, for afterload reduction, and possibly an intra-aortic balloon pump followed by surgical repair.

○   **When does cardiac rupture usually occur in patients who have suffered acute MIs?**

Fifty percent arise within the first 5 days, and 90% occur within the first 14 days post MI.

○   **Which type of infarct commonly leads to papillary muscle dysfunction?**

Inferior wall MI. Signs and symptoms include a mild transient systolic murmur and pulmonary edema.

○   **A patient presents two weeks post AMI with chest pain, fever, and pleuropericarditis. A pleural effusion is detected by on CXR. What is the diagnosis?**

Dressler's (post myocardial infarction) syndrome. This syndrome is caused by an immunologic reaction to myocardial antigens.

○   **What percentage of patients over age 80 experience chest pain with an AMI?**

Only 50%. Twenty percent experience diaphoresis, stroke, syncope, and/or acute confusion.

○   **Which type of thrombolytic agent is fibrin-specific?**

Tissue plasminogen activator. This agent is a human protein with no antigenic properties.

○   **What are the most common causes of myocarditis in the US?**

Viruses. Other causes include post viral myocarditis, an autoimmune response to recent viral infection, bacteria (diphtheria and tuberculosis), fungi, protozoa (Chagas' disease), and spirochetes (Lyme disease).

○   **What percentage of non-anticoagulated patients with mitral stenosis experience systemic emboli?**

25%. Patients with chronic atrial fibrillation or mitral stenosis should be chronically anticoagulated to prevent atrial mural thrombi.

○   **What is the most common cause of mitral stenosis?**

Rheumatic heart disease. The most common initial symptom is dyspnea.

○   **What physical findings may be associated with mitral stenosis?**

Prominent a-wave, early-systolic left parasternal lift, loud and snapping first heart sound, and early-diastolic opening snap with a low-pitched mid-diastolic rumble that crescendos into S1.

○   **A mid-systolic click with a late systolic crescendo murmur is indicative of what cardiac disease?**

Mitral valve prolapse (MVP).

○   **Is mitral valve prolapse more common among men or women?**

Women have a stronger genetic link to the disease. However, only 2% to 5% of the entire population has symptomatic MVP.

○   **What age group typically develops MVP syndrome?**

Patients in their twenties and thirties. Most patients with MVP are asymptomatic. MVP syndrome is symptomatic with chest pain, fatigue, palpitations, postural syncope, and dizziness.

○   **What is the hallmark sign of MVP?**

A midsystolic click, sometimes accompanied by a late systolic murmur. MVP is largely a clinical diagnosis. An ECG is performed to assess the degree of prolapse. Other clinical findings include a laterally-displaced, diffuse apical pulse; decreased S1; split S2; and a holosystolic murmur radiating to the axilla.

○   **How do the fixed-rate and demand modes of pacemakers differ?**

Fixed-rate mode produces an impulse at a continuous specific rate, regardless of the patient's own cardiac activity. Demand mode detects the patient's electrical activity and triggers only if the heart is not depolarizing.

○   **Describe the 3-lettered pacing code used in cardiac pacemakers.**

Letter 1: Chamber paced
Letter 2: Chamber sensed
Letter 3: Pacing function

O:	None		
A:	Atrial		
V:	Ventricular		
D:	Dual (A+V)	O:	None
A:	Atrial		
V:	Ventricular		
D:	Dual (A+V)	O:	None
I:	Inhibition		
T:	Triggering		
D:	Dual (I+T)		

○   **What is the treatment for ventricular fibrillation in a patient with a pacemaker?**

Defibrillation, but be sure to keep the paddles away from the pacer.

○   **A 25-year-old patient presents with splinted breathing and sharp, precordial chest pain that radiates to the back. The pain increases with inspiration and is mildly relieved by placing the patient in a forward sitting position. What might the ECG show?**

The ECG may reveal intermittent supraventricular tachycardias, ST- segment depression in aVR and VI, ST-segment elevation in all other leads, PR depression, and T wave inversion may arise. The patient probably has pericarditis.

○   **What is the most common cause of pericarditis?**

Idiopathic. Other causes are MI, post viral syndrome, aortic dissection that has ruptured into the pericardium, malignancy, radiation, chest trauma, connective tissue disease, uremia, and drugs, i.e., procainamide or hydralazine.

○   **What physical finding indicates acute pericarditis?**

Pericardial friction rub. The rub is best heard at the left sternal border or apex with the patient in a forward sitting position. Other findings include fever and tachycardia.

○   **Acute pyogenic pericarditis is most commonly caused by what organisms?**

Staphylococcus and *Haemophilus influenzae.*

○   **When diagnosing pericardial effusion, how much fluid must be present in the pericardial sac for visualization on an cardiac echocardiography and by x-ray?**

At least 15 mL for an echocardiography and 250 mL for an x-ray.

○   **What will be the appearance of a pericardial effusion on an x-ray?**

A water bottle silhouette.

○   **At what volume does pericardial effusion affect the intrapericardial pressure?**

80 to 200 mL. However, the rate of accumulation is more important than the amount of accumulation. If accumulated slowly the pericardium can tolerate up to 2000 mL of fluid.

○   **What is the treatment for pericarditis without effusion?**

A 2-week treatment of 650 mg aspirin every 4 hours, if no contraindictions exist. Ibuprofen, indomethacin, or colchicine are other alternatives. The use of corticosteroids is controversial, because recurrent pericarditis is common when doses are tapered.

○   **Rheumatic heart disease is the most common cause of stenosis of what 3 heart valves?**

Mitral, aortic (along with congenital bicuspid valve), and tricuspid.

○   **What is the 1-year recurrence rate for patients who have been resuscitated from sudden cardiac death?**

30%.

○   **Describe the Trendelenburg test for varicose veins.**

Raise the leg above the heart and then quickly lower it. If the leg veins become distended immediately after this test is performed, valvular incompetency is evident.

○   **What is a paradoxical embolus?**

A venous thrombus that goes through a right-to-left intra-cardiac shunt to the arterial side.

O   **Why is a paradoxical embolus able to cause septic end-organ disease?**

An infected venous thrombus can enter the arterial circulation via the right-to-left intra-cardiac shunt and be sent distal to affect end-organs.

O   **Splinter hemorrhages, Osler's nodes, Janeway lesions, petechiae, and Roth's spots can be indications of what process?**

They are physical signs associated with infective endocarditis.

O   **T/F: Osler's nodes are usually nodular and painful.**

True. In contrast, the macular Janeway lesions are painless plaques on soles and palms. Osler nodes are found on the tips of fingers and toes.

O   **What other conditions besides infective endocarditis can Osler's nodes be found with?**

Nonbacterial thrombotic endocarditis, gonococcal infections, and hemolytic anemia.

O   **What percentage of patients with infective endocarditis display peripheral manifestations of the disease?**

50%.

O   **What is bacterial endocarditis?**

Blood-borne bacteria that attach onto damaged or abnormal heart valves or on the endocardium near anatomic defects.

O   **How is bacterial endocarditis diagnosed?**

By evidence of valvular vegetations on echocardiogram combined with a positive blood culture.

O   **What is the sensitivity rate of a two-dimensional transesophageal echocardiograms for detecting vegetations?**

95%.

O   **What are the risk factors for endocarditis?**

Risk factors include Intravenous drug users, prosthetic valves, prior history of endocarditis, acquired valvular heart disease, hypertrophic cardiomyopathy, hemodialysis,peritoneal dialysis, indwelling venous catheters, postcardiac surgery, surgical systemic pulmonary shunts, rheumatic heart disease and uncorrected congenital heart disease. It is controversial as to whether mitral valve prolapse with significant regurgitation is a moderate risk factor.

O   **What are the most common organism associated with endocarditis?**

Streptococcus viridans, *Staph. aureus*, *Enterococcus* and fungal organisms. *Staph. aureus* is responsible for 75% of disease in IVDA's.

O   **Fungi cause what percent of prosthetic valve infective endocarditis?**

15%.

O   **What is more common in the general population: left-sided or right sided endocarditits?**

Left-sided (aortic and mitra involvement)

O   **What is more common in intravenous drug abusers; right-sided or left-sided diseae?**

Right-sided (60%) is most common.

O   **How is infective endocarditis treated?**

Intravenous antibiotics for 4-6 weeks. Close follow-up is necessary and the patient should have a series of two separate negative blood cultures to demonstrate resolution of the condition. If resolution of the infection does not occur promptly, embolization occurs, or fulminant CHF ensues and surgical valve replacement is indicated.

O   **What are the EKG changes associated with pericarditis?**

Concave upward ST elevation in at least seven leads except V1 and AVR. PR segment depression may also be present.

O   **What is the clinical picture of myocardial abscesses?**

Low-grade fevers, chills, leukocytosis, conduction system abnormalities, nonspecific ECG changes and signs and symptoms of acute MI .

O   **What is mural endocarditis?**

Inflammation and disruption of the nonvalvular endocardial surface of the cardiac chambers.

O   **What is the presentation of mural endocarditis?**

The presentation is similar to infective valvular endocarditis.

O   **What are the risk factors for mural endocarditis?**

Usually, mural endocarditis is from seeding of an abnormal area of endocardium during bacteremia or fungemia. Infectious thrombi from pulmonary veins, ventricular aneurysms, mural thrombi, chordal friction lesions, pacemaker lead insertion sites, idiopathic hypertrophic subaortic stenosis, jet lesions from ventriculoseptal defects, and other congenital defects are other factors. Immunocompromised patients are also at increased risks.

O   **What is the definitive treatment of an infected atrial myxoma?**

Urgent surgical removal.

O   **What is the risk for infection of a transvenous pacemaker during the first 3 years after insertion?**

1 to 6%.

○   **What are the risk factors associated with the development of pacemaker infections?**

Risk factors include: diabetes, malignancy, skin disorders, malnutrition, anticoagulants, steroids, and immunosuppressive medications.

○   **What are complications of pacemaker insertion?**

Post-insertion hematoma, seroma, or infection.

○   **What is a major risk factor for prosthetic vascular graft infection?**

Location. The incidence of infection is 1% to 1.5% for aorto-iliac grafts as opposed to 2% to 7% for femoral-popliteal arterial grafts.

○   **What is thought to be the cause of this infection?**

95% of the time, contamination at the time of insertion is thought to cause the infection.

○   **What is the clinical presentation of prosthetic vascular graft infection?**

Erythema, skin breakdown, or purulent drainage. Other symptoms may be thrombosis of the graft, fluid around the graft, or pseudoaneurysm formation.

○   **What are complications from arterial catheterization?**

Thrombosis (19-38%), infection (4-23%), pseudoaneurysm, and rupture.

○   **What is the most frequent cause of mitral stenosis?**

Rheumatic fever. Far less common causes include congenital, malignant carcinoid, SLE, rheumatoid arthritis, infective endocarditis with a large vegetation, and the muccopolysaccharidoses of the Hunter-Hurley phenotype.

○   **What percentage of patients with rheumatic mitral stenosis are female?**

66%.

○   **What percentage of patients with rheumatic heart disease have pure mitral stenosis?**

Twenty-five percent. An additional 40% have combined MS and MR.

○   **What are the principle symptoms in mitral stenosis?**

Dyspnea is most common. Patients with severe mitral stenosis can experience orthopnea, hemoptysis, chest pain, and frank pulmonary edema, often precipitated by exertion, fever, URI, sexual intercourse, pregnancy or the onset of rapid atrial fibrillation.

○   **What are the two most serious complications of mitral stenosis?**

Thromboembolism, most often occurring in the setting of atrial fibrillation, and pulmonary edema.

○   **What maneuvers can one do to differentiate the opening snap of mitral stenosis from a split S2 sound?**

Sudden standing widens the A2-opening snap interval whereas a split S2 narrows on standing. Progressive narrowing of the A2-OS interval on serial examinations suggests an increase in the severity of mitral stenosis.

❍ **What is the most accurate noninvasive technique for quantifying the severity of mitral stenosis?**

Doppler echocardiography.

❍ **What is the medical management strategy of rheumatic mitral stenosis?**

1) Penicillin prophylaxis for beta-hemolytic streptococcal infections and prophylaxis for infective endocarditis; 2) aggressive and prompt treatment of anemia and infections; 3) avoidance of strenuous exertion; 4) oral diuretics and sodium restriction in symptomatic patients; 5) beta-blockers to reduce heart rate; 6) cardioversion of atrial fibrillation, if possible; 7) aggressive slowing of refractory atrial fibrillation; and 8) anticoagulant therapy in patients who have experienced one or more thromboembolic episodes, or who have mechanical prosthetic valves.

❍ **What is the most common cause of mitral regurgitation?**

Rheumatic heart disease. It is more frequent in men than women. Other causes include infective endocarditis, mitral valve prolapse, ischemic heart disease, trauma, SLE, scleroderma, hypertrophic cardiomyopathy, dilated cardiomyopathy involving the left ventricle, and idiopathic degenerative calcification of the mitral annulus.

❍ **What percentage of patients with coronary artery disease considered for CABG have mitral regurgitation?**

Thirty percent. It is secondary to ischemic papillary muscle dysfunction.

❍ **What are the physical findings of patients with chronic mitral regurgitation?**

Harsh, pansystolic murmur heard best at the apex, radiating to the axilla or the base. The murmur is diminished by maneuvers that decrease preload or afterload, such as amyl nitrate inhalation, Valsalva or standing and increases with maneuvers that increase preload or afterload, such as squatting, handgrip or phenylephrine administration.

❍ **What are the most common causes of <u>acute</u> mitral regurgitation?**

Acute myocardial infarction with papillary muscle dysfunction (15% of acute MI results in acute mitral regurgitation) or papillary muscle rupture (.3% of acute MI), infective endocarditis, chordae tendineae rupture secondary to chest trauma, rheumatic fever, mitral valve prolapse, and hypertrophic cardiomyopathy with rupture of chordae tendinae.

❍ **Which is the best test to assess the detailed anatomy of rheumatic mitral valve disease and determine whether mitral valve replacement is necessary or whether reconstruction is feasible?**

Transesophageal echocardiography.

❍ **What is the appropriate medical management of mitral regurgitation?**

Vasodilator therapy with ACE inhibitors is the hallmark of therapy, even in patients who are asymptomatic. Diuretics are used in patients with severe MR. Cardiac glycosides, such as digoxin, are indicated in patients with severe MR and clinical evidence of heart failure. Endocarditis prophylaxis is indicated in all patients with MR. Anticoagulation should be given to all patients in atrial fibrillation.

○   **A 33-year-old female comes to you for a physical and you notice a harsh systolic murmur at the apex that is also heard at the base. The murmur increases on standing and Valsalva and decreases with handgrip. What is the most likely finding on echocardiography?**

Mitral valve prolapse. The murmur of pure mitral regurgitation decreases with Valsalva and standing and increases with handgrip or squatting.

○   **A 46-year-old male with a history of rheumatic fever at age 12 is admitted with an acute myocardial infarction. The patient's post-MI course is complicated by congestive heart failure. Echocardiogram reveals severe mitral regurgitation with rupture of one of the papillary muscles, prolapse of the posterior mitral valve leaflet without apparent calcification. Systolic function by echocardiogram is mildly reduced. What is the appropriate course of action in this patient?**

Mitral valve reconstruction and repair of the papillary muscle.

○   **What are the indications for operation in patients with severe, chronic mitral regurgitation?**

Patients with NYHA class II symptoms with end-systolic LV diameter of >45mm by echocardiography. Asymptomatic patients with severe MR under the age of 70 with ejection fractions less than 70% and end-systolic LV diameter >40mm by echocardiography who are likely to be candidates for mitral valve repair should also be strongly considered for surgery.

○   **What is the classic triad of symptoms of aortic stenosis?**

Syncope (often exertional), angina, and heart failure.

○   **What is the most common cause of aortic stenosis in patients *under* age 65?**

Calcification of congenitally bicuspid aortic valves (50%) followed by rheumatic heart disease (25%).

○   **What is the most common cause of aortic stenosis in patients over age 65?**

Calcific degeneration of the aortic leaflets.

○   **How does a heart murmur reflect the severity of aortic stenosis?**

The longer the duration of the murmur and the greater the increase in intensity of the murmur, the more severe the aortic stenosis. The degree of loudness of the murmur is not as important in assessing severity.

○   **What is the best pharmacologic agent for patients with asymptomatic aortic stenosis?**

Without contraindications, beta-blockers are the best agents as they are the most useful in treating the left ventricular hypertrophy and its sequelae that develop as a result of aortic stenosis.

○   **A 68-year-old female with severe asymptomatic aortic stenosis suddenly complains of dyspnea and palpitations. On EKG, she is found to be in atrial fibrillation with a ventricular rate of 130 beats per minute. What is the most appropriate action to be taken?**

Immediate DC cardioversion, followed by a search for previously unrecognized mitral valve disease. Once stabilized, the patient should be referred for cardiac catheterization and aortic valve replacement.

○   **What is the most common sustained tachyarrhythmia in patients with mitral valve prolapse?**

Paroxysmal supraventricular tachycardia.

○   **What is mitral valve prolapse syndrome?**

A symptom complex consisting of palpitations, chest pain, easy fatigability, exercise intolerance, dyspnea, orthostatic phenomena, and syncope or pre-syncope in patients with mitral valve prolapse, predominantly related to autonomic dysfunction.

❍   **What disorders are seen with increased frequency in patients with MVP syndrome?**

Graves' disease, asthma, migraine headaches, sleep disorders, fibromyositis, and functional gastrointestinal syndromes.

❍   **What is the most common cause of isolated severe aortic regurgitation?**

Aortic root dilatation resulting from medial disease. Other common causes include congenital (bicuspid) aortic valve, previous infective endocarditis, and rheumatic heart disease.

❍   **What murmur may be mistaken for mitral stenosis?**

The Austin-Flint murmur of severe aortic regurgitation, which occurs from a powerful regurgitant jet from the aorta, imparted to the anterior leaflet of the mitral valve, limiting the opening of the anterior leaflet of the mitral valve.

❍   **What is the survival of chronic aortic regurgitation after diagnosis?**

The five-year survival, after diagnosis, is 75%. The ten-year survival is 50%. Once symptoms begin, without surgical treatment, death occurs within 4 years after the development of angina, 2 years after the development of CHF.

❍   **What is the preferred pharmacologic agent in patients with asymptomatic chronic aortic regurgitation?**

Nifedipine, or ACE inhibitors. Both have shown major improvements in LVEF and major reduction in LV end-diastolic volume and mass with significantly lower incidence of the need for aortic valve replacement at 5 years.

❍   **What is the most common congenital abnormality producing tricuspid regurgitation?**

Tricuspid valve prolapse. Less common is Ebstein's anomaly.

❍   **What is the most common cause of acute tricuspid regurgitation and what is the preferred management of this situation?**

Tricuspid valve endocarditis, often as a result of intravenous drug abuse. The preferred management is complete removal of the valve with immediate or eventual replacement of the valve. Antibiotic therapy usually is futile in preventing valve surgery.

❍   **A 38-year-old Hispanic female with known mitral valve prolapse is scheduled for dental cleaning. Her dentist calls you asking for recommendations for endocarditis prophylaxis. She is not allergic to penicillin. What are your recommendations?**

Amoxicillin 3.0 gm po one hour before the procedure followed by 1.5 gm po six hours after the initial dose.

❍   **How does the sensitivity of transthoracic echocardiography compare with transesophageal echocardiography in the diagnosis of infective endocarditis?**

Transthoracic echocardiography carries a diagnostic sensitivity of 30-40%, whereas transesophageal echocardiography carries a diagnostic sensitivity between 90-100%.

O   **A 55-year-old gentleman who underwent a 4 vessel CABG three years ago has mild mitral and tricuspid regurgitation is scheduled for colonoscopy for rectal bleeding. What recommendations regarding endocarditis prophylaxis would you give the surgeon?**

No antibiotic prophylaxis is needed in this setting.

O   **How much myocardial damage from an acute myocardial infarction is necessary to result in congestive heart failure?**

Congestive heart failure is usually evident clinically if more than 25% of the left ventricle is infarcted.

O   **How much functional loss of left ventricular myocardium is required to result in cardiogenic shock?**

40%.

O   **What three secondary processes resulting in myocardial deterioration occur following acute myocardial infarction?**

Ventricular remodeling, typically following Q-wave infarctions; infarct expansion, occurring most frequently from anterior-apical infarctions and results in thinning of the left ventricular wall; and ventricular dilatation, an early and progressive response to acute myocardial infarction that is an important predictor of increased mortality following myocardial infarction.

O   **What factors play a role in the peak incidence of myocardial infarction being from 6 AM to noon?**

Blood pressure, coronary arterial tone, blood viscosity, circulating catecholamines and platelet aggregability increase on awakening and assumption of an erect posture.

O   **What is the most common cause of death related to acute myocardial infarction?**

Ventricular fibrillation, occurring within the first hour following symptoms.

O   **What percentage of patients with acute myocardial infarction develop cardiogenic shock?**

10%.

O   **What percentage of arteries successfully opened with thrombolytic therapy for acute myocardial infarction, reocclude?**

15% of arteries successfully opened reocclude during the first few days following thrombolytic therapy.

O   **What is the mortality benefit from aspirin alone in acute myocardial infarction with thrombolytic therapy and in subsequent reinfarction?**

Aspirin reduced mortality from acute myocardial infarction by 23% and reduced non-fatal reinfarction by 49%. When used with thrombolytic therapy, there was a 40-50% reduction in mortality from acute myocardial infarction.

O   **A 63-year-old gentleman presents to the Emergency department with moderate substernal chest pressure and lightheadedness for 90 minutes. His BP on admission is 80/40 and his HR is 110/min and regular. Physical exam reveals JVD to the angle of the jaw, a right parasternal S3 gallop, an apical S4 gallop and clear lungs on auscultation. ECG reveals 2 mm ST elevation in leads**

II, III, and aVF with reciprocal ST depression in V1-V3. What is the most likely diagnosis and what is the most appropriate initial therapy?

Inferior myocardial infarction with right ventricular infarction. Following 160-325 mg of aspirin administration, thrombolytic therapy, and a large bolus of intravenous saline followed by a moderately high infusion rate of saline are indicated. If the patient remains hypotensive despite adequate intravenous saline (as measured by the development of lung congestion on auscultation) intravenous Dobutamine is indicated.

○   **A 60-year-old patient suffers an acute inferior myocardial infarction. Three hours after he arrives in the hospital, he develops ventricular fibrillation and is successfully defibrillated back to normal sinus rhythm within 30 seconds. He makes a full recovery and has no further post-MI complications. What does his ventricular fibrillation episode indicate with regard to his subsequent risk of sudden death?**

This episode has no bearing on his subsequent risk of sudden death. Ventricular fibrillation in the immediate setting of an acute myocardial infarction has no prognostic significance.

○   **A 65-year-old female presents to the hospital with sudden crushing chest discomfort and moderate shortness of breath. Her initial ECG reveals 2mm ST depression in leads V1-V4 with inverted T waves. She has bibasilar rales in the lower half of both lungs on auscultation. CXR reveals moderate pulmonary edema. Serial ECG's and CPK's confirm a non-Q wave myocardial infarction. With diuretics, her pulmonary edema resolves within 24 hours. What is the most appropriate management strategy at this point?**

Cardiac catheterization with coronary angiography. A non-Q wave MI that results in pulmonary edema signifies a large amount of myocardium at risk for reinfarction within the next year.

○   **What arrhythmias that occur in patients with acute myocardial infarction require temporary pacing?**

Complete heart block (3° AV block); new LBBB; new bifascicular block; marked sinus bradycardia with ischemic pain, hypotension, CHF, frequent PVC's or syncope despite atropine; and Mobitz II type 2° AV block.

○   **A 54-year-old gentleman, admitted two days ago with an acute anterolateral myocardial infarction, suddenly develops atrial fibrillation with a ventricular rate of 135/min. He subsequently complains of substernal chest discomfort. His BP is 135/70. What is the most appropriate immediate action to be taken?**

Synchronized DC cardioversion.

○   **What percentage of patients with acute myocardial infarction develop paroxysmal atrial fibrillation?**

10-15%.

○   **What are the major complications of left ventricular aneurysms?**

LV thrombus formation (with the subsequent risk of thromboembolic events), CHF, and ventricular arrhythmias.

○   **What is the recommended therapy for patients with large anterior myocardial infarctions?**

Reperfusion therapy with thrombolytics, beta-blockers, intravenous nitroglycerin, and ACE inhibitors to limit and retard ventricular remodeling. Intravenous heparin in a sufficient dose to prolong the APTT to

1.5 to 2.0 times control should be started on admission and continued to discharge. In patients with large akinetic apical segments or mural thrombi, oral anticoagulation with warfarin is indicated for 3-6 months.

O **What is the significance of pericarditis following acute myocardial infarction?**

Pericarditis occurs in about 20% of patients with acute myocardial infarction. It is more likely in Q-wave infarcts than non-Q wave infarcts. Patients with pericarditis usually have significantly larger infarcts, lower ejection fractions, and a higher incidence of congestive heart failure. The presence of pericarditis and/or pericardial effusion following acute myocardial infarction is associated with a higher mortality.

O **A 68-year-old male with diabetes and a 60 pack-year history of smoking presents with sudden, severe substernal chest discomfort, radiating through to the interscapular area. BP is 150/80 mm Hg in the right arm and 135/65 mm Hg in the left arm. He complains of right arm numbness and weakness and you hear a II/VI diastolic murmur along the left sternal border. ECG reveals 1.5 mm ST elevation in the inferior leads. What is the diagnosis?**

Acute proximal thoracic aortic dissection, with involvement of the right coronary artery and brachiocephalic artery, as well as acute aortic regurgitation.

O **In the patient described in the last question, what other life-threatening complication must one look for, both on auscultation and on CXR?**

Pericardial effusion with cardiac tamponade. Listen for a pericardial rub on auscultation and look for marked cardiomegaly on CXR. Pulsus paradoxus of >10 mm Hg is virtually diagnostic of cardiac tamponade in this setting.

O **What CXR findings occur with a dissecting thoracic aortic aneurysm?**

Tortuosity of the proximal aorta with an enlarged aortic knob, mediastinal widening, pleural effusion (most common on the left), extension of the aortic shadow, displaced trachea to the right, cardiomegaly, and separation of the intimal calcification from the outer contour that is greater than 5 mm.

O **What is the prognosis for an untreated dissecting aortic aneurysm?**

Twenty-five percent die within 24 hours, 50% die within one week, 75% percent die within one month and 90% die within 3 months. With surgical treatment, the 10 year survival is 50%, the five year survival is 75-80%. Redissection occurs in 25% within 10 years of the original dissection.

O **What are the most common causes of MAT (multifocal atrial tachycardia)?**

COPD with exacerbation is the most common cause, followed by CHF, sepsis and methylxanthine toxicity. Treatment consists of treatment of the underlying disorder as well as the use of verapamil, magnesium, or digoxin for slowing the arrhythmia.

O **What are the most common causes of atrial fibrillation?**

Coronary artery disease, with myocardial ischemia, and hypertensive heart disease are the most common causes. Mitral or aortic valvular heart disease, cor pulmonale, dilated cardiomyopathy, hypertrophic cardiomyopathy (particularly the obstructive type), alcohol intoxication "holiday heart syndrome", hypo- or hyperthyroidism, pulmonary embolism, sepsis, hypoxia, pre-excitation syndrome and pericarditis are also common causes.

O **What percentage of patients with atrial fibrillation converted to sinus rhythm will revert back into atrial fibrillation?**

50% will revert back to atrial fibrillation within one year of cardioversion, regardless of medical therapy.

○   **What is the risk of CVA in patients with atrial fibrillation, with and without anticoagulation?**

Patients with atrial fibrillation, not anticoagulated with warfarin, have a 25% incidence of CVA within 5 years (5% per year). Those patients anticoagulated to therapeutic levels have a 4% incidence of CVA within 5 years (0.8% per year). Aspirin is a clearly inferior substitute to warfarin, but is much more preferable to no anticoagulant or antithrombotic therapy.

○   **What is the most common mechanism responsible for supraventricular tachycardia (SVT)?**

AV node re-entry.

○   **What are the common causes of SVT?**

Myocardial ischemia, myocardial infarction, congestive heart failure, pericarditis, rheumatic heart disease, mitral valve prolapse, pre-excitation syndromes, COPD, ethanol intoxication, hypoxia, pneumonia, sepsis and digoxin toxicity.

○   **What is the key feature of Mobitz I 2° AV block (Wenkebach)?**

A progressive prolongation of the PR interval until the atrial impulse is no longer conducted through to the ventricle, resulting in a dropped QRS. Almost always transient, atropine and transcutaneous/transvenous pacing is required for the rare instances of symptoms or cardiac instability.

○   **What is the feature of Mobitz II 2° AV block?**

A constant PR interval until one sinus beat fails to conduct through to the ventricle, resulting in a dropped QRS. Since this rhythm is indicative of His bundle damage, and 85% of patients with this rhythm eventually develop complete heart block, temporary followed by permanent pacing is usually required.

○   **A 57-year-old male is scheduled for a total colectomy for ulcerative colitis. He has stable angina for several years and has hypertension. His pre-op ECG reveals NSR, LVH and 1° AV block. What is the likelihood of high degree AV block occurring in the perioperative period?**

Patients with 1° AV block have an extremely low incidence of developing high degree AV block in the perioperative period or any other period. Thus, no temporary pacing in the perioperative period is required.

○   **A 26-year-old male presents to your clinic for an insurance physical. An ECG reveals Wolff-Parkinson-White syndrome. He is asymptomatic and has no history of palpitations or arrhythmia. What is the most appropriate management of this patient?**

No therapy or work-up is required at this time since there is no evidence that the risk of sudden death can be safely mitigated or that individuals with asymptomatic WPW can be reliably risk stratified with regard to sudden death.

○   **What is the most commonly occurring form of ventricular tachycardia?**

Ventricular tachycardia (VT) occurring in patients with healed myocardial infarction. Other causes include bundle branch reentry VT, VT of right ventricular outflow tract origin, idiopathic left ventricular tachycardia, drug-induced VT (proarrhythmia), and VT due to right ventricular dysplasia. Rare causes include long QT syndrome and lymphocytic myocarditis.

○   **A 48-year-old male with no history of angina, MI or other cardiac symptoms is referred to you for evaluation of palpitations. A 24-hour Holter monitor reveals four three-beat runs of ventricular tachycardia without any symptoms. The patient has no risk factors for coronary artery disease, is a**

non-smoker, and has a normal resting ECG. His echocardiogram is normal. What is the best management strategy for this patient?

No therapy or further work-up is required. The patient should be reassured that the risk of sudden death is very low and that medical therapy will either worsen his arrhythmia or be of no significant benefit.

○   **What is the agent of choice in diabetic patients with hypertension?**

ACE inhibitors.

○   **What drugs have been shown to regress LV hypertrophy and reduce LV mass?**

Beta-blockers, verapamil, alpha-methyldopa (Aldomet), ACE inhibitors, and thiazide diuretics.

○   **Which agent is more likely to cause bradycardia, verapamil or diltiazem?**

Diltiazem. Diltiazem blocks conduction through both the SA and AV node, whereas verapamil blocks only the AV node.

○   **Which drugs can precipitate digoxin toxicity?**

Quinidine, procainamide, verapamil, amiodarone, diltiazem, cyclosporin, diuretics, corticosteroids, erythromycin, and tetracycline, to name a few.

○   **What medications, used to maintain sinus rhythm in a patient recently cardioverted from atrial fibrillation, should be avoided in patients with stress-test proven myocardial ischemia?**

Class 1C antiarrhythmics, such as flecainide and propafenone and class 1A agents, such as quinidine and procainamide. They can lead to lethal proarrhythmia in patients with active myocardial ischemia. Amiodarone, an agent that has anti-ischemic properties, is the preferred agent.

○   **What antihypertensive agents are preferred agents to use in a 63-year-old obese, African-American male?**

Diuretics and/or ACE inhibitors.

○   **Non-traumatic cardiac arrest patients are most likely to be successfully resuscitated from what abnormal rhythm?**

Ventricular fibrillation. Success is time dependent, generally declining at a rate of 2-10% per minute.

○   **If a defibrillator is available, what is the immediate treatment of a patient with ventricular fibrillation?**

Unsynchronized countershock at 200J, then 200-300J, then 360J.

○   **What is the differential diagnosis of pulseless electrical activity (PEA)?**

Hypoxia
Hypovolemia
Hyperkalemia/hypokalemia
Hyperthermia

Acute MI
Acidosis

Tension preumothoray
Tamponade (cardiac)
Thrombosis (pulmonary)
Tablets (drug OD)

○   **What is the differential diagnosis of asystole?**

Drug overdose, acidosis, hyperkalemia, hypothermia, hypokalemia, hypoxia.

○   **What is the treatment for <u>unstable</u> supraventricular tachycardia?**

Synchronized cardioversion. (100J, 200J, 300J then 360J)

○   **A patient in the ED suddenly demonstrates ventricular fibrillation on the monitor. The patient is alert and has a pulse. What should you do?**

Check the monitor leads.

○   **Inferior wall MI's commonly lead to what two types of heart block?**

First degree AV block and Mobitz Type I (Wenckebach) second degree AV block. Sinus bradycardia can also occur. Progression to complete AV block is not common. The mechanism for this is damage to autonomic fibers in the atrial septum giving increased vagal tone impairing AV node conduction.

○   **Anterior wall MI's may directly damage intracardiac conduction. This may lead to which type of arrhythmias?**

The dangerous type! A Mobitz II second degree AV block can suddenly progress to complete AV block.

○   **Which type of drug is contraindicated for the treatment of Torsade de pointes?**

Any drug that prolongs repolarization (QT interval). For example, class Ia antiarrhythmics, such as quinidine and procainamide, are contraindicated for treating Torsade de pointes. Other drugs that share this effect include TCA's, disopyramide, and phenothiazine.

○   **What are the classic ECG findings associated with posterior MI?**

A large R wave in leads V1 and V2, ST depression in leads V1 and V2, Q waves in the inferior leads and, occasionally, ST elevation in the inferior leads.

○   **What is the classic ECG finding for Wolff-Parkinson-White syndrome?**

The delta wave, a change in the upstroke of QRS.

○   **Which valve is most commonly injured during blunt trauma?**

The aortic valve.

○   **What is the most likely cause of a new systolic murmur and ECG infarct pattern in a patient with chest trauma?**

Ventricular septal defect.

❍   **What is the most common complication of extracorporeal circulation?**

Stroke occurs in 1 to 2% of patients after open-heart operations. Other postoperative complications are arrhythmias, bleeding, renal failure, and respiratory complications.

❍   **What drug is used to reverse heparin after open-heart surgery?**

Protamine.

❍   **The left main coronary artery gives rise to which two coronary arteries?**

The left anterior descending artery and the left circumflex coronary artery.

❍   **What is the vessel of preference in coronary bypass grafting?**

The internal mammary artery. This artery has a much higher rate of patency at 10 years than venous grafts (95% versus 50%). Also, venous grafts tend to be more prone to atherosclerosis.

❍   **Which nerve should be located and avoided during pericardiotomy?**

Phrenic nerve. The phrenic nerve runs along the superolateral aspect of the pericardium.

❍   **A radial pulse on examination indicates a BP of at least what level?**

80 mm Hg.

❍   **A femoral pulse on examination indicates a BP of at least what level?**

70 mm Hg.

❍   **A carotid pulse indicates a BP of at least what level?**

60 mm Hg.

❍   **Where is the most common location of left ventricular aneurysms?**

Anterolateral left ventricle (80%). Left ventricular aneurysms result from transmural infarctions and subsequent replacement of muscle with fibrous tissue. Unlike atherosclerotic aneurysms, these aneurysms progressively enlarge but rarely rupture.

❍   **What is the cardiac arrhythmia?**

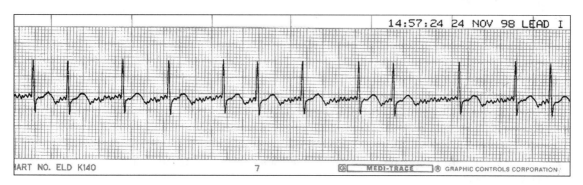

Atrial fibrillation.

○ **What is the cardiac arrhythmia?**

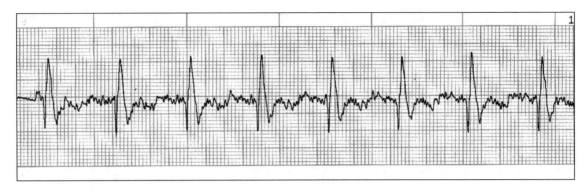

Ventricular paced rhythm with artifact.

○ **What is the cardiac arrhythmia?**

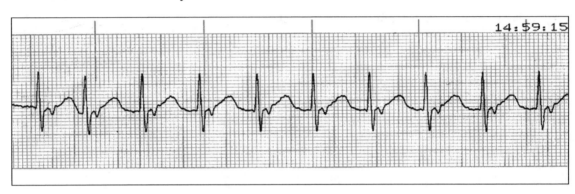

Accelerated junctional rhythm with retrograde P waves.

○ **What is the cardiac rhythm seen below?**

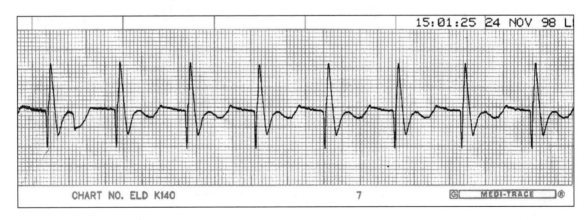

Ventricular pacemaker rhythm.

○   **What is the ECG rhythm abnormality seen below?**

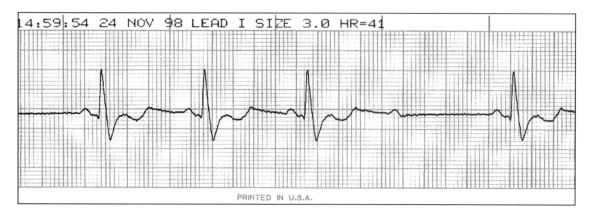

Mobitz II second degree AV block.

○   **What is the ECG rhythm abnormality seen below?**

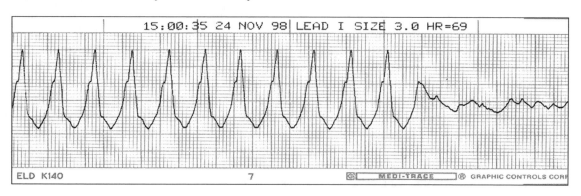

Ventricular tachycardia evolving into ventricular fibrillation.

○   What is the cardiac arrhythmia below?

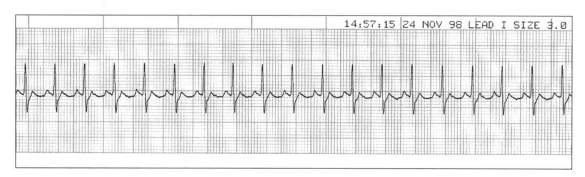

Atrial tachycardia with 2:1 conduction.

○   **What is the abnormality in the ECG seen below?**

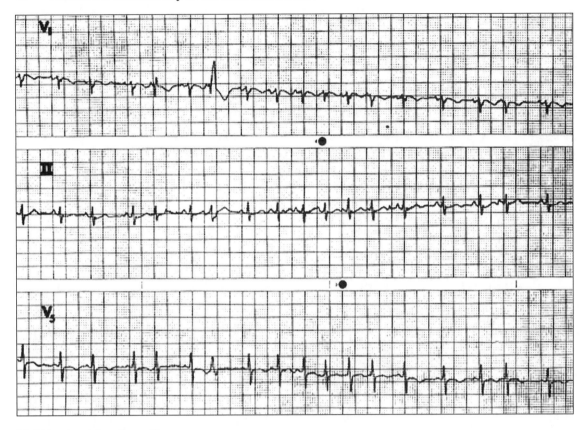

Multifocal atrial tachycardia.

○   **What is the abnormality seen in the rhythm below?**

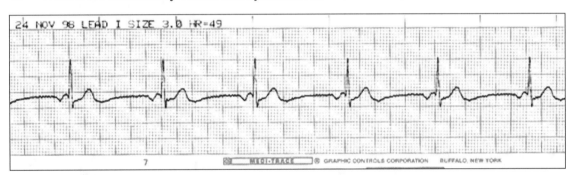

Junctional rhythm.

○   **What is the abnormality seen in the rhythm below?**

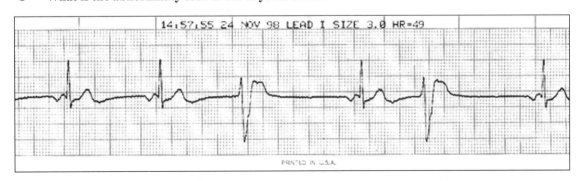

Junctional rhythm with escape ventricular beats.

⭕   **What is the abnormality seen in the rhythm below?**

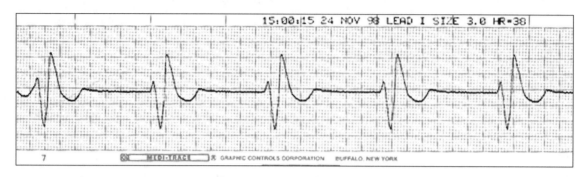

Idioventricular rhythm.

⭕   What is the abnormality seen in the rhythm below?

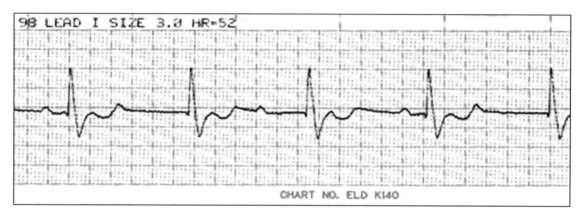

2:1 AV block.

⭕   **What is the abnormality seen in the rhythm below?**

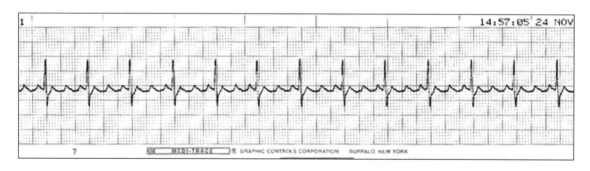

Atrial flutter.

○ **What is the abnormality seen in the rhythm below?**

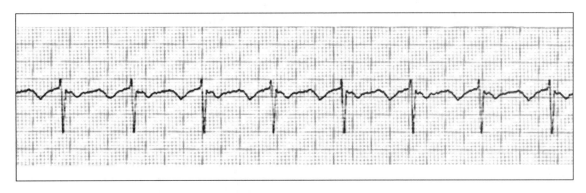

Rhythm strip erroneously mounted upside down. When viewed right-side up, it shows normal sinus rhythm.

○ **What is the rhythm abnormality seen below?**

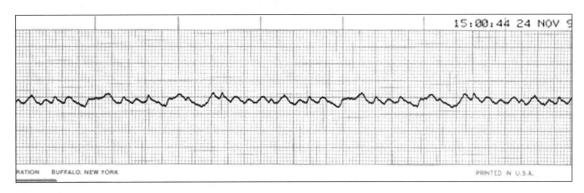

Ventricular fibrillation.

○ **What is the interpretation of this ECG shown below?**

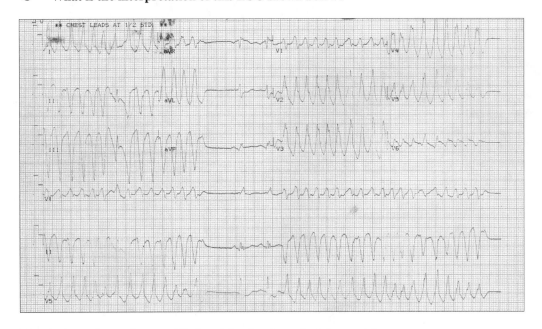

Ventricular tachycardia, most likely originating from the left ventricle.

❍   **What is the interpretation of this ECG shown below?**

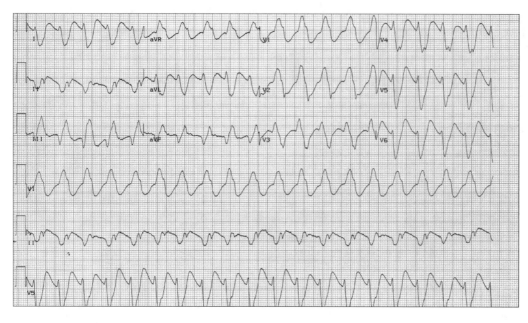

Ventricular tachycardia with hyperkalemia. Note the very wide QRS complex with the early stages of a "sine wave".

❍   **What is the interpretation of the ECG shown below?**

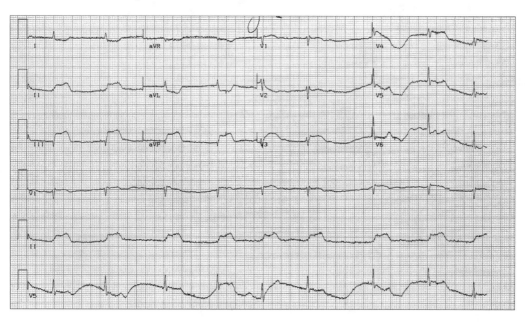

Acute inferior myocardial infarction with posterior wall involvement, atrial fibrillation with slow ventricular rate.

○   **What is the interpretation of the ECG shown below?**

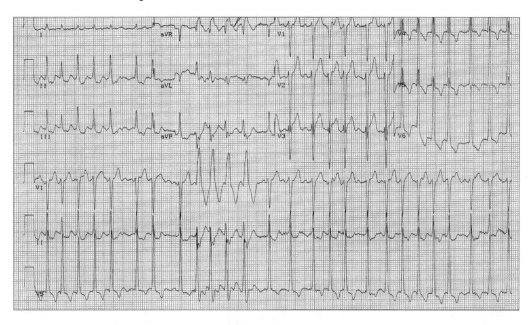

Atrial fibrillation with rapid ventricular rate of 155, LVH, and ischemic-type ST depression in the inferior and lateral leads.

○   **What is the interpretation of the ECG shown below?**

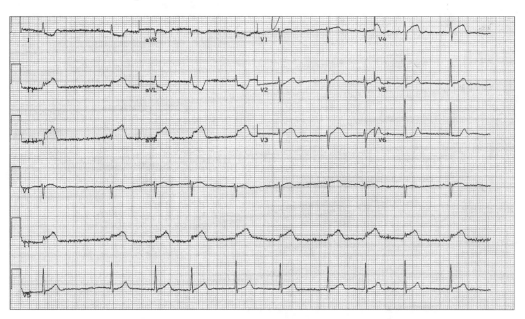

Acute inferior myocardial infarction, atrial fibrillation with slow ventricular rate.

○   **In the above ECG, does this patient absolutely have myocardial ischemia?**

Not necessarily. Patients with supraventricular tachycardia of any type with ST depression can have "ischemic" appearing ST depression without having myocardial ischemia. The ST depression can be as a result of abnormal repolarization that occurs in any tachyarrhythmia. Nonetheless, it would be incorrect to automatically assume that this patient's ST depression is not due to myocardial ischemia.

○   **What is the interpretation of the ECG shown below?**

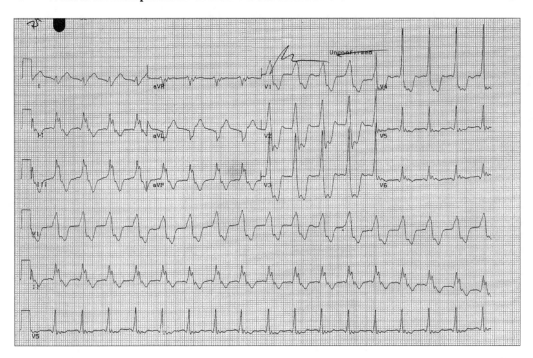

Ventricular tachycardia with a ventricular rate of 103. Note the VA conduction evidenced by the retrograde P waves, which occur in the early part of the ST segment.

○   **What is the abnormality in the echocardiogram shown below?**

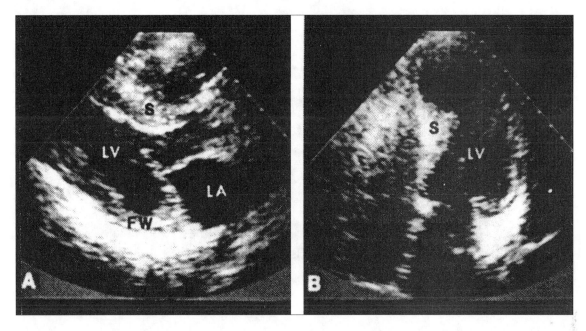

Hypertrophic cardiomyopathy. Note the very thickened septum and anterior systolic motion of the mitral valve.

○   **What is the interpretation of the ECG seen below?**

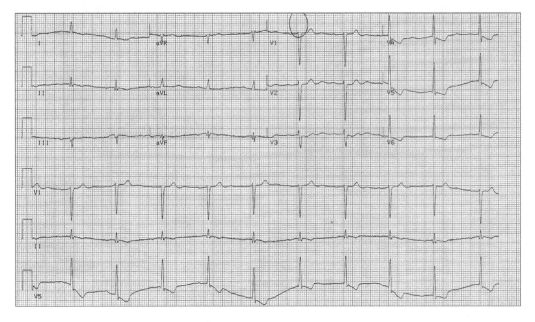

Ectopic atrial rhythm with an old inferior infarction and non-specific ST-T abnormality.

❍   **What is the interpretation of the ECG seen below?**

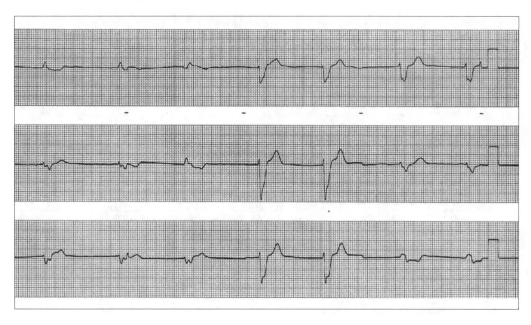

Idioventricular rhythm, rate of 40/min.

❍   **What is the interpretation of the ECG seen below?**

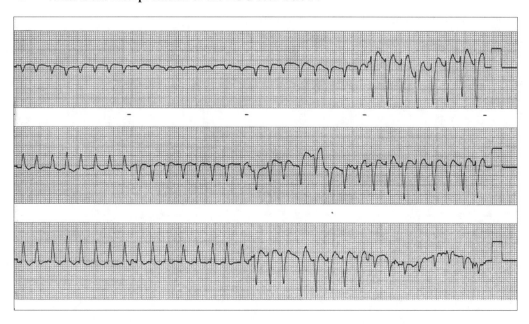

Supraventricular tachycardia.

❍   **How do you treat V-Fib?**

Defibrillate at 200J then 300 J then 360J. Give 1 mg of epinephrine IV push q 3-5 minutes **OR** Vasopressin 40 U IV x 1. Continue defbrillation at 360J. Consider other antiarrythmics (amiodarone, lidocaine, magnesium, procainamide). These are the American Heart Association's guidelines for 2001.

❍   **How do you treat pulseless V-tach?**

Using the same algorithm as V-fib. See above.

○   **How do you treat Pulseless electrical activity?**

Treat the underlying causes first (hypovolemia, hypoxia, hyper/hypokalemia, hypothermia, acidosis, acute MI, tamponade (cardiac), tension pneumothorax, thrombus (pulmonary), tablets). If unknown cause or unsuccessful treat with 1 mg of epinephrine IV push q 3-5 minutes. If the PEA rate is slow use atropine 1 mg IV q 3-5 minutes to a total dose of .04 mg/kg.

○   **How do you treat stable, narrow complex, paroxysmal supraventricular tachycardia?**

First attempt vagal maneuvers, then adenosine 6 mg IV push followed by a repeated doses of 12 mg. If the heart function is preserved (EF>40%) then consider the following drugs in this order of priority: Calcium chanenel blockers, Beta blockers, digoxin, DC cardioversion, procainamide, amiodarone and sotalol. If the heart function is not preserved (EF<40%) there is not priority order. Use digoxin, amiodarone, or diltiazem. Do **NOT** DC Cardiovert these patients. These are the American Heart Association's guidelines for 2001.

○   **What is an ABI, and why is it significant?**

An ankle/brachial index. The ankle systolic pressure (numerator) is compared to the higher of the 2 brachial arterial pressures (denominator). It is used to determine if arterial obstruction is present.

○   **What technical factors can affect the accuracy of the ABI?**

Probe pressure, rapid deflation of the BP cuff, arterial wall calcifications, and probe placement, which should be longitudinal to the vessel and at a 30 to 60 degree angle to the skin surface.

PULMONARY

○ **What should be suspected if a very young, non-smoking patient has symptoms similar to those associated with emphysema?**

α -1-antitrypsin deficiency. Without a-1-antitrypsin, excess elastase accumulates, resulting in lung damage. Treatment for this condition is the same as that emphysema. An α -1 proteinase inhibitor may also be useful.

○ **List two drugs that can cause ARDS.**

Heroin and aspirin.

○ **A 14-year-old boy was exposed to asbestos for three days and has a non-productive cough and chest pain. Does this boy have asbestosis?**

No. Although a non-productive cough and pleurisy are symptoms of asbestosis, other signs, such as exertional dyspnea, malaise, clubbed fingers, crackles, cyanosis, pleural effusion and pulmonary hypertension, should be displayed before making a diagnosis of asbestosis. In addition, asbestosis does not develop until 10 to 15 years after regular exposure to asbestos.

○ **Asbestosis increases the risk of what two diseases?**

Lung cancer and malignant mesothelioma.

○ **Where does aspiration generally occur as revealed by chest x-ray?**

The lower lobe of the right lung. This is the most direct path for foreign bodies into the lung.

○ **What is the pH of aspirated fluid that suggests a poor prognosis?**

pH < 2.5.

○ **What x-ray markings may be observed in a patient with a long history of bronchial asthma?**

Increased bronchial wall markings and flattening of the diaphragm. The bronchial wall markings are caused by epithelial inflammation and thickening of the bronchial walls.

○ **What is the "best" pulmonary function test for the diagnosis of asthma?**

FEV1/FVC. This test determines the amount of air exhaled in 1 minute compared to the total amount of air in the lung that can be expressed. A ratio under 80% is diagnostic of asthma. Peak flow monitors are helpful in monitoring asthma at home, or during an acute exacerbation.

○ **Is wheezing an integral part of asthma?**

No. Thirty-three percent of children with asthma will only have cough variant asthma with no wheezing.

○ **Which is more effective for relieving an acute exacerbation of bronchial asthma in a conscious patient: nebulized albuterol or albuterol MDI administered via an aerosol chamber?**

They are both equally effective.

O   **What are the chances that a child born to two asthmatic parents will also have asthma?**

Up to 50%.

O   **What extrinsic allergens most commonly affect asthmatic children?**

Dust and dust mites.

O   **What treatment should be initiated for a patient with acute asthma who does not improve with humidified O$_2$, albuterol nebulizers, steroids, or anticholinergics?**

Subcutaneous epinephrine (1:1000), 0.3 cc administered every 5 minutes.

O   **Asthmatics will most likely have a family history of what?**

Asthma, allergies, or atopic dermatitis.

O   **What medications should be avoided for a pregnant patient with asthma?**

Epinephrine and parenteral ß-adrenergic agonists.

O   **What is a normal peak expiratory flow rate in adults?**

Males: 550 to 600 L/minute. Females: 450 to 500 L/minute. However, this varies somewhat with body size and age.

O   **Sympathomimetic agents are used to treat asthma. What enzyme do they activate?**

Adenyl cyclase.

O   **What reaction is catalyzed by adenyl cyclase?**

Adenyl cyclase catalyzes ATP to cyclic AMP.

O   **What effects do increased levels of cAMP have on bronchial smooth muscle and the release of chemical mediators, such as histamine, proteases, platelet activation and chemotactic factors, from airway mast cells?**

Smooth muscles are relaxed and release of mediators is decreased. Recall that the effects of cAMP are opposed by cGMP. Thus, another treatment approach can be provided by decreasing the levels of cyclic GMP via the use of anticholinergic (antimuscarinic) agents, such as ipratropium bromide.

O   **Right upper lobe cavitation with parenchymal involvement is a classic indicator** for what?

TB. Lower lung infiltrates, hilar adenopathy, atelectasis, and pleural effusion are also common.

O   **Which ß-adrenergic receptors primarily control bronchiolar and arterial smooth muscle tone?**

ß-2-adrenergic receptors.

❍   **Terbutaline is administered subcutaneously for asthma in what dose?**

0.01 mL/kg of 1 mg/mL terbutaline up to 0.25 mL, i.e., 0.25 mg, which may be repeated once in 20 to 30 minutes.

❍   **Is theophylline useful in the emergency management of a severely asthmatic pediatric patient?**

No. It has not been shown to affect further bronchodilatation in patients fully treated with ß-adrenergic agents. However, theophylline can be used successfully for inpatient management of asthma and may be started in the hospital.

❍   **If corticosteroids are prescribed for acute asthma exacerbation, how should prednisone be dosed?**

1 to 2 mg/kg/day in 2 divided doses. Tapering is not necessary if the duration of therapy is 5 days or less.

❍   **What effect does pre-existing acidosis have on the efficacy of treatment with ß-adrenergic agonists?**

Decreased efficacy.

❍   **What is the appropriate parenteral dose of methylprednisolone (Solu-Medrol) to administer to a pediatric patient with status asthmaticus?**

1 to 2 mg/kg every 6 hours.

❍   **What is the most common postoperative respiratory complication?**

Atelectasis. Respiratory failure and aspiration pneumonia are other postoperative complications.

❍   **Atelectasis accounts for what percentage of postoperative fevers?**

90%.

❍   **Why do we care about postoperative atelectasis?**

If it persists for more than 72 hours, pneumonia may develop. Perioperative mortality rates are then 20%. Incentive spirometry is an important therapy for the prevention of atelectasis.

❍   **A chest x-ray shows honeycombing, atelectasis, and increased bronchial markings. What is the diagnosis?**

Bronchiectasis, an irreversible dilation of the bronchi that is generally associated with infection. Bronchography shows dilations of the bronchial tree, but this method of diagnosis is not recommended for routine use.

❍   **Bronchiectasis occurs most frequently in patients with what conditions?**

Cystic fibrosis, immunodeficiencies, lung infections, or foreign body aspirations.

❍   **Which is the most common type of pathogen in bronchiolitis?**

RSV. It generally affects infants under age 2. Bronchiolitis rarely develops in adults.

O   **What is the treatment for severe RSV documented bronchiolitis?**

Ribavirin.

O   **Where in the US is coccidioidomycosis most prevalent?**

The Southwest. If severe, treat the afflicted patient with amphotericin B.

O   **Which populations are predisposed to progressive infection with coccidioidomycosis?**

African Americans and diabetics.

O   **What is the hallmark symptom of COPD?**

Exertional dyspnea.

O   **What percentage of cigarette smokers develop chronic bronchitis?**

10 to 15%. Chronic bronchitis generally develops after 10 to 12 years of smoking.

O   **Other than smoking, what are the risk factors for COPD?**

Environmental pollutants, recurrent URI's (especially in infancy), eosinophilia or increased serum IgE, bronchial hyperresponsiveness, a family history of COPD, and protease deficiencies.

O   **Is there any hope for patients with COPD who quit smoking?**

Yes. Symptomatically speaking, coughing stops in up to 80% of these patients. Fifty-four percent of COPD patients find relief from coughing within a month of quitting.

O   **If a patient with chronic bronchitis suffers an acute exacerbation of his illness, such as dyspnea, cough, or purulent sputum, what type of O2 therapy should be initiated?**

We have forever been warned against overriding the COPD patient's drive to breathe by over-oxygenating him. Patients with COPD are no longer prompted to breathe by hypercarbia, but by hypoxia alone. However, in the case of acute exacerbation of bronchitis, oxygen therapy should be guided by pO_2 levels. Adequate oxygen must be maintained at a pO_2 above 60 mm Hg. This should be accomplished with the minimal amount of oxygen necessary. The pO_2 must be kept above 60 mm Hg even if the patient loses the drive to breathe.

O   **Which pulmonary function test shows an increase in COPD?**

Residual volume. All other tests (FEV1, FEV1/FVC, and FEV25%–75%,) indicate decreases and diffusion capacity.

O   **Which part of the lung is affected by emphysema? By chronic bronchitis?**

Emphysema: Terminal bronchi
Chronic bronchitis: Large airways

O   **What is the risk of placing a patient with COPD on a high FIO_2?**

Suppression of the hypoxic ventilatory drive.

O   **What is the definition of chronic bronchitis?**

A productive cough for 3 months out of each year for 2 years straight.

○ **What is a "blue bloater" ?**

An overweight patient with COPD, bronchitis, and central cyanosis. These individuals have normal lung capacity and are hypoxic.

○ **What is a "pink puffer" ?**

A patient with COPD and emphysema. These patients are generally thin and non-cyanotic. They have an increased total lung capacity and a decreased FEV1.

○ **In treating a patient with a common cold, you prescribe an oral decongestant. Is it necessary to also suggest an antitussant?**

No. Most coughs, arising from a common cold, are caused by the irritation of the tracheobronchial receptors in the posterior pharynx as a result of postnasal drip. Postnasal drip can be relieved with decongestant therapy, thus eliminating the need for cough suppressant therapy.

○ **What are the most common etiologies of a chronic cough?**

Postnasal drip (40%), asthma (25%), and gastroesophageal reflux (20%). Other etiologies include bronchitis, bronchiectasis, bronchogenic carcinoma, esophageal diverticula, sarcoidosis, viruses, and drugs.

○ **What drugs can induce a chronic cough?**

ACE inhibitors cause chronic cough as a result of the accumulation of prostaglandins, kinins, or substances that excite the cough receptors (Remember that ACE sitting next to you at the boards!!). ß-Blockers evoke bronchoconstriction, and thus coughing, by blocking ß-2 receptors. Never give ß-Blockers to asthmatics or other patients with an airway disease.

○ **Hoarseness can herald far greater problems than viral laryngitis. At what point is a more thorough workup indicated?**

If hoarseness persists for over 6 to 8 weeks or is accompanied by a mass, chest pain, weight loss, aspiration dyspnea, or any other signs of malignancy. You should be suspicious of smokers with chronic cough or hoarseness if there is a change in either.

○ **Your vitamin-crazed father insists that his "vitamin C a day" regime has helped him avoid colds for the past 53 years. Is there any validity to this statement?**

No. Studies have failed to show a prophylactic effect of vitamin C. However, it has been shown that consuming 1 g of vitamin C per day decreases the severity and duration of symptoms associated with the common cold by 23%.

○ **What condition must be ruled out when childhood nasal polyps are found?**

Cystic fibrosis.

○ **What age group is afflicted with the most colds per year?**

Kindergartners win the top billing with an average of 12 colds/year. Second place goes to preschoolers with 6 to 10 per year. School children contract an average of 7 colds/year. Adolescents and adults average only 2 to 4 colds/year.

○ **What is the duration of a common cold?**

3 to 10 days (self-limited).

○ **A 2-year-old presents with wheezing, rhonchi, inspiratory stridor, and a sudden, harsh cough which worsens at night. What is the diagnosis?**

Croup, also known as laryngotracheitis. This condition is usually preceded by a URI and is frequently caused by the parainfluenza virus.

○ **What age group usually contracts croup?**

6 months to 3 years. Croup is characterized by cold symptoms; a sudden, barking cough; inspiratory and expiratory stridor; and a slight fever.

○ **A newborn presents with poor weight gain, steatorrhea, and a GI obstruction arising from thick meconium ileus. What test should be performed?**

The sweat test, which detects electrolyte concentrations in the sweat. The infant may have cystic fibrosis, an autosomal recessive defect that affects the exocrine glands, producing higher electrolyte concentrations in the sweat glands.

○ **What is the classic triad of cystic fibrosis?**

1) COPD
2) Pancreatic enzyme deficiency
3) Abnormally high concentration of sweat electrolytes

○ **What is the most common lethal, inheritable disease in the Caucasian population?**

Cystic fibrosis, an autosomal recessive disease that occurs in 1 in 2,000 births.

○ **Empyema is most often caused by what organism?**

Staphylococcus aureus. Gram-negative organisms and anaerobic bacteria may also cause empyema.

○ **What percentage of effusions are associated with malignancy?**

25%.

○ **What is the difference between the cough of croup and the cough of epiglottitis?**

Croup has a seal-like barking cough, while epiglottitis is accompanied by a minimal cough. Children with croup have a hoarse voice, while those with epiglottitis have a muffled voice.

○ **What is the "thumb print sign"?**

A soft tissue inflammation of the epiglottis seen on a lateral x-ray of the neck. The epiglottis, normally long and thin, appears swollen + flat at the base of the hypopharynx in patients with epiglolttitis.

○ **What is the "steeple sign"?**

Subglottic edema, which creates a symetrically tapered configuration in the subglottic portion of the trachea when imaged in a frontal soft tissue x-ray of the neck. This is consistent with croup.

○ **How is fetal lung maturity assessed?**

By measuring the ratio of lecithin to sphingomyelin (L/S). An L/S ratio greater than 2 and the presence of phosphatidyl glycerol verifies that the fetal lungs are mature.

○ **Hantavirus occurs most commonly in what geographic location?**

Southwestern US, especially in areas with deer mice.

○ **What is the definition for massive hemoptysis?**

Coughing of more than 600 mL of blood in 24 hours.

○ **What are the most common causes of hemoptysis in non-hospitalized patients?**

Bronchitis, bronchogenic carcinoma, tuberculosis, pneumonia, abscess, trauma and idiopathic causes.

○ **What systemic illnesses cause hemoptysis?**

Lung cancer, amyloidosis, CHF, mitral stenosis, sarcoidosis, SLE, vasculitis, coagulation disorders, and pulmonary-renal syndromes.

○ **Life threatening hemoptysis should be suspected when there is:**

1) A large volume of blood
2) Appearance of a fungus ball in a pulmonary cavity on chest x-ray
3) Hypoxemia

○ **What percentage of people in the Ohio and the Mississippi valleys are infected with histoplasmosis?**

100% in endemic areas. However, only 1% of these individuals develop the active disease. The spores of *H. capsulatum* can remain active for 10 years. For unknown reasons, bird and bat feces promote the growth of the actual fungus. The disease is transmitted when the spores are released and inhaled.

○ **What is Pancoast syndrome?**

Tumor of the apex of the lung that gives rise to Horner's syndrome and shoulder pain. The tumor invades the bronchial plexus.

○ **What is Horner's syndrome?**

Miosis, ptosis, and anhydrosis (lack of sweat).

○ **What are Kerley B lines?**

Short horizontal linear densities found on the chest x-ray in patients with pulmonary edema. Fluid in the lung causes waterlogged interlobular septa that then become fibrotic.

○ **What antibiotic is the most effective for treating uncomplicated lung abscesses?**

Clindamycin.

○ **T/F: Flora of lung abscesses are usually polymicrobial.**

True.

○   **What is the most common cancer in the US?**

Lung cancer.

○   **What cancers generally metastasize to the lungs?**

Breast, colon, prostate, and cervical cancers.

○   **What routine program is recommended for screening lung cancer in the adult population?**

None. Screening programs for lung cancer have not demonstrated a decrease in morbidity or mortality. Practitioners must be aware of the signs and symptoms associated with lung cancer, including chronic non-productive cough, increased sputum production, hemoptysis, dyspnea, recurrent pneumonia, hoarseness, pleurisy, weight loss, shoulder pain, SVC syndrome, exercise fatigue, and anemia. Incidental findings on a chest x-ray should also be investigated.

○   **Where do the following cancers most commonly develop within the lung: adenocarcinoma and large cell; and squamous cell and small cell?**

Adenocarcinoma and large cell carcinomas are usually located peripherally, while squamous and small cell carcinomas are located centrally.

○   **Which form of lung cancer is the most common?**

Squamous cell carcinoma (40 to 50%), followed by adenocarcinoma (35%) and small-cell (oat cell) carcinoma (25%).

○   **Name 5 HIV-related pulmonary infections.**

PCP, TB, histoplasmosis, *Cryptococcus*, and CMV.

○   **Describe the chest x-ray of a patient with PCP.**

A reticular patern ranging from fine to course, ill defined patchy areas, segmental and subsegmental consolidation.

○   **What diagnostic test is helpful for the identification of a sub-clinical PCP infection?**

Exertional pulse oximetry is indicative of PCP if after 3 minutes of exercise the O_2 saturation decreases by 3% or the A-a gradient increases by 10 mm Hg from rest.

○   **The initial therapy for PCP includes what antibiotics?**

Trimethoprim-sulfamethoxazole (Bactrim) or pentamidine.

○   **What other medication should be prescribed to a patient with PCP?**

Corticosteroids when the pO_2 is < 70 mm Hg or an A-a gradient > 35 mm Hg.

○   **What two drugs are used as prophylactic treatment to prevent PCP in HIV patients?**

Aerosolized pentamidine (Pentam) or trimethoprim/sulfamethoxazole (Bactrim).

○   **What age group is usually afflicted by pertussis?**

Infants younger than 2 years of age.

○   **Where does pain from pleurisy radiate to?**

The shoulder, as a result of diaphragmatic irritation.

○   **Pneumatoceles (thin-walled air-filled cysts) on an infant's x-ray are a sign of which type of pneumonia?**

Staphylococcal.

○   **What are the most common causes of Staphylococcal pneumonias?**

Drug use and endocarditis. This pneumonia produces high fever, chills, and a purulent productive cough.

○   **What are the extrapulmonary manifestations of mycoplasma?**

Erythema multiforme, pericarditis, and CNS disease.

○   **What is the most frequent etiology of nosocomial pneumonia?**

Pseudomonas aeruginosa. There is a high mortality associated with pneumonia caused by Pseudomonas. It most frequently occurs in immunocompromised patients or patients on mechanical ventilation.

○   **A 67-year-old alcoholic was found in an alley, covered in his own vomit and beer. Upon examination, he is shaking, has a fever of 103.5 °F, and is coughing up currant jelly sputum. What is the diagnosis?**

Pneumonia induced by *Klebsiella pneumoniae*. This is the most probable etiology in alcoholics, the elderly, the very young, and immunocompromised patients. Other gram-negative bacteria, such as *E. coli* and other *Enterobacteriaceae*, may cause pneumonia in alcoholics who have aspirated.

○   **Match the pneumonia with the treatment.**

1) *Klebsiella pneumoniae*	a) **Erythromycin, azithromycin, tetracycline, or**
2) *Streptococcus pneumoniae*	**doxycycline**
3) *Legionella pneumophila*	b) **Penicillin G**
4) *Haemophilus influenzae*	c) **Cefuroxime and clarithromycin**
5) *Mycoplasma pneumoniae*.	d) **Erythromycin and rifampin**

Answers: (1) c, (2) b, (3) d, (4) c, and (5) a.

○   **Describe the classic chest x-ray findings in a patient with mycoplasma pneumonia.**

Patchy diffuse densities involving the entire lung. Pneumatoceles, cavities, abscesses, and pleural effusions can occur, but are uncommon. Treat the patient with erythromycin.

○   **Describe the classic chest x-ray finding associated with *Legionella* pneumonia.**

Dense consolidation and bulging fissures. Expect elevated liver enzymes and hypophosphatemia. The patient with *Legionella* pneumonia classically presents with a relative bradycardia.

○   **A 43 year old male presents with pleurisy, sudden onset of fever and chills, and rust colored sputum. What is the probable diagnosis?**

Pneumococcal pneumonia caused by *Streptococcus pneumoniae*, the most common community-acquired pneumonia. It is a consolidating lobar pneumonia and can be treated with penicillin G or erythromycin.

O   **A 20 year old college student is home for winter break and presents complaining of a 10 day history of a non-productive dry hacking cough, malaise, a mild fever, and no chills. What is a possible diagnosis?**

Mycoplasma pneumoniae, also known as walking pneumonia. Although this is the most common pneumonia that develops in teenagers and young adults, it is an atypical pneumonia and most frequently occurs in close contact populations, i.e., schools and military barracks.

O   **A 56 year old smoker with COPD presents with chills, fever, green sputum, and extreme shortness of breath. An x-ray shows a right lower lobe pneumonia. What is expected from the sputum culture?**

Haemophilus influenzae. This organism is generally found in pneumonia and bronchitis patients with underlying COPD. The next most common organism detected in this patient population is *Moraxella catarrhalis*. Ampicillin/clavulanate (Augmentin) is the drug of choice, but patients at high risk should have yearly influenza vaccinations.

O   **Describe the different presentations of bacterial and viral pneumonia.**

Bacterial pneumonia is typified by a sudden onset of symptoms, including pleurisy, fever, chills, productive cough, tachypnea, and tachycardia. The most common bacterial pneumonia is Pneumococcal pneumonia.

Viral pneumonia is characterized by gradual onset of symptoms, no pleurisy, chills or high fever, general malaise, and a non-productive cough.

O   **What is the most common cause of pneumonia in children?**

Viral pneumonia. Infecting viruses include influenza, parainfluenza, RSV, and adenoviruses.

O   **What percent of upper respiratory infectious agents are non-bacterial?**

Non-bacterial agents account for over 90% of pharyngitis, laryngitis, tracheal bronchitis, and bronchitis.

O   **Name two anti-viral medications that are used for viral pneumonia.**

Amantadine, for influenza A, and aerosolized Ribavirin, for RSV.

O   **If a patient has a patchy infiltrate on a chest x-ray and bullous myringitis, what antibiotic should be prescribed?**

Erythromycin for *Mycoplasma*.

O   **What secondary bacterial infection often occurs following a viral pneumonia?**

Staphylococcal pneumonia.

O   **In what season does Legionella pneumonia most commonly occur?**

Summer. *Legionella pneumophila* thrive in environments such as the water cooling towers that are used in large buildings and hotels. Staphylococcal pneumonias also occur more frequently in summer.

O   **An older patient with GI symptoms, hyponatremia, and a relative bradycardia probably has which type of pneumonia?**

Legionella.

O   **What is the indication for a chest tube in a patient with a pneumothorax?**

Over 15% pneumothorax or a clinical indication, such as respiratory distress or enlarging pneumothorax.

O   **What therapy may increase the body's absorption of a pneumothorax or pneumomediastinum?**

A high FiO_2.

O   **What is the profile of a classic patient with a spontaneous pneumothorax?**

Male, athletic, tall, slim and 15 to 35 years of age.

O   **What is the recurrence rate of spontaneous pneumothoraxes?**

30 to 50%.

O   **Which types of pneumonia are commonly associated with pneumothorax?**

Staphylococcal, TB, *Klebsiella*, and PCP.

O   **What is the anticoagulant treatment schedule for a PE?**

IV heparin until PTT is 2 to 2.5 times normal. After a day, warfarin is added until the INR is greater than 2.0. If clots recur, consider a Greenfield filter in the IVC. Pulmonary embolectomy is only necessary in cases of massive embolisms. Lovenox may also be used instead of heparin.

O   **What three syndromes are associated with the various degrees of pulmonary embolism?**

1) Acute cor pulmonate: Occurs with massive embolism that obstructs over 60% of the pulmonary
                          circulation
2) Pulmonary infarction: Occurs with embolization to the distal branches of the pulmonary circulation
3) Acute dyspnea: Milder obstruction not enough to warrant infarction

O   **What is the equation for the A-a gradient?**

$A\text{-}a = (713 \text{ mm Hg} \times FiO_2)\text{-}pCO_2\text{-}pO_2/0.8)$.

The normal A-a gradient is 5 to 15 mm Hg (though it increases with age). The A-a gradient increases with PE and diffusion defects (i.e., pulmonary edema and right to left cardiac shunts).

O   **Most pulmonary embolisms arise from what veins?**

The iliac and femoral veins.

O   **Primary pulmonary hypertension is most common in what population?**

Young females. PPH is rapidly fatal within a few years.

O   **What heart sounds accompany pulmonary hypertension?**

A narrowed second heart sound split and a louder P2.

❍   **What is the major etiology of pulmonary hypertension?**

Chronic hypoxia, most commonly from COPD.

❍   **T/F: Pulse oximetry is a reliable method for estimating oxyhemoglobin saturation in a patient suffering from CO poisoning.**

False. COHb has light absorbance that can lead to a falsely elevated pulse oximeter transduced saturation level. The calculated value from a standard ABG may also be falsely elevated. The oxygen saturation should be determined by using a co-oximeter that measures the amounts of unsaturated O_2Hb, COHb, and metHb.

❍   **A newborn is breathing rapidly and grunting. Intercostal retractions, nasal flaring, and cyanosis are noted. Auscultation shows decreased breath sounds and crackles. What is the diagnosis?**

Newborn respiratory distress syndrome, also known as hyaline membrane disease. X-rays show diffuse atelectasis. Treatment involves artificial surfactant and O2 administration through CPAP.

❍   **Other than avoiding prematurity, what can be done to prevent newborn respiratory distress syndrome?**

If the fetus is older than 32 weeks, administer betamethasone 48 to 72 hours before delivery to augment surfactant production.

❍   **Sarcoidosis is most common in what race and age group?**

African Americans between 20 and 40 years of age.

❍   **What will the chest x-ray of a patient with sarcoidosis classically reveal?**

Bilateral hilar and paratracheal adenopathy with diffuse nodular appearing infiltrate. Sarcoidosis can be staged by the chest x-ray:

Stage 0:   Normal
Stage 1:   Hilar adenopathy
Stage 2:   Hilar adenopathy and parenchymal infiltrates
Stage 3:   Parenchymal infiltrates only
Stage 4:   Pulmonary fibrosis

❍   **What other systems can be affected by sarcoidosis?**

The cardiovascular, gastrointestinal, immunological, integumental, lymphatics, and the ocular systems.

❍   **Upper lobe nodules and eggshell hilar node calcification are displayed on x-rays of an individual with what disease?**

Silicosis.

❍   **What is the indication for long-term tracheostomy?**

When intubation is expected to exceed 3 weeks.

❍   **Differentiate between transudate and exudate.**

Transudate: Pleural: Serum protein < 0.5

Pleural: Serum LDH is < 0.6
Most common with CHF, renal disease, and liver disease.

Exudate: Pleural: Serum protein > 0.5
Pleural: Serum LDH > 0.6
Most common with infections, malignancy, and trauma.

○   **What are the side effects of INH?**

Neuropathy, pyridoxine loss, lupus-like syndrome, anion-gap acidosis and hepatitis.

○   **What percentage of tuberculosis cases are drug resistant?**

About 15%.   The rate is highly dependent upon geographic location.

○   **What are the classic signs and symptoms of TB?**

Night sweats, fever, weight loss, malaise, cough, and a greenish yellow sputum most commonly observed in the mornings.

○   **Name some common extrapulmonary TB sites.**

The lymph nodes, bone, GI tract, GU tract, meninges, liver, and the pericardium.

○   **T/F: Patients under 35 years of age with positive TB skin tests should undergo at least 6 months of isoniazid chemoprophylaxis.**

True.

○   **A patient presents with cough, lethargy, dyspnea, conjunctivitis, glomerulonephritis, fever, and purulent sinusitis.   What is the probable diagnosis?**

Wegener's granulomatosis. This is a necrotizing vasculitis and pulmonary granulomatosis that attacks the small artery and veins. Treat the patient with corticosteroids and cyclophosphamide.

○   **What serological test is diagnostic for Wegener's granulomatosis?**

c-ANCA in association with appropriate clinical evidence. A renal, lung, or sinus biopsy may also be helpful in making the diagnosis.

○   **What is the mechanism of alveolar hypoventilation (manifested by high PCO$_2$) in myxedema?**

Depression of the hypoxic and hypercapnic respiratory drive. Respiratory muscle myopathy and phrenic neuropathy are uncommon.

○   **Should all individuals with chronic unexplained alveolar hypoventilation be tested for hypothyroidism?**

Yes.

○   **Is obstructive sleep apnea common in hypothyroidism?**

Yes. Contributing factors include enlarged tongue and myopathy. Hypothyroidism should be excluded in most patients with sleep apnea.

○   **What other endocrine disorder is associated with an increased frequency of sleep apnea?**

Acromegaly. Sleep apnea may be central or obstructive in origin.

○   **Can beta-adrenergic agonists result in tolerance?**

Yes. Repeated administration of beta agonist bronchodilators can result in hyposensitization of the receptors, but this should not preclude their use. Glucocorticoids have been shown to restore the depressed receptor responsiveness.

○   **Prior steroid administration can precipitate adrenal insufficiency under conditions of stress. How long can this effect last?**

Up to one year.

○   **What is the common mechanism of hyponatremia in pulmonary tumors and infections?**

SIADH.

○   **What type of lung cancer is commonly associated with hypercalcemia?**

Squamous cell carcinoma. The production of parathormone related peptide can produce hypercalcemia even without bony metastases.

○   **Which non-neoplastic pulmonary disease is often associated with hypercalcemia and hypercalciuria?**

Sarcoidosis.

○   **What type of lung tumors can cause excessive ACTH production and Cushing's syndrome?**

Small cell carcinoma and carcinoid tumors.

○   **What are the pulmonary manifestations in Paget's Disease?**

High output cardiac failure with pulmonary edema, impaired respiratory control from bony involvement at base of skull, vertebral fractures leading to kyphosis and restrictive lung disease.

○   **What is acute chest syndrome in sickle cell disease?**

The syndrome includes fever, chest pain, leukocytosis and pulmonary infiltrate. The major dilemma is in distinguishing infarction from pneumonia. Acute chest syndrome can also be caused by fat embolism and pulmonary edema.

○   **What is sickle cell chronic lung disease?**

It is thought to be the result of years of uncontrolled and often asymptomatic sickling and characterized by pulmonary hypertension, cor pulmonale and ventilatory defects.

○   **What is the most common cause of pneumonia in sickle cell disease?**

Streptococcus pneumoniae.

○   **What are the preventive measures commonly employed in sickle cell disease?**

Pneumococcal vaccine, *Haemophilus influenzae* b vaccine and yearly influenza vaccine in those with chronic pulmonary symptoms.

○ **Which type of pneumonia is often associated with cold agglutinins?**

Mycoplasma pneumoniae.

○ **Name some of the hypercoagulable states predisposing individuals to thrombosis and pulmonary embolism.**

Deficiencies of protein C, protein S and antithrombin III; factor V mutation; antiphospholipid syndrome; malignancy particularly adenocarcinoma; nephrotic syndrome; protein losing enteropathy; extensive burns; paroxysmal nocturnal hemoglobinuria; and oral contraceptives.

○ **What are the pulmonary manifestations of polycythemia?**

Pulmonary embolism related to hyperviscosity and pulmonary hemorrhage related to an increased bleeding tendency.

○ **What is the normal PCO^2 in pregnancy?**

30-34 mm Hg from chronic mild hyperventilation, presumably as a result of progesterone.

○ **What is the predominant change in the lung volumes in pregnancy?**

Decrease in functional residual capacity by as much as 15-25%..

○ **Why is the incidence of thromboembolism increased in pregnancy?**

Venous stasis from the uterine pressure on the inferior vena cava, increase in clotting factors, increased fibrinogen and decreased fibrinolysis.

○ **What are some of the risk factors for thromboembolism in pregnancy?**

C-Section, multiparity, bed rest, obesity, increased maternal age, and surgical procedures.

○ **What are the potential mechanisms of cardiorespiratory collapse?**

Mechanical obstruction of pulmonary vasculature, alveolar capillary leak, pulmonary edema from LV failure, anaphylaxis.

○ **What is the mortality rate in amniotic fluid embolism?**

About 80%.

○ **What is the classic presentation of venous air embolism?**

Sudden hypotension with a mill wheel murmur audible over the precordium.

○   **What is the preferred patient position in suspected venous air embolism?**

Left lateral decubitus and Trendelenburg.

○   **What are some of the common misconceptions about the management of asthma during pregnancy?**

That dyspnea is common in pregnancy and that medications should be sparsely used. Uncontrolled asthma causes more fetal harm than medications.

○   **What drug will produce hilar and mediastinal adenopathy as a toxic reaction?**

Methotrexate.

○   **T/F: Generally the cough related to ACE inhibitors resolves within a few days of withdrawal of the drug.**

False. The resolution of cough may be slow, taking several weeks.

○   **What is the incidence of aspirin-induced bronchospasm in patients with nasal polyps?**

Up to 75%.

○   **T/F: In aspirin-induced bronchospasm, there can be cross-reactivity with non-steroidal anti-inflammatory drugs.**

True.

○   **What laboratory finding distinguishes patients with primary SLE and drug-induced lupus?**

Drug-induced lupus has a positive ANA, but a <u>negative</u> ds-DNA.

○   **T/F: Beta-adrenergic antagonists in massive overdose may cause severe bronchospasm in normal individuals.**

False.

○   **T/F: Cardioselective beta-blockers avoid precipitation of bronchospasm in asthmatic individuals.**

False.

○   **What is the therapeutic drug of choice for beta-blocker-induced bronchospasm?**

Inhaled ipratropium bromide. If severe, parenteral glucagon can reverse effects.

❍ **Name 4 antibiotics known to have <u>in vitro</u> activity against anaerobic bacteria in virtually all cases.**

Metronidazole, chloramphenicol, imipenem and beta-lactam/beta-lactamase inhibitors.

❍ **Which gram-negative aerobes are known to cause lung abscess?**

Pseudomonas and *Klebsiella*.

❍ **What are the two major risk factors for the development of anaerobic lung infection?**

Periodontal disease and predisposition to aspiration.

❍ **What is the drug of choice for pneumonias acquired in the outpatient setting due to anaerobic bacteria?**

Clindamycin.

❍ **What factor determines the magnitude of injury in gastric acid aspiration?**

The gastric pH. A pH less than 3 produces the most severe injury.

❍ **Empyema in the absence of parenchymal lung infiltrate suggests what underlying process?**

Subphrenic or other intra-abdominal abcess.

❍ **What is the recommended duration of antibiotic therapy for necrotizing anaerobic pneumonia, lung abcess or empyema?**

4 - 8 weeks.

❍ **Under what circumstances is aspiration of vomitus, oral secretions or foreign material likely?**

Anything producing an altered level of consciousness (e.g. alcohol, overdose, general anesthesia, stroke), impaired swallowing or abnormal gastro-intestinal motility, or disruption of the esophageal sphincters predisposes to aspiration.

❍ **What are the signs of a large obstructing foreign body in the larynx or trachea?**

Respiratory distress, stridor, inability to speak, cyanosis, loss of consciousness, and death.

❍ **What are the symptoms of a smaller (distally lodged) foreign body?**

Cough, dyspnea, wheezing, chest pain and fever.

❍ **What is the procedure of choice for foreign body removal in the lung?**

Rigid bronchoscopy. Fiberoptic bronchoscopy is an alternate procedure in adults, not in children. If bronchoscopy fails, thoracotomy may be required.

❍ **What are the common radiographic findings in foreign body aspiration?**

Normal film, atelectasis, pneumonia, contralateral mediastinal shift (more marked during expiration), and visualization of the foreign body.

❍ **What are the common directly toxic (non-infected) respiratory tract aspirates?**

Gastric contents, alcohol, hydrocarbons, mineral oil, animal and vegetable fats. All of these produce an inflammatory response and pneumonia. Gastric contents are the most common offender.

○   **What are the consequences of aspirating acid?**

The response is rapid, with near immediate bronchitis, bronchiolitis, atelectasis, shunting and hypoxemia. Pulmonary edema may occur within 4 hours. The clinical manifestations are dyspnea, wheezing, cough, cyanosis, fever and shock.

○   **Under what circumstances are antibiotics used in aspiration?**

Aspiration of infected material, intestinal obstruction, immune compromised host, and evidence of bacterial superinfection after a non-infected aspirate (new fever, infiltrates, or purulence after the initial 2 to 3 days).

○   **What are the radiographic manifestations of acid aspiration?**

Varied, may be bilateral diffuse infiltrates, irregular "patchy" infiltrates, or lobar infiltrates.

○   **What outcomes occur in patients who do not rapidly resolve gastric acid aspiration pneumonitis?**

ARDS (adult respiratory distress syndrome), progressive respiratory failure and death; bacterial superinfection.

○   **What is the frequency of ARDS (adult respiratory distress syndrome) after near drowning?**

40%.

○   **What are the invasive therapies for massive hemoptysis?**

Thoracotomy, embolization, balloon tamponade (via bronchoscopy), double-lumen tube for lung separation and independent ventilation, and laser bronchoscopy.

○   **What is the most feared complication of bronchial artery embolization?**

Anterior spinal artery embolization.

○   **What is the most common cause of hemoptysis in patients with leukemia?**

Fungal infections, often *Aspergillus*.

○   **Which bacterial pneumonias frequently cause frank hemoptysis?**

Pseudomonas aeruginosa, Klebsiella pneumoniae, and Staphylococcus aureus.

○   **What are the major cardiovascular causes of hemoptysis?**

Mitral stenosis, pulmonary hypertension, Eisenmenger's complex.

○   **Calculate the alveolar-arterial oxygen (A-aO_2) gradient given the following arterial blood gas obtained at sea level: pH 7.24, PaCO_2 60 PaO_2 45.**

30 mmHg.
To calculate the alveolar-arterial oxygen gradient, first calculate the expected alveolar partial pressure of oxygen (PaO_2) using the alveolar gas equation: $PAO_2 = PIO_2 - PaCO_2/R$, where PIO_2 is the partial pressure of oxygen in the inspired gas and R is the respiratory exchange ratio, commonly estimated at 0.8. PIO_2 is calculated as follows: $PIO_2 = FIO_2 (P_B - P_{H2O})$ where FIO_2 is the inspired concentration of oxygen (0.21 at sea

level), P_B is the atmospheric pressure (760 mm Hg at sea level) and P_{H2O} is the partial pressure of water (47 mmHg). At sea level, P_{IO_2} is equal to 150 mmHg. Thus, for this example, P_{AO_2} = 150 - 60/0.8 or 75 mmHg.

The A-aO2 gradient is P_{AO_2} - P_{aO_2}. Therefore, in this example, the A-aO_2 gradient is 75 - 45 or 30 mmHg.

❍   **What is the age related decline in PaO_2?**

The PaO_2 declines by 2.5 mmHg per decade. Given that a PaO_2 of 95-100 mmHg is normal for a 20-year-old, a PaO_2 of 75-80 would be normal for a 80-year-old.

❍   **What are the four principal mechanisms that lead to hypoxemia?**

Hypoventilation, diffusion limitation, shunt and ventilation-perfusion inequality. A fifth mechanism, low inspired oxygen concentration, is important only at altitudes above 8000 feet..

❍   **Which of the four above mechanisms is the most common?**

Ventilation-perfusion inequality.

❍   **What are the 3 major mechanisms of hypoventilation and what clinical conditions are associated with each?**

1.   Failure of the central nervous system ventilatory centers - drugs (narcotics, barbiturates), stroke.
2.   Failure of the chest bellows - chest wall diseases (kyphoscoliosis), neuromuscular diseases (amyotrophic lateral sclerosis), diaphragm weakness.
3.   Obstruction of the airways - asthma, chronic obstructive pulmonary disease.

❍   **How can hypoxemia secondary to hypoventilation alone be distinguished from the other causes of hypoxemia?**

If the hypoxemia is from hypoventilation alone, the A-aO_2 gradient is normal. It is elevated in all other causes.

❍   **What are the most common clinical conditions in which shunt is the primary mechanism for hypoxemia?**

Alveolar filling with fluid (pulmonary edema) and pus (pneumonia) are the most commonly seen clinically. Any condition that fills or closes the alveoli preventing gas exchange can lead to shunt.

❍   **How can shunt be distinguished from the other causes of hypoxemia?**

If given 100% oxygen, the hypoxemic patient with shunt will not have a significant increase in their PaO_2. There will be a significant increase in PaO_2 when 100% oxygen is given to patients with hypoventilation or ventilation-perfusion inequality.

❍   **A leftward shift in the oxyhemoglobin dissociation curve indicates an increased or decreased hemoglobin affinity for oxygen?**

Increased.

❍   **Changes in temperature, $PaCO_2$ or pH, or the level of 2,3-diphosphoglycerate (2,3-DPG) cause a shift in the oxyhemoglobin dissociation curve. To cause a rightward shift, what are the changes that must occur?**

Increased temperature, increased $PaCO_2$, decreased pH, and increased 2,3-DPG level. An easy way to remember this is that these conditions are often associated with decreased tissue oxygen levels. By right-shifting the curve, more oxygen is released from the hemoglobin to the tissues.

O   **What is the Bohr effect?**

The rightward shift of the oxyhemoglobin desaturation curve, secondary to decreased pH.

O   **Which types of hemoglobin are associated with an leftward shift of the oxyhemoglobin dissociation curve?**

Hemoglobin F (fetal hemoglobin), carboxyhemoglobin, and methemoglobin.

O   **Which drugs cause methemoglobinemia?**

Oxidant drugs, such as antimalarials, dapsone, nitrites/nitrates (nitroprusside) and local anesthetics (lidocaine). Methemoglobinemia occurs when the iron moiety of hemoglobin is oxidated from the ferrous to the ferric state.

O   **Which common enzyme deficiency predisposes to the development of methemoglobinemia in the presence of the above drugs?**

G-6-PD deficiency.

O   **What is the treatment of methemoglobinemia?**

Methylene blue.

O   **What are the determinants of the oxygen content of blood?**

Hemoglobin concentration, the PaO_2 and SaO_2. The equation to determine the oxygen content of blood is: $CaO_2 = (1.34 \times [Hgb] \times SaO_2) + (PaO_2 \times 0.003)$. The first term is the hemoglobin bound oxygen and the second is the dissolved oxygen. Dissolved oxygen content is a minor portion of total oxygen content unless PaO_2 is very high.

O   **How does the shape of the oxyhemoglobin dissociation curve effect the oxygen content of blood?**

Since SaO_2 does not increase significantly if the $PaO_2 > 60$ mmHg, the oxygen content of blood will increase significantly above this level only by increasing the hemoglobin concentration.

O   **What are the determinants of oxygen delivery to the peripheral tissues?**

Oxygen content of the blood (CaO_2) and cardiac output. An increase in either will increase oxygen delivery to the tissues.

O   **What is the difference between anatomic and physiologic dead space?**

Dead space refers to areas of lung that are ventilated but not perfused. Anatomic dead space refers to the conducting airways (trachea, bronchi and bronchioles) where there is no gas exchange because there are no alveoli. Physiologic dead space includes the anatomic dead space and any diseased lung in which there is ventilation but no perfusion.

O   **What is the normal dead space in an average 70 kg subject?**

150 ml.

○ **Which pulmonary diseases are most associated with an increased physiologic dead space?**

Asthma and chronic obstructive pulmonary disease (COPD).

○ **How is the minute ventilation related to alveolar and dead space ventilation?**

Minute ventilation (V_E) is the product of tidal volume multiplied by breathing frequency ($V_E = V_T$ X f). Alveolar ventilation (V_A) is that portion of the minute ventilation that contributes to gas exchange while dead space ventilation (V_D) is that portion that does not contribute to gas exchange. Thus, $V_E = V_A + V_D$.

○ **What is the effect of increased alveolar ventilation (V_A) on $PaCO_2$?**

$PaCO_2$ will decrease as V_A increases.

○ **What is the relationship between alveolar ventilation, minute ventilation and the dead space ratio (V_D/V_T)?**

Alveolar ventilation is proportional to both minute ventilation and the term ($1 - V_D/V_T$). Any process that decreases minute ventilation or increases the dead space will decrease alveolar ventilation.

○ **Why do asthmatics eventually have an increased $PaCO_2$ if untreated?**

As the asthma attack continues untreated, the work of breathing will continue to increase. Eventually, the diaphragm fatigues and the patient hypoventilates. The hypoventilation, in association with the increased dead space and increased CO_2 production, increases the $PaCO_2$.

○ **What is the normal $PaCO_2$ and does it vary with age?**

Normal $PaCO_2$ is 35-45 mmHg and does not vary with age.

○ **What is the normal expected change in pH if there is an acute change in the $PaCO_2$?**

The pH will increase or decrease 0.8 units for every 10 mmHg decrease or increase (respectively) in $PaCO_2$.

○ **What is the expected change in serum bicarbonate in chronic respiratory acidosis or alkalosis?**

Bicarbonate increases by approximately 3 mEq/l for each 10 mmHg increase in $PaCO_2$ in chronic respiratory acidosis. Bicarbonate decreases by 4-5 mEq/l for each 10 mmHg decrease in $PaCO_2$ in chronic respiratory alkalosis.

○ **What are the consequences of hypercapnia?**

Acute hypercapnia has physiologic consequences due to the increased $PaCO_2$ itself and the decreased pH. Physiologic effects of the $PaCO_2$ increase include:
1. Increases in cerebral blood flow.
2. Confusion, headache ($PaCO_2 > 60$ mmHg), obtundation and seizures ($PaCO_2 > 70$ mmHg).
3. Depression of diaphragmatic contractility.
The primary consequences of the decreased pH are on the cardiovascular system with changes in cardiac contractility (decreased), the fibrillation threshold (decreased), and vascular tone (predominantly vasodilatation).

○ **What are the consequences of hypocapnia?**

Acute hypocapnia has physiologic consequences due to the decreased $PaCO_2$ itself and the increased pH. Physiologic effects of the $PaCO_2$ decrease include:

1. Decreases in cerebral blood flow. This reflex is used in the management of neurologic disorders with high intracranial pressures as a short-term measure to decrease the increased intracranial pressure.
2. Confusion, myclonus, asterixis, loss of consciousness and seizures.

The primary consequences of the increased pH are, again, primarily on the cardiovascular system with increased cardiac contractility and vasodilatation.

❍   **A 25-year-old male presents to the emergency room obtunded. Examination is significant for a respiratory rate of 8 breaths/min and pinpoint pupils. An arterial blood gas reveals a pH of 7.28, a $PaCO_2$ of 55, and a PaO_2 60. What is a likely cause of the hypoxemia and hypercapnia?**

Acute narcotic overdose leading to hypoventilation. Give the man some narcan!

❍   **The chest x-ray reveals no pulmonary parenchymal lesions but does show prominent hila and an enlarged right ventricle. What diagnostic test should be performed?**

The patient has no pulmonary parenchymal lesions to cause a shunt; therefore, she most likely has an intracardiac right-to-left shunt (most likely a previously undiagnosed atrial septal defect). An echocardiogram should be performed.

❍   **A 45-year-old obese male presents with dyspnea, peripheral edema, snoring, and excessive daytime sleepiness. A room air arterial blood gas in drawn and the pH is 7.34, $PaCO_2$ 60 mmHg, the PaO_2 is 58 mmHg, and the calculated HCO_3^- is 28 mEq/l. What is acid-base disturbance?**

Chronic, compensated respiratory acidosis. If this was acute respiratory acidosis, the pH would be 7.24 with a normal HCO_3^-.

❍   **What is the cause of the hypoxemia?**

Hypoventilation is one cause. However, since the $A-aO_2$ gradient is elevated, there is another cause in addition to the hypoventilation. In an obese patient, both ventilation-perfusion inequality and shunt (secondary to atelectasis) can contribute to the development of hypoxemia.

❍   **A 50-year-old woman presents with a pneumonia in the right lower and middle lobes. On 50% oxygen by face mask, her PaO_2 is 75 mmHg. Should the patient be positioned right side down or up?**

Right side up. Blood flow is gravity dependent. If the patient is positioned right side down, blood flow will preferentially go to the right side. However, because of the pneumonia, this will increase the amount of shunt, lowering the PaO_2 further.

❍   **T/F: If a patient presents with a $PaCO_2$ of 75, he/she should be emergently intubated.**

False. There is no $PaCO_2$ level at which a patient must be intubated. Intubation is based upon the total clinical condition of a patient, not just upon a blood gas result.

❍   **A 45-year-old presents to the ER after being rescued from a fire. He is dyspneic and cyanotic. SaO_2 on 50% mask is 84%. The blood gas, however, reveals a PaO_2 of 125 mmHg. Why the discrepancy?**

A fire victim is likely to have carbon monoxide poisoning. The carbon monoxide has converted the hemoglobin to carboxyhemoglobin, which decreases the binding of oxygen to hemoglobin and prevents an accurate pulse oximetry reading. However, carbon monoxide does not affect dissolved oxygen, which is what is measured in the arterial blood gas.

❍   **What is the treatment for carbon monoxide poisoning?**

100% oxygen, which increases carbon monoxide clearance by competing for binding to hemoglobin. If there is no significant response to 100% oxygen, hyperbaric oxygen (oxygen provided at higher than atmospheric pressure) is an alternative therapy.

○ **A 25-year-old woman with a history of mitral valve prolapse presents with 'nervousness', chest tightness, hand numbness and mild confusion. Arterial blood gas reveals: pH 7.52, $PaCO_2$ 25 mmHg, PaO_2 108 mmHg. What is the diagnosis?**

Acute anxiety attack. She is hyperventilating.

○ **Why is the PaO_2 elevated?**

Because the lower $PaCO_2$ means a higher PAO_2 (see alveolar gas equation above).

○ **What is the treatment?**

The acute hyperventilation can be terminated by having the patient breathe in and out of a bag. Anxiolytics can also be provided.

○ **T/F: Oxygen should never be given to a hypoxemic patient with COPD who has chronic CO_2 retention.**

False. Oxygen should always be given to a patient who is hypoxemic.

○ **What is the major side effect associated with the inhalation of N-acetylcysteine?**

Cough and bronchospasm, most likely due to irritation from the low pH (2.2) of the aerosol solution.

○ **What is the effect of macrolide antibiotics (erythromycin, clarithromycin) on mucus hypersecretion?**

Some macrolide antibiotics have the ability to down regulate mucus secretion by an unknown mechanism. This is thought to be due to an anti-inflammatory activity.

○ **Exposure to what mineral, used as insulation, greatly enhances the carcinogenic potential of exposure to cigarette smoke?**

Asbestos.

○ **What other exposures are also factors contributing to the development of bronchogenic carcinoma?**

Radon, uranium, nickel, arsenic, bis (chloromethyl) ether, ionizing radiation, vinyl chloride, mustard gas, polycyclic aromatic hydrocarbons, and chromium.

○ **Second hand cigarette smoke exposure is a risk factor for the development of what two major lung diseases?**

Lung cancer and COPD.

○ **Which primary lung cancer is most frequently associated with paraneoplastic syndromes?**

Small cell undifferentiated carcinoma.

○ **The incidence of lung cancer is increasing in the USA among members of which gender?**

Females.

❍ **What accounts for this increase?**

Increased cigarette smoking prevalence.

❍ **Which vitamin has been associated with a protective effect against the development of lung cancer?**

Vitamin A.

❍ **What myopathic syndrome is associated with lung cancer?**

Eaton-Lambert Syndrome.

❍ **What finding on physical examination can be used to differentiate Eaton-Lambert Syndrome from Myasthenia Gravis?**

Muscle function improves with repeated activity in the former, but degrades in the latter.

❍ **Radiographic stability for what period is assumed to indicate benign origin of a solitary pulmonary nodule?**

Two years.

❍ **What is the initial diagnostic test in a clinically stable patient suspected of having lung cancer?**

Sputum cytologic examination.

❍ **What finding indicates emergent radiation therapy for superior vena cava syndrome?**

Cerebral edema.

❍ **What is the major indication for laser bronchoscopy in the treatment of bronchogenic carcinoma?**

Tumor obstruction of large airways.

❍ **What is the 5 year survival of all patients diagnosed with primary lung cancer?**

<15%.

❍ **Which primary lung cancer is most likely to cavitate?**

Squamous cell carcinoma.

❍ **The best 5-year survival for non-small cell carcinoma of the lung is achieved by what therapy modality?**

Surgical resection.

❍ **The increase in death rate from lung cancer among smokers, as opposed to non-smokers, is how high?**

8 to 20-fold.

○ **Do low tar cigarettes decrease the risk of lung cancer?**

No.

○ **The risk of lung cancer following smoking cessation approaches that of lifelong non-smokers after how many years?**

15.

○ **The incidence of lung cancer among urban residents is how many times than among rural residents?**

About 1.5 times higher among urban residents.

○ **The most common malignancy associated with asbestos exposure is which of the following: esophageal carcinoma, primary lung cancer, mesothelioma, or gastric carcinoma ?**

Primary lung cancer.

○ **A solitary pulmonary nodule in an HIV-infected patient may represent which of the following: PCP, histoplasmosis, cryptococcosis, or bronchogenic carcinoma?**

All of the above.

○ **What happens to minute ventilation at submaximal work rates in Interstitial lung disease?**

It increases due to increased dead space ventilation. Respiratory rate increases, tidal volume decreases.

○ **What is the incidence of post-operative respiratory complications in patients with COPD?**

50% or more.

○ **Is cessation of smoking 24 hours pre-operatively beneficial?**

Yes, by reduction in pulse, blood pressure, and carboxyhemoglobin level.

○ **Which neuromuscular diseases and spinal diseases can lead to ventilatory insufficiency?**

Muscular dystrophy, polymyositis, myotonic dystrophy, polyneuritis, Eaton Lambert Syndrome, myasthenia gravis, amyotrophic lateral sclerosis, injury, Guillain-Barre syndrome, multiple sclerosis, Parkinson's disease and stroke.

○ **Adequacy of alveolar ventilation is reflected by which component of arterial blood gas analysis?**

PaCO2.

○ **Patients on mechanical ventilation can develop hypoventilation based on what factors?**

Increased dead space (including length of ventilator circuit proximal to the "Y" piece separating the inspiratory and expiratory limbs), decreased tidal volume, overdistention of lung, air leaks, and massive pulmonary embolism.

○ **What is the principle mechanism of increased PaCO2 with increased FiO2?**

Worsening V/Q mismatch and the Haldane effect.

○   **How does malnutrition contribute to respiratory failure?**

Increase in the oxygen cost of breathing and respiratory muscle weakness.

○   **What conditions or commonly used medications result in an increase in serum theophylline concentration?**

Fever, congestive heart failure, and liver failure; Cimetidine, macrolides, quinolones, and verapamil.

○   **How can the work of breathing with mechanical ventilation associated with intrinsic PEEP be reduced?**

Add CPAP, reduce tidal volume, reduce inspiratory time, and increase expiratory time.

○   **Through what mechanism does PEEP decrease cardiac output?**

Reduced preload.

○   **Through what mechanism does positive pressure ventilation increase cardiac output?**

Decreased afterload.

○   **How can compliance of the lung/chest wall be approximated from airway pressure measurements during mechanical ventilation?**

Compliance =tidal volume/(Inspiratory plateau pressure - End expiratory pressure).

○   **What evidence of barotrauma can be observed on chest x-ray?**

Pneumomediastinum, pneumothorax, pneumopericardium, subcutaneous emphysema, and pulmonary interstitial emphysema.

○   **What is the primary determinant of the oxygen content of arterial blood?**

The product of hemoglobin concentration and the % hemoglobin oxygen saturation of arterial blood. The amount of oxygen dissolved in the plasma (a function of the PaO2) is negligible at one atmosphere of pressure.

○   **What is bronchiectasis?**

Bronchiectasis is an abnormal dilatation of the proximal medium sized bronchi greater than 2 mm in diameter. It is due to the destruction of the muscular and elastic components of their walls, usually associated with chronic bacterial infection and fowl smelling sputum.

○   **Which lung segments are most frequently involved in bronchiectasis?**

Posterior basal segments of the left or right lower lobes.

○   **What are the symptoms of bronchiectasis?**

Chronic cough, purulent sputum, fever, weakness, weight loss, dyspnea in some patients, and hemoptysis. Hemoptysis is generally mild, originates from bronchial arteries, and is not a common cause of death (< 10% of deaths attributed to hemoptysis).

❍ **What are the most common complications of bronchiectasis?**

Recurrent attacks of pneumonia, empyema, pneumothorax, and lung abscess.

❍ **What is the mainstay of treatment of bronchiectasis?**

Antibiotics.

❍ **What are the adjunctive treatment measures that may be beneficial in patients with bronchiectasis?**

Chest physiotherapy, nutritional support, inhaled Indomethacin (shown to decrease bronchial hypersecretion by inhibiting neutrophil recruitment) bronchodilators, supplemental oxygen, immunoglobulin administration for Immunoglobulin deficiency, replacement treatment for patients with alpha-1-anti-trypsin deficiency, and recombinant DNAase to reduce sputum viscosity in patients with Cystic fibrosis (CF).

❍ **What is Kartagener's syndrome?**

Triad of: (1) Situs inversus, (2) Bronchiectasis, and (3) Nasal polyps or recurrent sinusitis.

❍ **What are the possible manifestations of alpha-1-anti-trypsin deficiency?**

Panlobular emphysema and bronchiectasis and hepatic cirrhosis.

❍ **Pathology in Cystic Fibrosis is confined predominantly to what part of the lung?**

The conducting airways.

❍ **Why is a pneumothorax more common in advanced Cystic Fibrosis?**

Subpleural cysts often occur on the mediastinal surfaces of the upper lobes and are thought to contribute to pneumothorax in patients with advanced disease.

❍ **What is the most common site of non-pulmonary pathology in Cystic Fibrosis?**

The GI tract, with striking changes seen in the exocrine pancreas. Islets of Langerhans are spared.

❍ **What are the reproductive abnormalities in Cystic Fibrosis?**

In males: The Vas deferens, tail and body of the epididymis and the seminal vesicles are either absent or rudimentary.
In females: Uterine cervical glands are distended. The mucous and cervical canals are plugged with tenacious mucus secretions. Endocervicitis also seen.

❍ **What are the most frequent respiratory pathogens in patients with Cystic Fibrosis?**

Staphylococcus aureus and *Pseudomonas aeruginosa*.

❍ **What are the immunological defects in Cystic Fibrosis?**

CF patients have low levels of serum IgG in the first decade of life which increase dramatically once chronic infection is established. T-lymphocyte numbers are adequate. With advancing severity of pulmonary disease, lymphocytes of CF patients proliferate less briskly in response to *P. aeruginosa* and other gram-negative organisms. Deficient opsonic activity of alveolar macrophages are seen in patients with established *P. aeruginosa* infection. Major IgG subclass in serum and lungs in CF patients is IgG.

O   **What are the various radiographic manifestations of Cystic Fibrosis?**

Hyperinflation, peribronchial cuffing, mucous impaction in airways seen as branching finger like shadows, bronchiectasis, subpleural blebs, (most prominent along the mediastinal border), and prominent pulmonary artery segments with advanced disease.

O   **What is the immediate mortality with massive hemoptysis?**

~ 10%.

O   **What are the diagnostic criteria for Cystic Fibrosis?**

Primary:
Characteristic pulmonary manifestations and/or,
Characteristic gastrointestinal manifestations and/or,
A family history of CF
          Plus
Sweat Cl (concentration > 60 mEq/L) [repeat measurement if sweat Cl is 50 - 60 mEq/ L].
Secondary Criteria:
Documentation of dual CFTR mutations, and
Evidence of one or more characteristic manifestations.

O   **What are the conditions associated with an elevated sweat chloride?**

CF, Hypothyroidism, Pseudohypoaldosteronism, Hypoparathyroidism, Nephrogenic Diabetes Insipidus, Type I glycogen storage disease, Mucopolysaccharidosis, Malnutrition, PGE administration, Hypogammaglobulinemia, and Pancreatitis.

O   **What is the test recognized by the Cystic Fibrosis foundation to be the definitive diagnostic test for Cystic Fibrosis?**

Collection of sweat (at least 50 mg in a 45 minute period) by pilocarpine iontophoresis, coupled with chemical determination of the chloride concentration (> 60 mEq/L, >80 mEq/L in adults).

O   **What is the effect of nutritional supplementation on the disease?**

Patients with adequate nutrition experience a slower rate of decline of lung function.

O   **What is the life expectancy of a patient with Cystic Fibrosis?**

50% patients survive to 28 - 30 years of age.

O   **Stridor is observed in what phase of respiration?**

Inspiratory.

O   **What is stridor due to?**

With extrathoracic airway obstruction, the pressure inside the extrathoracic part of the airway is much more negative relative to atmospheric pressure. This results in further narrowing of the larynx during inspiration and therefore, stridor.

O   **Grunting is observed during what phase of respiration?**

Expiratory. Exhalation against a closed glottis.

O   **How do retropharyngeal abscesses arise?**

Lymphatic spread of infections in the nasopharynx, oropharynx, or external auditory canal.

O   **What is the most common type of tracheo-esophageal fistula?**

Blind esophageal pouch with a fistulous connection of the trachea to the distal esophagus.

O   **What is the narrowest part of the adult airway?**

The glottic opening.

O   **A 24-year-old female has a high fever, hoarseness, and increased stridor of 3 hours duration. She also has a low fever and sore throat. Examination shows an ill appearing woman with a temperature of 40° C, inspiratory stridor, drooling and mild intercostal retractions. She prefers to sit up. The most likely diagnosis is:**

Epiglottitis.

O   **In the diagnosis of a radioluscent foreign body lodged in the right mainstem bronchus, producing incomplete obstruction, inspiratory and expiratory films will show air-trapping and increased luscency of the lung on the involved side. This phenomenon is due to:**

Ball-valve airtrapping. Air enters around the foreign body during inspiration, but is trapped as the airway closes around the foreign body during expiration, preventing emptying of that side.

O   **What are the clinical features associated with pleural effusion?**

A pleural rub (may be the only finding in the early stages), pleuritic chest pain due to involvement and inflammation of parietal pleura, cough (distortion of lung), dyspnea (mechanical inefficiency of respiratory muscles stretched by outward movement of chest wall and downward movement of diaphragm), diminished chest wall movements, dull percussion, decreased tactile and vocal fremitus, decreased breath sounds and whispering pectoriloquy. With large amounts, there may be contralateral shift of the mediastinum.

O   **What is the minimum amount of pleural liquid that can be detected roentgenographically?**

Approximately 400 ml in upright views of the chest. A lateral decubitus film taken with the patient lying on the affected side can detect as little as 50 ml of liquid.

O   **What is the most common cause of exudative effusion?**

Parapneumonic effusion is the most common cause of exudative effusion. .

O   **What is the typical eosinophil count of a tuberculous pleural effusion?**

An eosinophil count of greater than 10% usually excludes tubercular effusion. The eosinophil count in pleural fluid can be elevated after pneumothorax and thoracentesis.

O   **What is the treatment of tuberculous pleural effusion?**

A nine month course of Isoniazid 300 mg and Rifampin 600 mg, daily. A therapeutic thoracentesis is recommended only to relieve dyspnea. Corticosteroids can decrease the duration of fever and time required for fluid absorption, but do not decrease the amount of pleural thickening at 12 months after treatment is initiated. They are therefore recommended only for patients who are markedly symptomatic and only after institution of appropriate antimicrobial therapy.

○   **What is the most common cause of transudative pleural effusions?**

Congestive heart failure.

○   **What are the radiological features of pleural effusion associated with cirrhosis?**

They are small to massive right-sided effusion in 70%, left sided in 15%, and bilateral in 15% with normal heart size.

○   **What is the mechanism of a pleural effusions are associated with atelectasis?**

Atelectasis leads to decreased perimicrovascular pressure, resulting in a pressure gradient. Fluid moves from the parietal pleural interstitium into the pleural space due to decreased perimicrovascular pressure.

○   **What is the primary mechanism of pleural effusion in nephrotic syndrome?**

Decreased plasma oncotic pressure due to hypoalbuminemia.

○   **What is the incidence of pleural effusion associated with malignancy?**

Malignant pleural effusions are the second most common exudative effusions after parapneumonic effusions. The most common malignancies are lung and breast cancer.

○   **What are the conditions associated with malignant transudative effusions?**

Lymphatic obstruction, endobronchial obstruction, and hypoalbuminemia due to the primary malignancy.

○   **What type of effusions are suggestive of malignancy?**

Massive effusions, large effusions without contralateral mediastinal shift or bilateral effusions with normal heart size suggest malignancy.

○   **What type of pleural effusion is associated with malignant mesothelioma?**

Large unilateral effusions. Contralateral pleural plaques are present in 20% of the cases. Loculated pleural masses may be evident after thoracentesis.

○   **What factors play a role in the pathogenesis of pleural effusions associated with pulmonary embolism?**

Effusions are present in 40-50% of cases of pulmonary embolism. Increased capillary permeability, due to ischemia and leak of protein rich fluid into pleural space, are the main factors. Atelectasis may contribute to transudate and lung necrosis can lead to hemorrhage.

○   **What is the incidence of pleural involvement in systemic lupus erythematosus?**

50% to 75% of patients with systemic lupus erythematosus develop pleural effusion or pleuritic pain during the course of their disease.

○   **What are the clinical features of lupus pleuritis?**

Pleuritic chest pain is the most common presentation. Other features are cough, dyspnea, pleural rub, and fever. An episode of pleuritis usually indicates exacerbation of lupus.

○   **What are the radiological features of lupus pleuritis?**

Small to moderate bilateral effusions are most common. Unilateral and massive effusion can occur. Other radiographic abnormalities such as alveolar infiltrates, atelectasis, and increasing cardiac silhouette can occur.

○   **What are some drugs reported to be associated with pleural effusion?**

Procainamide, Nitrofurantoin, Dantrolene, Methysergide, Procarbazine, Methotrexate, Amiodarone, Mitomycin, and Bleomycin.

○   **What respiratory rate should be used in CPR during a respiratory or cardiac arrest?**

10-12 breaths per minute. After resuscitation, when circulation has been restored, the rate should be 12-15 breaths per minute.

○   **When may end-tidal carbon dioxide detectors prove inaccurate?**

In patients with very low blood flow to the lungs, or in those with a large dead space (i.e. following a pulmonary embolism).

○   **What is the most common complication of endotracheal intubation?**

Intubation of a bronchus. Other complications include lacerations of the lip, tongue, pharyngeal or tracheal mucosa resulting in bleeding, hematoma, or abscess. Tracheal rupture, avulsion of an arytenoid cartilage, vocal cord injury, pharyngeal-esophageal perforation, intubation of the pyriform sinus, aspiration of vomitus, hypertension, tachycardia, or arrhythmias can also occur.

○   **What oxygen concentration will be supplied by nasal cannula with a flow rate of 1 L/min?**

24%. For each 1 L/min increase in flow, a 4% increase in oxygen concentration will occur. 6 L/min produces a 44% oxygen concentration.

○   **What oxygen flow rate is recommended for face mask ventilation?**

At least 5 L/min. Recommended flow is 8-10 L/min, which will produce oxygen concentrations as high as 40% to 60%.

○   **What oxygen concentration can be supplied with a face mask and oxygen reservoir?**

6 L/min provides approximately 60% oxygen concentration, and each liter increases the concentration by 10%. 10 L/min is almost 100%.

○   **What degree of leukocytosis is considered a risk factor for poor outcome among patients with bacterial pneumonia?**

Greater than 30,000 cells/mm^3.

○   **What bacteria are associated with pneumonia following influenza?**

Streptococcus pneumoniae, *Staphylococcus pneumoniae*, and *Haemophilus influenzae*.

❍   **What is the leading identifiable cause of acute community-acquired pneumonia in adults?**

Streptococcus pneumoniae.

❍   **What two underlying medical conditions are associated with *Hemophilus influenzae* pneumonia?**

Chronic obstructive lung disease and HIV infection.

❍   **At what age should the pneumococcal vaccine be administered among healthy adults with no comorbid conditions?**

Age 65 or greater..

❍   **What is the most common etiologic agent of atypical pneumonia?**

Mycoplasma pneumoniae. Chlamydia pneumoniae is the second most common.

❍   **Of the following organisms, which is commonly spread by person-to-person contact: *Legionella pneumoniae* or *Mycoplasma pneumoniae?***

Mycoplasma pneumoniae.

❍   **What is the most common cause of community-acquired bacterial pneumonia among patients infected with HIV?**

Streptococcus pneumoniae.

❍   **What three x-ray findings are associated with a poor outcome in patients with pneumonia?**

Multi-lobe involvement, pleural effusion, and cavitation.

❍   **What are the two most important risk factors for the development of anaerobic lung abscess?**

Poor oral hygiene and a predisposition toward aspiration.

❍   **Which lung segments are most often the site of lung abscess formation?**

The posterior segments of the upper lobe and the superior segments of the lower lobes.

❍   **What anaerobic respiratory infection is associated with slowly enlarging pulmonary infiltrates, pleural effusions, rib destruction and fistula formation?**

Actinomycosis.

❍   **What proportion of the patients with pneumonia develop pleural effusions?**

40%.

❍   **What pathological process is suggested by an air-fluid level in the pleural space?**

Bronchopleural fistula.

○   **What is the definition of nosocomial pneumonia?**

Pneumonia occurring in patients who have been hospitalized for at least 72 hours.

○   **What are the two most important routes of transmission of nosocomial bacterial pneumonia?**

Person-to-person transmission via healthcare workers and contaminated ventilator tubing.

○   **You are at a restaurant and the person at the table next to you begins coughing loudly. She stands up and begins wheezing between coughs, but she is still able to eke out a "Help! I'm choking." How should you help?**

Encourage her to cough deeper and keep breathing. Do not interrupt her spontaneous attempts at expulsion if she still has good air exchange, as evidenced by her state of consciousness and the degree of coughing and wheezing. Should she display severe respiratory difficulty with a weakening cough and the inability to talk, perform the Heimlich maneuver.

○   **What should be done if the above patient is markedly obese and in severe respiratory distress?**

The normal Heimlich maneuver will not be as effective. Instead of positioning your fists above the patient's navel, place your cupped fist on the patient's chest and deliver swift thrusts. This is also the method of choice for pregnant women.

○   **What is Virchow's triad?**

1) Injury to the endothelium of the vessels.
2) Hypercoagulable state.
3) Stasis.
These represent risk factors for pulmonary embolus. Other risk factors are smoking, birth control pills, history of prior clots, cancer, recent surgery, and prolonged sitting (eg, airplane flight).

○   **What does normal ventilation with decreased lung perfusion suggest?**

Pulmonary embolus.

○   **What are the most common signs and symptoms of PE?**

Tachypnea (92%), CP (88%), dyspnea (84%), anxiety (59%), tachycardia (44%), fever (43%), DVT (32%), hypotension (25%), and syncope (13%).

○   **Can a patient with a PE have a pO2 greater than 90 mm Hg?**

Yes, but rarely (5%).

○   **What is the most common CXR finding in PE?**

Elevated dome of one hemidiaphragm. This finding is caused by decreased lung volume, which occurs in 50% of patients with PE. Other common findings include a lack of lung markings in the area perfused by the occluded artery, pleural effusions, atelectasis, and pulmonary infiltrates.

○   **What are two relatively specific CXR findings in PE?**

Hampton's hump: Area of lung consolidation with a rounded border facing the hilus.

Westermark's sign: Dilated pulmonary outflow tract proximal to the emboli with decreased perfusion distal to the lesion.

○   What test is considered the gold standard for the diagnosis of DVT? For the diagnosis of PE?

1) DVT: venography.
2) PE: pulmonary angiography.

○   **When treating DVT/PE, when should warfarin therapy be initiated?**

On the first or second day after initiation of heparin therapy. Although heparin should be administered immediately, it can be discontinued when the PTT is 1.5 to 1.8 times normal for at least 3 days.

○   **How long should chronic warfarin therapy, as a prophylaxis for DVT, be given?**

Warfarin should be administered for at least 3 to 6 months after a DVT to maintain an INR at 2 to 3 times the normal.

○   **What historical findings suggest an embolus as opposed to a thrombosis in a lower extremity?**

Embolus: Associated with a history of arrhythmia, valvular disease, MI, no skin changes from chronic arterial insufficiency, and no symptoms in the opposite extremity.

Thrombosis: Opposite extremity shows evidence of chronic arterial occlusive disease with history of rest pain, claudication, etc.

○   **What is the risk factor for PE in a patient with an axillary or subclavian vein thrombus?**

About 15%.

○   **At what percentage of an airway obstruction will inspiratory stridor become evident?**

70% occlusion.

○   **What is the initial treatment for a tension pneumothorax?**

Large bore IV catheter placed in the anterior second intercostal space (not a chest tube).

○   **What is the most important cause of hypoxia in a patient with flail chest?**

Underlying lung contusion.

○   **How much fluid must collect in the chest to be detected on decubitus or upright chest x-rays?**

200 to 300 mL. If supine, greater than 1 L may be necessary to be seen on AP CXR.

○   **A foreign body is suspected in the lower airways. What will plain films show?**

Air trapping on the affected side. Inspiration and expiration views demonstrate mediastinal shift away from the affected side.

GASTROINTESTINAL

○   A patient states that food sticks in his mid-chest and then is regurgitated as a putrid, undigested mess. A barium study shows a dilated esophagus with a distal "beak." What is the diagnosis?

Achalasia.

○   What is the gold standard for diagnosing achalasia?

Esophageal manometry.

○   What are the possible findings of an upper GI series from a woman with telangiectasias, tight knuckles, and acid indigestion?

Aperistalsis, which is characteristic of scleroderma.

○   What is the typical profile of a patient with anorexia nervosa?

Female, adolescent, upper class, perfectionist.

○   Name some common conditions that mimic acute appendicitis.

Mesenteric lymphadenitis, PID, Mittlesmertz, gastroenteritis, and Crohn's disease.

○   What conditions are associated with an atypical presentation of acute appendicitis?

Situs inversus viscerum, malrotation, hypermobile cecum, long pelvic appendix, and pregnancy.

○   What are the most frequent symptoms of acute appendicitis?

Anorexia and abdominal pain. The classical presentation of anorexia and periumbilical pain with progression to constant RLQ pain is present in only 60% of the cases.

○   What percentage of patients with acute appendicitis cases have an elevated WBC count?

An elevated leukocyte count and an elevated absolute neutrophil count are present in only 85% of the cases.

○   Until discounted, what intra-abdominal pathology should be assumed for a pregnant woman with right upper quadrant pain?

Acute appendicitis.

○   Rovsing's, psoas, and obturator signs can all indicate an inflamed posterior appendix. Describe these signs.

Rovsing's sign:	RLQ pain with palpation over the LLQ
Psoas sign:	RLQ pain with right thigh extension
Obturator sign:	RLQ pain with internal rotation of the flexed right thigh

❍   **What does an ultrasound show in acute appendicitis?**

A fixed, tender, non-compressible mass, but only in 75 to 90% of cases. CT is the prefered imaging test for appendicitis.

❍   **Barrett's esophagitis is associated with which type of cancer?**

Esophageal adenocarcinoma. Squamous cell carcinoma is the predominant cancer of the upper esophagus.

❍   **Which method is more sensitive for locating the source of GI bleeding, a radioactive Tc-labeled red cell scan or angiography?**

A bleeding scan can detect a site bleeding at a rate as low as 0.12 mL/minute, while angiography requires rapid bleeding, i.e., greater than 0.5 mL/min.

❍   **A patient with an "acid stomach" develops melena and vomits copious amounts of bright red blood. Is esophagitis a feasible cause?**

No. Capillary bleeding rarely causes impressive acute blood loss. Arterial bleeding from a complicated ulcer, foreign body, Mallory-Weiss tear or variceal bleeding are much more probable.

❍   **Repeated violent bouts of vomiting can result in both Mallory-Weiss tears and Boerhaave's syndrome. Differentiate between the two.**

Mallory-Weiss tears: Involve the submucosa and mucosa, typically in the right posterolateral wall of the gastroesophageal junction.

Boerhaave's syndrome: It is a full-thickness tear, usually in the unsupported left posterolateral wall of the abdominal esophagus.

❍   **Recurrent pneumonias, especially in the right middle lobe or the superior segments of the bilateral upper lobes, are indicative of what syndrome?**

Aspiration associated with motor diseases and gastroesophageal reflux.

❍   **A 6-month-old infant is constipated, flaccid, and only stares straight ahead. His mother states that he is not running a fever; however, she is especially worried because he won't take his bottle, not even for her honey on the tip of the bottle trick. What is the diagnosis?**

Infantile botulism. Infants ingest spores that are in the environment, most commonly in honey. The spores then grow and produce toxins within the host.

❍   **How does infantile botulism differ from food-borne botulism?**

Infantile botulism is caused by the spores of *C. botulinum* while adult food-borne botulism arises from the ingestion of *C. botulinum* neurotoxins.

❍   **What is the antidote for botulism poisoning?**

Trivalent A-B-E antitoxin. This antidote is not required for infantile botulism.

❍   **What is the most frequent complication of choledocholithiasis?**

Cholangitis (60%). Other complications are bile duct obstruction, pancreatitis, biliary enteric fistula, and hemobilia.

○   **Gallbladder stones are generally formed of what material?**

Cholesterol. The diagnostic test of choice is ultrasound. This technique may show stones, sludge, bile plugging, or dilated bile ducts.

○   **Acalculous cholecystitis commonly occurs in what type of patients?**

Postoperative, posttraumatic and burn patients secondary to dehydration, and hemolysis secondary to blood transfusions.

○   **A patient with a history of gallstones presents with acute, postprandial right upper quadrant pain. What's the KUB likely to show?**

Nothing specific. Only about 10% of gallstones are radiopaque. Complications of cholelithiasis, such as emphysematous cholecystitis, perforation, and pneumobilia, are uncommon but useful findings.

○   **A child with sickle-cell disease presents with fever, RUQ abdominal pain, and jaundice. What is the diagnosis?**

Charcot's triad suggests ascending cholangitis. The precipitating cause in this case is probably pigment stones resulting from chronic hemolysis.

○   **A postoperative patient develops right upper quadrant pain, nausea, and low-grade fevers. According to his surgeon, the gallbladder did not contain stones. What is the probable diagnosis?**

Acalculous cholecystitis.

○   **Eight years after her cholecystectomy, a woman develops right upper quadrant pain and jaundice. What is the chance of recurrent biliary tract stones developing?**

At least 10%, due either to retained stones or in-situ formation by biliary epithelium.

○   **List the ultrasound findings that are suggestive of acute cholecystitis.**

Formation of gall stones or sludge in acalculous cholecystitis, thickening of the gallbladder wall by more than 5 mm, and the presence of pericholecystic fluid. A dilated common bile duct, i.e. > 10 mm suggests common duct obstruction.

○   **Name two findings in acute cholecystitis that mandate an emergency laparotomy.**

Emphysematous cholecystitis and perforation. Otherwise, timing of surgery is somewhat dependent upon the institution and the surgeon.

○   **Can non-gallstone cholecystitis perforate?**

Yes. Up to 40% of gallbladder perforations are associated with acalculous cholecystitis.

○   **A 24-year-old male complains that he has endured two days of rice-water stools, muscle cramps and extreme fatigue. He looks pale, dehydrated, and very ill. The patient states that he has just returned from India. What is the diagnosis?**

Cholera. The incidence of cholera in the US is 1/10,000,000. This disease usually develops in people that have traveled to endemic areas, such as India, Africa, southeast Asia, southern Europe, Central and South America, and the Middle East. Infection occurs by consuming unpurified water, raw fruits and vegetables, and undercooked seafood.

○   **A patient presents with palmar erythema, spider angiomas, testicular atrophy, and asterixis. What other signs and symptoms may be exhibited?**

Hematemesis, encephalopathy, hepatomegaly, splenomegaly, jaundice, caput medusa, ascites, and gynecomastia may also occur. This patient has cirrhosis.

○   **A cirrhotic patient vomits bright red blood and has a systolic blood pressure of 90 mm Hg. After aggressive fluid resuscitation with 4 units of packed RBCs and a gastric lavage, his pressure is still 90 mm Hg. What's next?**

Assume a coagulopathy. Transfuse fresh frozen plasma, start a vasopressin or octreotide drip, and arrange for an emergency endoscopic evaluation/intervention, usually for sclerotherapy or banding.

○   **What are the peak ages for the onset of ulcerative colitis?**

15 to 35 years, with a smaller incident rate in the seventh decade.

○   **How does the pathology of Crohn's disease differ from that of ulcerative colitis?**

Crohn's is a trans-mucosal, segmental, granulomatous process, while ulcerative colitis is a mucosal, juxtapositioned, ulcerative process.

○   **At least one-third of the patients with Crohn's disease develop kidney stones. Why?**

Dietary oxalate is usually bound to calcium and then excreted. When terminal ileal disease leads to decreased bile salt absorption, the resulting fattier intestinal contents bind calcium by saponification. Free oxalate is "hyper-absorbed" in the colon, resulting in hyperoxaluria and calcium oxalate nephrolithiasis.

○   **Complications of Crohn's disease include perirectal abscesses, anal fissures, rectovaginal fistulas, and rectal prolapse. What percentage of patients with Crohn's disease have perirectal involvement?**

Approximately 90%.

○   **What are the odds that a patient with severe ileal disease will be cured by surgery?**

Virtually zero. Crohn's disease invariably recurs in the remaining GI tract. In contrast, total proctocolectomy with ileostomy is curative procedure for ulcerative colitis.

○   **What hereditary diseases evident in infancy may cause cirrhosis?**

Glycogen storage disease, cystic fibrosis, galactosemia, fructose intolerance, tyrosinemia, and acid cholesterol esterhydrolase deficiency.

○   **A cirrhotic patient presents with weakness and edema. What electrolyte imbalances might be present?**

Hyponatremia (dilutional or diuretic-induced), hypokalemia (from GI losses, secondary hyperaldosteronism, or diuretics), and hypomagnesemia.

○   **What diuretic is the optimal choice for treating most cirrhotics with ascites?**

Potassium-sparing agents. Treat the hyperaldosterone state specifically.

○   **A confused cirrhotic patient enters the hospital. She is afebrile and has asterixis. What should your examination include to determine the precipitant of hepatic encephalopathy?**

Assess her mental status and examine her for localizing neurologic signs suggestive of an occult head injury. Look for dry mucous membranes and a low jugular venous pressure, which are indicative of hypovolemia and azotemia. In addition, check a stool guaiac for GI bleeding. Focused lab testing can pinpoint other causes, including diuretic overuse and hypokalemia, hypoglycemia, anemia, hypoxia, and infection. Administer thiamine and folate.

○   **Aside from fixing the above, what therapy is useful for hepatic encephalopathy?**

Lactulose. This synthetic disaccharide produces an acidic diarrhea which traps nitrogenous wastes in the gut.

○   **Are there any useful therapies for the rapid renal failure that can accompany cirrhosis?**

Unfortunately there are not. The hepatorenal syndrome still has a mortality rate that approaches 100%.

○   **What is the most common neoplasm of the GI tract?**

Colon cancer. It is also the second most common cause of cancer death in the US.

○   **What are the current recommendations from the American Cancer Society for screening colon cancer?**

An annual digital examination for patients over 40 and an annual testing for occult blood in patients over 50. A flexible sigmoidoscopy should be performed every 3 to 5 years on individuals older than 50 years. Earlier screening is required in patients with familial polypoidosis.

○   **Which is the most common type of colon cancer?**

Adenocarcinoma (95%).

○   **Which is the most common type of rectal cancer?**

Adenocarcinoma (95%).

○   **To where on the body does colon cancer most commonly spread?**

The regional lymph nodes. Hematogenous spread occurs most often to the liver or lungs.

○   **Where is the most common site of colorectal cancer?**

For adenocarcinoma, 60 to 65% of cases occur in the distal colon or the rectum, and 35 to 40% occur in the proximal colon. The typical sites for carcinoid, squamous, and melanoma are the appendix or the rectum, the anal area, and the area adjacent to the dentate line, respectively.

○   **Clinically, differentiate between right-sided and left-sided adenocarcinoma of the colon.**

Right-sided: Pain and/or mass in RLQ, occult blood in stool, dyspepsia, fatigue secondary to anemia; stool appearance rarely changes.

Left-sided: Change in bowel habits, red blood in stool, reduced caliber of stool, and pencil thin stools.

○   **T/F: Serum CEA is a proficient screening tool for colorectal cancer.**

False. Although 70% of patients with colorectal cancer will have an elevated CEA, it is not specific for colorectal cancer. It is however, a good measure of recurrent colon cancer.

○   **Describe the Duke's stages.**

Duke's stage A: Mucosal involvement which may involve the submucosa
Duke's stage B1:   Cancer extends to muscularis propria but not through the serosa
Duke's stage B2:   Cancer extends beyond the serosa
Duke's stage C: Regional lymph node involvement
Duke's stage D: Distant metastases

○   **It has been conclusively determined that a 72-year-old female has cancer of the colon with involvement of the regional lymph nodes. What Duke's stage is this?**

Duke's stage C.

○   **What is the typical five year survival rate for a colon cancer Duke's stage A?**

95%. Duke's B1 is 85 to 90%, B2 is 60 to 70%, C is 15 to 25%, and D is 5%.

○   **What stool studies are crucial for evaluating acute diarrhea?**

None. Most cases require no testing, just oral rehydration. In patients at risk for complications, i.e., at the extremes of age, recently hospitalized, or immunocompromised, enteroinvasive infection should be ruled out with a stool guaiac and fecal leukocyte test. Also consider checking for ova and parasites.

○   **Which diarrheal illnesses cause fecal leukocytes?**

The usual culprits are *Shigella,* Campylobacter, and enteroinvasive *E. coli.* Others include *Salmonella, Yersinia, Vibrio parahaemolyticus*, and *C. difficile.* Fecal WBCs are absent in toxigenic and enteropathogenic infection, even with such a virulent organism as *Vibrio* cholera. Viral and parasitic infections rarely produce fecal WBCs.

○   **What is the most common cause of bacterial diarrhea?**

E. coli (enteroinvasive, enteropathogenic, enterotoxigenic).

○   **Which is the most common form of acute diarrhea?**

Viral diarrhea. It is generally self-limited, lasting only 1 to 3 days.

○   **Diarrhea that develops within 12 hours of a meal is most probably caused by what?**

An ingested pre-formed toxin.

○   **When does traveler's diarrhea typically occur?**

3 to 7 days after arrival in a foreign land.

○   **What is the treatment for traveler's diarrhea?**

Traveler's diarrhea is usually caused by *E. coli*; the preferable treatment is with Cipro.

○   **What is the definition of chronic diarrhea?**

Passage of > 200 g of loose stool per day for over three weeks.

○   **A 73-year-old women with no prior medical history presents with fever, chills, vomiting, nausea, and an acute onset of pain in her left lower quadrant. Her pain becomes worse after she eats and is mildly relieved after a bowel movement. Upon physical examination, you note that she has guarding, rebound tenderness, and a tender, firm, non-mobile mass in the left lower quadrant. What is the likely diagnosis?**

Diverticulitis.

○   **Where in the colon are diverticula most commonly found?**

The sigmoid and distal colon.

○   **If there is associated bleeding with the diverticulitis, where is the most likely etiology?**

The right side of the colon. Fifty percent of the bleeds originate in this area even though diverticulitis is more common in the left side.

○   **T/F: A barium enema is not a good diagnostic test if diverticulitis is suspected.**

True. If a patient is having an acute attack of diverticulitis, the risk of perforation is too great. Cat scan is the prefered diagnostic test for diverticulitis.

○   **Why is pentazocine, not morphine, the analgesic of choice for the treatment of diverticulitis?**

Morphine increases colonic pressure.

○   **Prescribe an outpatient antibiotic regimen for uncomplicated diverticulitis.**

TMP-SMX-DS or ciprofloxacin plus metronidazole. Argmentin is an alternative.

○   **Is diverticulitis the probable diagnosis for a patient with low abdominal pain and bright red blood per rectum?**

No. Typically diverticulosis bleeds, while diverticulitis doesn't. Diverticular bleeding is usually painless. If the patient has bleeding diverticulitis, remember that 50% of bleeding diverticula originates on the right side.

○   **What barium findings distinguish colonic obstruction caused by acute diverticulitis from that caused by colon cancer?**

Diverticulitis is extraluminal. Thus, the mucosa appears intact and involved bowel segments are longer. Adenocarcinoma distorts the mucosa, involves a short segment of bowel, and has overhanging edges.

○   **What symptoms are usually associated with neuromuscular dysphagia?**

Nasopharyngeal regurgitation and hoarseness.

○   **A 40-year-old smoker describes an acute crescendo substernal chest tightness penetrating to his back. The pain is not relieved by antacids. An ECG shows ST changes, and his pain resolves 7 to 10 minutes after a nitroglycerin tablet. Is this angina?**

Maybe, although the delayed response to nitrates characterizes "esophageal colic" which is caused by segmental esophageal spasm and is often triggered by reflux. (Admiting him to rule out an MI is still your best plan.)

❍   **An elderly woman has trouble swallowing solids and later develops difficulty with liquids. She presents with sudden drooling after dinner.   What is the concern?**

A peptic stricture or esophageal cancer complicated by bolus obstruction.

❍   **Name the most common symptom of esophageal disease.**

Pyrosis (heartburn).

❍   **What classical features distinguish chest pain of esophageal origin from cardiac ischemia?**

None. Exertional pain and palliation with rest or NTG occur in both groups. Pain relief from nitroglycerin in the GI group usually takes 7 to 10 minutes while ischemic pain usually responds in 2 to 3 minutes.

❍   **What is the most common benign esophageal neoplasm?**

Leiomyoma. Papilloma and fibrovascular polyps also occur, but benign esophageal neoplasms are rare.

❍   **What percentage of patients with esophageal cancer are also afflicted with distant metastasis?**

80%. The 5 year survival rate is 5%. If the cancer is squamous and there is no lymph node involvement, the survival rate is 15 to 20%.

❍   **What is the most common location of esophageal cancer?**

The lower third (50%), followed by the upper third (30%) and the middle third (20%).

❍   **Objects bigger than what size rarely pass the stomach?**

5cm x 2cm.

❍   **A child swallows a coin and it gets lodged in the esophagus. How will the coin appear on an AP chest x-ray?**

Coins in the esophagus lie in the frontal plane, it will be seen as a round object. Coins in the trachea lie in the sagittal plane, they will be seen as a narrow line (edge view).

❍   **What is the appropriate management for an ingested button battery that is in the stomach?**

In asymptomatic patients, repeat radiographs. Endoscopic retrieval is required if symptoms occur or if the battery does not pass the pylorus after 48 hours.

❍   **Foreign bodies tend to lodge at what esophageal level in the pediatric patient?**

Foreign bodies most commonly lodge at the level of the cricopharyngeus muscles. The level of the thoracic inlet, aortic arch, tracheal bifurcation, and lower esophageal sphincter are also possible lodging sites.

❍   **In children, what physical findings suggest that a foreign body has been swallowed?**

Distress, a red or scratched oropharynx, dysphagia, a high fever, or peritoneal signs may be evident. In addition, subcutaneous air suggests perforation.

❍   **Most objects, even sharp ones, pass thorough the GI tract without incident. When should such objects be removed?**

Remove if they obstruct or perforate, if longer than 5cm x 2cm, and if they are toxic (such as batteries). Sharp or pointed objects, including sewing needles and razor blades, should be removed if they haven't yet passed the pylorus.

○   **What is the best way to remove a meat bolus causing esophageal obstruction?**

Endoscopy. However, IV glucagon, 1 mg IV push after a small test dose, then repeated as a 2 mg dose at 20 minutes. Glucagon relaxes esophageal smooth muscle. Meat tenderizer should be avoided because perforation has occurred.

○   **What test must be performed after the food bolus is cleared?**

Either a barium study or endoscopy. This confirms the passage or removal of the foreign body and checks for underlying pathology which is present in most adults with obstructing food boluses.

○   **People who live in what countries are at greatest risk for gastric carcinoma?**

Japan, Chile, and Costa Rica. Risk factors include a diet high in additives, achlorhydria, intestinal metaplasia, polyps or dysplasia, *H. pylori* infection (disputed), familial polyposis, and pernicious anemia.

○   **What is the most common type of gastric carcinoma? What percentage of these are ulcerative, polypoid or linitis plastica?**

Adenocarcinomas account for 90% of gastric carcinomas. Of these, 75% are ulcerative, 10% are polypoid, and 15% are diffuse infiltrative scirrous (linitis plastica).

○   **What percentage of gastric carcinomas produce a positive hemoccult test?**

50%.

○   **What percentage of gastric carcinomas are associated with a palpable mass?**

25%.

○   **What is a Krukenberg tumor?**

A gastric carcinoma that has metastasized to the ovary.

○   **Stomach cancer is associated with the enlargement of what lymph nodes?**

Supraclavicular nodes. These are called Virchow's nodes.

○   **What is the treatment of choice for gastric carcinoma?**

A radical subtotal gastrectomy with gastrojejunostomy or gastroduodenostomy. Chemotherapy is not very effective and can only be used for some palliation.

○   **Which type of hepatitis is characterized by an SPGT greater than the SGOT?**

Hepatitis A. The SGPT is usually greater than 1,000.

○   **Which type of hepatitis is usually contracted through blood transfusions?**

Hepatitis C accounts for 85% of hepatitis infections via this route.

○   **A poor prognosis is associated with which two LFTs in acute viral hepatitis?**

A total bilirubin > 20 mg/dL and a prolongation of the prothrombin time > 3 seconds. The extent of transaminase elevation is not a useful marker.

○   **Match the following hepatitis serologies with the correct clinical description.**

1) HBsAg (-) and anti-HBs (+)   a) Ongoing viral replication, highly infectious
2) IgM HBcAg (+) and anti-HBs (-)   b) Remote infection, not infectious
3) IgG HBcAg (+) and anti-HBs (-)   c) Recent or ongoing infection (a high titer means high
                                          infectivity, while a low titer suggests chronic, active infection)
4) HBeAg (+)   d) Prior infection or vaccination, not infectious

Answers: (1) d, (2) c, (3) b, and (4) a.

○   **T/F: The d-agent can cause hepatitis D in a patient without active hepatitis B.**

False. The d-agent is an incomplete, "defective" RNA virus that is responsible for hepatitis D. It is an obligate covirus and requires hepatitis B for replication.

○   **You stick yourself with a needle withdrawn from a chronic hepatitis B carrier. You've been vaccinated but have never had your antibody status checked. What is the appropriate post-exposure prophylaxis?**

Measure your anti-HB titer. If it's adequate (> 10 mIU), treatment is not required. If it is inadequate, you need a single dose of HBIG as soon as possible and a vaccine booster.

○   **List three types of internal hernias.**

1) Diaphragmatic hernia
2) Lesser sac hernia, i.e., through the foramen of Winslow
3) Omental or mesenteric hernia

○   **Are small or large hernias more dangerous?**

Small, because incarceration is more likely.

○   **What are the borders of Hesselbach's triangle?**

The inguinal ligament, the inferior epigastric vessels, and the lateral border of the rectus abdominis.

○   **Which type of hernia passes through Hesselbach's triangle?**

Direct hernias.

○   **Among women, which is more common, inguinal or femoral hernia?**

Inguinal. Femoral hernias occur more commonly among women than men, but inguinal hernias are the most common type of hernias in women.

○   **Distinguish between a groin hernia, a hydrocele, and a lymph node.**

Hydroceles transilluminate and are not tender. Lymph nodes are freely moving and firm. Hernias don't transilluminate and may produce bowel sounds.

○ **A patient's groin bulged two days ago. He then developed severe pain with progressive nausea and vomiting. He has a tender mass in his groin. What should you NOT do?**

Don't try to reduce a long-standing, tender, incarcerated hernia! The abdomen is no place for dead bowel.

○ **What simple test can distinguish between conjugated and unconjugated hyperbilirubinemia?**

A dipstick test for urobilinogen, which reflects conjugated (water soluble) hyperbilirubinemia.

○ **In addition to conjugated hyperbilirubinemia, what liver function abnormalities suggest biliary tract disease?**

Elevated alkaline phosphatase levels that are out of proportion to transaminases.

○ **Portal hypertension produces internal hemorrhoids through what veins?**

The superior rectal and inferior mesenteric veins. Internal hemorrhoids are proximal to the fabled dentate line in the 2, 5, and 9 o'clock positions in the prone patient and are typically not palpable on rectal examination.

○ **Currant jelly stool in a child indicates what?**

Intussusception.

○ **What is the most common cause of bowel obstruction in children under age 2?**

Intussusception. Usually the terminal ileum slides into the right colon. The cause remains unknown but hypertrophied lymph nodes at the junction of the ileum and colon are suspected.

○ **What is the treatment for intussusception?**

A barium enema is both a diagnostic tool and often curative (i.e., it can reduce the intussusception). If the barium enema is unsuccessful, surgical reduction may be required.

○ **List four contraindications to the introduction of a nasogastric tube.**

1) Suspected esophageal laceration or perforation
2) Near obstruction due to stricture
3) Esophageal foreign body
4) Severe head trauma with rhinorrhea

○ **What test should be performed when an elderly patient is suffering from pain that is out of proportion to the physical examination?**

Angiography. This test is the gold standard for diagnosing mesenteric ischemia.

○ **What is the defining characteristic for obesity?**

A weight 20% above the height/weight recommendation.

○ **In order of prevalence, what are the three most common causes of colonic obstruction?**

Cancer, diverticulitis, and volvulus.

❍ **An elderly man is constipated but does not have tenesmus, abdominal pain, nausea, or vomiting. A rectal examination determines that he has hard stool in the vault. A KUB shows a colon "full of stool." Is an enema all he needs?**

No. Fecal impaction with "obstipation" is both common and benign; however, it is usually associated with tenesmus. The patient must also be evaluated for a colorectal tumor.

❍ **A KUB suggests a large bowel obstruction. What are the next steps in this examination?**

An unprepped sigmoidoscopy to confirm obstruction, followed by a barium study to determine the cause. If a pseudo-obstruction is suspected, don't order a barium study because of the possibility of concretion and obstruction. Colonoscopy can be diagnostic as well as therapeutic.

❍ **Pseudo-obstruction is typically caused by medications. Name three classes of drugs that give rise to pseudo-obstruction.**

Anticholinergics, antiparkinsonian drugs, and tricyclic antidepressants.

❍ **What is the most frequent cause of small bowel obstruction?**

Adhesions, followed by incarcerated hernias, are the most common causes of extraluminal obstruction. Gallstones and bezoars are the most common causes of intraluminal obstruction.

❍ **An elderly woman has a recurrent small bowel obstruction with a unilateral pain in one thigh. What occult process may be present?**

An obturator hernia incarceration. This condition often presents with pain down the medial thigh to the knee.

❍ **What disease is indicated by epigastric pain that radiates to the back and is relieved, to some extent, by sitting up?**

Pancreatitis.

❍ **What are the major causes of acute pancreatitis?**

Alcohol and biliary stone disease.

❍ **Is a nasogastric tube always required for acute pancreatitis?**

No, only if nausea and vomiting are severe. In fact, one study showed that NG tubes contributed to more complications, including aspiration.

❍ **When are antibiotics useful in acute pancreatitis?**

Because pancreatitis is a chemical disease, antibiotics are only useful for treating complications, such as abscess or sepsis, and those cases that are associated with choledocholithiasis.

❍ **Where is the most common site of pancreatic cancer?**

The pancreatic duct system (90 to 95%). If an ultrasound and CT are negative, an ERCP may still verify the presence of cancer.

❍ **With regards to pancreatic cancer, distinguish between periampullary lesions and lesions of the body and tail.**

Periampullary lesions most commonly develop at the head of the pancreas. These lesions are usually adenocarcinomas and are associated with jaundice, weight loss, and abdominal pain.

Lesions of the body and tail tend to be much larger at presentation because of their retroperitoneal location and their distance from the common bile duct. Weight loss and pain are typical.

O **What is the most common cause of lower GI perforation?**

Diverticulitis, followed by tumor, colitis, foreign bodies, and instrumentation.

O **Which types of patients are at risk for gallbladder perforation?**

The elderly, diabetics, and those with recurrent cholecystitis.

O **What does burning epigastric pain shooting to the back, hypovolemic shock, and a high amylase level suggest?**

A posterior perforation of a duodenal ulcer.

O **Enteric coated potassium tablets, typhoid, tuberculosis, tumors, and a strangulated hernia can all cause what rare process?**

Non-traumatic small bowel perforation.

O **What percentage of patients with a perforated viscus also have radiographic evidence of a pneumoperitoneum?**

60 to 70%. Therefore, one-third of patients will not have this sign. Maintain the patient in either the upright or the left lateral decubitus position for at least 10 minutes prior to taking x-rays.

O **After a high-speed motor vehicle accident, an unrestrained driver develops abdominal and chest pain radiating to the neck. An upper chest film shows left-sided pleural fluid. What gastroesophageal catastrophe might have occurred?**

Impact against a steering wheel can result in Boerhaave's syndrome with esophageal perforation and mediastinitis.

O **What test should be ordered if a perforated esophagus is suspected?**

A water-soluble contrast study. In the mean time, start broad-spectrum antibiotics and consult a surgeon immediately.

O **A former IV drug user with sickle-cell disease and a history of splenectomy presents with unremitting fever, crampy abdominal pain, and meningismus. He has no diarrhea but has recently purchased a pet turtle. What bacteria may be the culprit?**

Salmonella typhi, the causative agent of typhoid fever. The infection rate is remarkably high for HIV, asplenic, and sickle-cell disease patients. Rose spots occur in 10 to 20% of these cases. Relative bradycardia with a high fever and a low to normal WBC with a pronounced left shift are suggestive findings.

O **What is the treatment for the above patient?**

IV fluoroquinolone, ceftriaxone, or chloramphenicol. Check blood cultures for the presence of bacteremia. Avoid antimotility agents.

O **Is peptic ulcer disease more common in males or in females?**

Males, (3:1).

O   **What percentage of PUD patients are afflicted with duodenal ulcers? Gastric ulcers?**

75% and 25%, respectively.

O   **Are patients with duodenal PUD usually younger or older?**

Younger. Duodenal PUD is more often associated with H. pylori. Older people tend to develop gastric ulcers as a result of NSAID use.

O   **In what percentage of patients will a visible vessel in the base of an ulcer result in a rebleed?**

50%. A clean ulcer base will rebleed in only 1% of patients.

O   **What are some indications for surgery in a bleeding ulcer?**

A visible vessel in the ulcer bed, more than 6 units of blood transfused in 24 hours, or more than 3 to 4 units transfused per day for three days.

O   **Do gastric or duodenal ulcers heal faster?**

Duodenal.

O   **Are "stress ulcers" a surgical problem?**

Typically not. The diffuse gastric bleeding that results from CNS tumors, head trauma, burns, sepsis, shock, steroids, aspirin, or alcohol is usually mucosal and can be life-threatening. However, this condition can usually be managed medically. Endoscopic diagnosis is key.

O   **Are gastric and duodenal perforations more commonly associated with malignant ulcers or with benign ulcers?**

Benign ulcers.

O   **What medical conditions are related to an increased incidence of PUD?**

COPD, cirrhosis, and chronic renal failure.

O   **Where is the most common location of a perforated peptic ulcer?**

The anterior surface of the duodenum or pylorus and the lesser curvature of the stomach.

O   **After the fluid and blood resuscitation of a bleeding ulcer, what is the most useful diagnostic test?**

Endoscopy, which can also be therapeutic, with cryo- or electrocautery of an arterial bleeder.

O   **What clinical finding essentially eliminates a gastric outlet obstruction in a patient with early satiety and ulcer symptoms?**

Bilious vomitus.

O   **Name two endocrine problems that can cause peptic ulcer disease.**

Zollinger-Ellison syndrome and hyperparathyroidism (hypercalcemia).

○ **T/F: H2-blockers decrease the risk of perforation and rebleeding in peptic ulcer disease.**

False. However, cimetidine reduces the need for surgery, improves the rate of ulcer healing, and lowers the mortality rate from the initial bleeding episode.

○ **A patient with "half a stomach", as a result of a bleeding ulcer, presents with weight loss, epigastric burning, and diarrhea. What are potential reasons?**

An obstructed afferent loop (Billroth II), bile reflux gastritis, dumping syndrome, malabsorption, remnant carcinoma. Anemia (from B12, iron, and folate malabsorption) and osteoporosis (from vitamin D and calcium malabsorption) are also common.

○ **T/F: Antibiotics are not required after an uncomplicated perirectal abscess is incised and drained.**

True, assuming the patient has no underlying immunoincompetence, such as HIV, diabetes, or malignancy. Primary aftercare includes sitz baths beginning the next day.

○ **Do pilonidal abscesses communicate with the anal canal?**

No. They are virtually always midline and overlie the lower sacrum. Posterior-opening, horseshoe-type anorectal fistulas can find their way to the lower sacrum but are rarely in the midline.

○ **Should pilonidal cysts be excised in the office?**

Probably not. Incision and drainage are okay, followed by a bulky dressing, analgesics, and hot sitz baths, which should be initiated the next day. Antibiotics are not typically necessary. Excision should be completed in the OR once the acute infection clears up.

○ **In adults, pruritus ani develops because of dietary factors contributing to liquid stool, such as caffeine and mineral oil, sexually transmitted infections, fecal contamination, overzealous hygiene, and vitamin deficiencies. What is the most common cause in children?**

Enterobius vermicularis, or pinworm. Test for pinworms by applying a piece of scotch tape, sticky-side down, to the perineal area, and then use a cotton swab to smooth the tape on to a glass slide. Examine the slide for eggs with a low-power microscope. Treat the pediatric patient with mebendazole, 100 mg in a single dose, and repeat in 2 weeks if necessary.

○ **A patient with new diarrhea and abdominal pain has been on antibiotics for sinusitis for two weeks. What might be revealed by sigmoidoscopy?**

Yellowish superficial plaques. This finding is indicative of pseudomembranous colitis. Stool studies will implicate the *C. difficile* toxin.

○ **What is the treatment for pseudomembranous colitis?**

Oral vancomycin, 125 mg qid, or oral metronidazole, 500 mg qid. Either regimen should be administered for 7 to 10 days. Cholestyramine, which binds the toxin, can help relieve the diarrhea. Perform follow-up stool studies to confirm clearance of the toxin.

○ **Procidentia in adults mandates what intervention?**

Proctosigmoidoscopy and surgical repair. In children, rectal prolapse can be manually reduced with good results.

❍   **What is the most common presenting symptom of rectal cancer?**

Persistent hematochezia. Other symptoms include tenesmus and the feeling of incomplete voiding after a bowel movement.

❍   **What organism is usually responsible for causing SBP.**

E. coli. Streptococcus pneumoniae is second.

❍   **What is the best therapy for SBP?**

Intravenous ampicillin. An aminoglycoside is a reasonable empiric therapy pending culture results.

❍   **What two therapies can reduce the risk of recurrence of SBP?**

Diuretics, which decrease ascitic fluid, and nonabsorbable oral antibiotics, which decrease the gut bacterial load thereby limiting bacterial translocation.

❍   **A patient with chronic and occasionally bloody diarrhea develops severe diarrhea and abdominal pain with marked distention. What "can't miss" diagnosis is confirmed by these signs?**

Toxic megacolon. This condition is a life-threatening complication of ulcerative colitis.

❍   **Watery diarrhea with profuse rectal discharge and weakness might suggest which type of "uncommon" tumor?**

Villous adenoma.

❍   **A double bubble on an x-ray or a "bird's beak" and dilated colon on a barium enema are indicative of what?**

Volvulus.

❍   **A patient presents with tremor, ataxia, dementia, cirrhosis, and grey-green rings around the edge of his cornea. What is the diagnosis?**

Wilson's disease. Kayser-Fleischer rings, i.e., golden brown or grey-green pigmentation around the cornea, CNS disturbances, chronic hepatitis, and cirrhosis are all caused by copper retention as a result of impaired copper excretion.

❍   **In Wilson's disease, what are the levels of copper in the urine and serum?**

Serum copper levels are low because there is a deficiency in ceruloplasmin, the copper-binding protein. However, urine copper is high. Treatment for this disease is penicillamine, which chelates copper.

❍   **What are the most common cancers of the small bowel?**

Adenocarcinoma, followed by carcinoid, lymphoma, and leiomyosarcoma. The small bowel is not a common site for malignancy and accounts for only 2% of all GI malignancies.

❍   **What carcinoid tumors have the highest rate of metastasis?**

Ileal carcinoids. Malignancy is highly dependent on the size of the tumor: only 2% of tumors under 1 cm in diameter are malignant, while 80 to 90% of tumors > 2 cm are malignant.

○   **A patient complains of severe pain when defecating. He is constipated, has blood-streaked stools and a bloody discharge following bowel movements. What is the diagnosis?**

Anal fissure. Ninety percent of anal fissures are located in the posterior midline. If fissures are found elsewhere in the anal canal, then anal intercourse, TB, carcinoma, Crohn's disease, and syphilis should be considered.

○   **Differentiate between mucosal rectal prolapse, complete rectal prolapse, and occult rectal prolapse.**

Mucosal rectal prolapse-involves only a small portion of the rectum protruding through the anus and have the appearance of radial folds.
Complete rectal prolapse-involves all the layers of the rectum protruding through the anus. Clinically, this condition appears as concentric folds.
Occult rectal prolapse-does not involve protrusion through the anus but rather intussusception.

○   **Which are more painful, internal or external hemorrhoids?**

External. The nerves above the pectinate or dentate line are supplied by the autonomic nervous system and have no sensory fibers. The nerves below the pectinate line are supplied by the inferior rectal nerve and have sensory fibers.

○   **Differentiate between first, second, third, and fourth degree hemorrhoids.**

First degree: Appear in the rectal lumen, but do not protrude past the anus
Second degree: Protrude into the anal canal if the patient strains only
Third degree: Protrude into the anal canal, but can be manually reduced
Fourth degree: Protrude into the canal and cannot be manually reduced
Treatment for degrees one and two is a high-fiber diet, Sitz baths, and good hygiene. The treatment of choice for third or fourth degree hemorrhoids is rubber band ligation. Other treatments are photocoagulation, electrocauterization, and cryosurgery.

○   **What percentage of patients with diverticula are symptomatic?**

20%.

○   **What are some extraintestinal manifestations of ulcerative colitis?**

Ankylosing spondylitis, sclerosing cholangitis, arthralgias, ocular complications, erythema nodosum, aphthous ulcers in the mouth, thromboembolic disease, pyoderma gangrenous, nephrolithiasis, and cirrhosis of the liver.

○   **If blood is recovered from the stomach after an NG tube is inserted, where is the most likely location of the bleed?**

Above the ligament of Treitz.

○   **Where do the majority of Mallory-Weiss tears occur?**

In the stomach (75%), gastroesophageal junction (20%), and distal esophagus (5%).

○   **Where is angiodysplasia most frequently found?**

In the cecum and proximal ascending colon. Lesions are generally singular; bleeding is intermittent and seldom massive.

○   **Are tumors located in the jejunum and ileum more likely malignant or benign?**

Benign. Tumors of the jejunum and ileum comprise only 5% of all GI tumors. The majority are asymptomatic.

○   **What is the most common remnant of the omphalomesenteric duct?**

Meckel's diverticulum.

○   **What is the Meckel's diverticulum rule of 2's?**

2% of the population has it, it is 2 inches long, 2 feet from the ileocecal valve, occurs most commonly in children under 2, and is symptomatic in 2% of patients.

○   **What is the difference in the prognosis between familial polyposis and Gardner's disease?**

Although both are inheritable conditions of colonic polyps, Gardner's disease rarely results in malignancy, where as familial polyposis virtually always results in malignancy.

○   **How much blood must be lost in the GI tract to cause melena?**

50 ml. Healthy patients normally lose 2.5 ml/day.

○   **What are the most common causes of upper GI bleeding?**

PUD (45%), esophageal varices (20%), gastritis (20%), and Mallory-Weiss syndrome (10%).

○   **What percentage of patients with upper GI bleeds will stop bleeding within hours of hospitalization?**

85%. About 25% of these patients will re-bleed within the first 2 days of hospitalization. If no re-bleeding occurs in five days, the chance of re-bleeding is only 2%.

○   **What percentage of patients with PUD bleed from their ulcers?**

20%.

○   **How soon after an episode of bleeding has occurred can an ulcer patient be fed?**

12 to 24 hours after the bleeding has stopped.

○   **Which type of ulcer is more likely to re-bleed?**

Gastric ulcers are three times more likely to re-bleed compared to duodenal ulcers.

○   **Where is the most common site of duodenal ulcers?**

The duodenal bulb (95%). Surgery is indicated only if perforation, gastric outlet obstruction, intractable disease, or uncontrollable hemorrhage occur.

○   **What is the most common site for gastric ulcers?**

The lesser curvature of the stomach. Surgery is considered earlier in gastric ulcers because of the higher recurrence rate after medical treatment, and because of the higher potential for malignancy.

○   **What is the most common cause of portal hypertension?**

Intrahepatic obstruction (90%), which is most often due to cirrhosis. Other causes of portal hypertension are increased hepatic flow without obstruction, i.e., fistulas, and extrahepatic outflow obstruction.

○   **What organism causes amebic liver abscesses?**

Entamoeba histolytica. Amebic liver abscesses are primarily found in middle-aged men living in, or who have traveled to, tropical areas. Ninety percent occur in the right lobe of the liver. Treatment is with oral metronidazole.

○   **What are the most commonly isolated organisms in pyogenic hepatic abscesses?**

E. coli and other gram-negative bacteria. The source of such bacteria is most likely an infection in the biliary system.

○   **What clinical sign can assist in the diagnosis of cholecystitis?**

Murphy's sign: pain on inspiration with palpation of the RUQ. As the patient breaths in, the gallbladder is lowered in the abdomen and comes in contact with the peritoneum just below the examiner's hand. This will aggravate an inflamed gallbladder, causing the patient to discontinue breathing deeply.

○   **What is the difference between cholelithiasis, cholangitis, cholecystitis, and choledocholithiasis?**

Cholelithiasis:	Gallstones in the gallbladder
Cholangitis:	Inflammation of the common bile duct, often secondary to bacterial infection or choledocholithiasis
Cholecystitis:	Inflammation of the gallbladder secondary to gallstones
Choledocholithiasis:	Gallstones, which have migrated from the gallbladder to the common bile duct

○   **What percentage of people with asymptomatic gallstones will develop symptoms?**

Only 50%.

○   **Which ethnic group has the largest proportion of people with symptomatic gallstones?**

Native Americans. By the age of 60, 80% of Native Americans with previously asymptomatic gallstones will develop symptoms, as compared to only 30% of Caucasian Americans and 20% of African Americans.

○   **What percentage of patients with cholangitis are also septic?**

50%. Chills, fever, and shock can occur.

○   **What percentage of gallstones can be visualized on ultrasound?**

95%. Ultrasound is the diagnostic procedure of choice in patients with suspected cholecystitis.

○   **What is Charcot's triad?**

1) Fever
2) Jaundice
3) Abdominal pain
This is the hallmark of acute cholangitis.

○   **What is Reynolds' pentad?**

Charcot's triad plus shock and mental status changes. This is the hallmark of acute toxic ascending cholangitis.

○   **What is the diagnostic test of choice for acute cholecystitis?**

HIDA scan (technetium-99-labeled N-substituted iminodiacetic acid scan). The HIDA scan uses a gamma-ray-emitting isotope that is selectively extracted by the liver into bile. The labeled bile can then be used to determine if there is cystic duct obstruction or extrahepatic bile duct obstruction, which is based whether the bile fills the gall bladder or enters the intestine. For practical reasons, the diagnosis is frequently make using clinical impressions, CBC and ultrasound.

○   **How effective is oral dissolution therapy with bile acids for those with symptomatic gallstones?**

Oral therapy with bile acids can dissolve up to 90% of stones. However, therapy works only on stones smaller than 0.5 mm, made of cholesterol, and floating in a functioning gallbladder. Patients are then treated for 6 to 12 months and 50% have recurrence of gallstones within 5 years.

○   **What are the contraindications to lithotripsy?**

Stones > 2.5 cm, more than 3 stones, calcified stones, stones in the bile duct, and poor overall condition of the patient.

○   **What electrolyte disturbances are associated with acute pancreatitis?**

Hypocalcemia and hypomagnesemia.

○   **Serum amylase is frequently elevated in acute pancreatitis. What other conditions can cause a similar rise in amylase?**

Bowel infarction, cholecystitis, mumps, perforated ulcer, and renal failure. Lipase is more specific. A two-hour urine amylase is a more accurate test in pancreatitis.

○   **What are the most common causes of acute pancreatitis?**

Alcoholism (40%) and gallstone disease (40%). The remaining cases of acute pancreatitis are due to familial pancreatitis, hypoparathyroidism, hyperlipidemia, iatrogenic pancreatitis, and protein deficiency.

○   **What are some abdominal x-ray findings associated with acute pancreatitis?**

A sentinel loop (either of the jejunum, transverse colon, or duodenum); a colon cutoff sign, (an abrupt cessation of gas in the mid or left transverse colon due to inflammation of the adjacent pancreas); or calcification of the pancreas. About two-thirds of patients with acute pancreatitis will have x-ray abnormalities.

○   **What is the treatment for pancreatic pseudocysts?**

Initial therapy is to wait for regression (4 to 6 weeks). If no improvement occurs, or if superinfection occurs, surgical drainage or excision is required.

○   **What are Ranson's criteria?**

A means of estimating prognosis for patients with pancreatitis.

At initial presentation	Developing within 24 hours
Age > 55	Hematocrit falling > 10%
WBC > 16,000/mm^3	Increase in BUN > 5 mg/dL
AST > 250 UI/L	Serum Ca^c < 8 mg/dl

Serum glucose > 200 mg/dl	Arterial PO$_2$ < 60 mm Hg
LDH > 700 iu/L	Base deficit > 4 mEq/L
	Fluid sequestration > 6 L

0 to 2 criteria = 2% mortality
3 to 4 criteria = 15% mortality
5 to 6 criteria = 40% mortality
7 to 8 criteria = 100% mortality

❍   **What is the most common cause of pancreatic pseudocysts in adults?**

Chronic pancreatitis. Pseudocysts are generally filled with pancreatic enzymes and are sterile. They present about 1 week after the patient has a bout with acute pancreatitis displayed as upper abdominal pain with anorexia and weight loss. Forty percent will regress spontaneously.

❍   **What are some other causes of pancreatitis?**

Surgery, trauma, ERCP, viral and mycoplasma infections, hypertriglyceridemia, vasculitis, drugs, penetrating peptic ulcer, anatomic abnormalities about the ampulla of Vater, hyperparathyroidism, end stage renal disease and organ transplantation.

❍   **What are some of the drugs known to cause pancreatitis?**

Sulfonamides, estrogens, tetracyclines, pentamidine, azathioprine, thiazides, furosemide and valproic acid.

❍   **What are some of the infectious causes of pancreatitis?**

Mumps, viral hepatitis, Coxsackievirus group B, and mycoplasma.

❍   **What are the common symptoms of acute pancreatitis?**

Epigastric or diffuse abdominal pain radiating to the back, nausea and vomiting.

❍   **What are the common signs of acute pancreatitis?**

Fever, tachycardia, hypotension, distended abdomen, guarding with diminished or absent bowel sounds. Rarely seen signs include tender subcutaneous nodules from fat necrosis, and hypocalcemic tetany.

❍   **What is the mechanism of hypotension in severe cases of acute pancreatitis?**

Fluid sequestration in the intestine and retroperitoneum, systemic vascular effects of kinins, vomiting and bleeding.

❍   **What is Cullen's sign?**

Periumbilical ecchymosis indicative of pancreatitis, severe upper bowel bleeding or ruptured ectopic pregancy.

❍   **Does acute pancreatitis commonly progress to chronic pancreatitis?**

No. Only rarely.

❍   **What are the pathological spectra in acute pancreatitis?**

Edematous pancreatitis (mild cases), and necrotizing pancreatitis (severe cases). Hemorrhagic pancreatitis may evolve from either of them.

O   **What is the mechanism of necrosis and vascular damage in acute pancreatitis?**

Autodigestion of the pancreas by various proteolytic and lipolytic enzymes.

O   **What are the laboratory abnormalities in pancreatitis?**

Leukocytosis, hemoconcentration followed by anemia, hyperglycemia, prerenal azotemia, hypoxemia, hyperamylasemia, LFT abnormalities, and elevated lipase.

O   **What are some other causes of hyperamylasemia besides pancreatitis?**

Pancreatic pseudocyst, pancreatic trauma, pancreatic carcinoma, ERCP, perforated duodenal ulcer, mesenteric infarction, renal failure, intestinal obstruction, salivary gland origin, ovarian disorders, prostate tumors, DKA, macroamylasemia.

O   **Does the level of amylase elevation correlate with severity?**

No. Higher levels are seen in biliary pancreatitis.

O   **What is the role of serum lipase determinations?**

It is slightly less sensitive than amylase but much more specific. It is also elevated in renal failure and non-pancreatic acute abdominal conditions. Lipase levels are elevated longer than amylase levels.

O   **When is surgery indicated in pancreatitis?**

When a patient has an infected pancreatic necrosis or an abscess that cannot be adequately drained and treated.

O   **Should immediate surgery be performed in gallstone pancreatitis?**

No. It should be performed after the pancreatitis has subsided

O   **What is Hamman's sign?**

Air in the mediastinum following an esophageal perforation. This condition produces a crunching sound over the heart during systole.

O   **What is the most common site of rupture in Boerhaave's syndrome?**

The posterior distal esophagus. Boerhaave's syndrome is rupture of the esophagus that occurs after binge drinking and vomiting. Patients experience sudden, sharp pain in the lower chest and epigastric area. The abdomen becomes rigid, then shock may follow.

METABOLIC AND ENDOCRINE

○ **What are the signs and symptoms of hyponatremia?**

Weakness, nausea, anorexia, vomiting, confusion, lethargy, seizures, and coma.

○ **What are some causes of factitious hyponatremia?**

Hyperglycemia, hyperlipidemia, and hyperproteinemia.

○ **How does hyperglycemia lead to hyponatremia?**

Because glucose stays in the extracellular fluid, hyperglycemia draws water out of the cell into the extracellular fluid thus diluting the sodium. Each 100 mg/dL increase in plasma glucose decreases the serum sodium by 1.6 to 1.8 mEq/L.

○ **What is the most common cause of euvolemic hyponatremia in children?**

Syndrome of inappropriate secretion of antidiuretic hormone (SIADH). Other causes include CNS disorders, medications, tumors, and pulmonary disorders.

○ **What is central pontine myelinolysis (osmotic demyelination syndrome)?**

The complication of brain dehydration following the rapid correction of severe hyponatremia. Correct hyponatremia slowly, i.e., < 12 mEq/day for chronic hyponatremia.

○ **What are the signs and symptoms of hypernatremia?**

Confusion, muscle irritability, seizures, respiratory paralysis, and coma.

○ **What are the most common causes of hypotonic fluid loss leading to hypernatremia?**

Diarrhea, vomiting, hyperpyrexia, and excessive sweating.

○ **What are the ECG findings of a patient with hypokalemia?**

Flattened T waves, depressed ST segments, prominent P and U waves, and prolonged QT and PR intervals.

○ **What are the ECG findings of a patient with hyperkalemia?**

Peaked T waves, prolonged QT and PR intervals, diminished P waves, depressed T waves, QRS widening, and with levels near 10 mEq/L, a classic sine wave.

○ **What are the causes of hyperkalemia?**

Acidosis, tissue necrosis, hemolysis, blood transfusions, GI bleed, renal failure, Addison's disease, primary hypoaldosteronism, excess po K^+ intake, RTA IV, and medication, such as succinylcholine, ß-blockers, captopril, spironolactone, triamterene, amiloride, and high-dose penicillin.

○ **What is the treatment for sever hyperkalemia?**

Kayexalate, glucose, insulin, sodium bicarbonate, calcium gluconate or calcium chloride, dialysis, and high dose nebulized albuterol.

○   **What are the causes of hypocalcemia?**

Shock, sepsis, multiple blood transfusions, hypoparathyroidism, vitamin D deficiency, pancreatitis, hypomagnesemia, alkalosis, fat embolism syndrome, phosphate overload, chronic renal failure, loop diuretics, hypoalbuminemia, tumor lysis syndrome, and medication, such as Dilantin, phenobarbital, heparin, theophylline, cimetidine, and gentamicin.

○   **In order of prevalence, what are the three most common causes of hypercalcemia?**

Malignancy, primary hyperparathyroidism, and thiazide diuretics.

○   **What are the signs and symptoms of hypercalcemia?**

The most common gastrointestinal symptoms are anorexia and constipation. Remember:

Stones: Renal calculi
Bones: Osteolysis
Abdominal groans: Peptic ulcer disease and pancreatitis
Psychic overtones: Psychiatric disorders

○   **What is the initial treatment for hypercalcemia?**

Restoration of the extracellular fluid with 5 to 10 L of normal saline within 24 hours. After the patient is rehydrated, administer furosemide in doses of 1 to 3 mg/kg. Patients with hypercalcemia are dehydrated because high calcium levels interfere with ADH and the ability of the kidney to concentrate urine.

○   **A patient with a history of alcohol abuse presents after a recent tonic-clonic seizure. What particular electrolyte abnormality should be considered and treated during evaluation?**

Hypomagnesemia. Treat the patient with $MgSO_4$, 2 g IV over 1 hour. Total deficit is often 5-10 grams.

○   **What is the most common cause of secondary adrenal insufficiency and adrenal crisis?**

Iatrogenic adrenal suppression from prolonged steroid use. Rapid withdrawal of steroids may lead to collapse and death.

○   **What are the most common causes of hyperphosphatemia?**

Acute and chronic renal failure.

○   **What is thyrotoxicosis? What causes it?**

A hypermetabolic state occurring secondary to excess circulating thyroid hormone. Thyrotoxicosis is caused by thyroid hormone overdose, thyroid hyperfunction, or thyroid inflammation.

○   **What are the hallmark clinical features of myxedema coma?**

Hypothermia (75%) and coma.

○   **What is the most common cause of hypoglycemia seen in the ED?**

An insulin reaction in a diabetic patient.

○ **What is the most important initial step in treating DKA?**

Volume replacement, with the first liter administered over about 60 minutes.

○ **In the first two years of life, what is the most common cause of drug-induced hypoglycemia?**

Salicylates. Between ages 2 and 8, alcohol is the most likely cause, and between ages 11 and 30, insulin and sulfonylureas are the primary causes.

○ **What principle hormone protects the human body from hypoglycemia?**

Glucagon.

○ **How is sulfonylurea induced hypoglycemia treated?**

IV glucose alone may be insufficient. It may require diazoxide, 300 mg slow IV over 30 minutes, repeated every 4 hours.

○ **Which is the most common type of hypoglycemia in children?**

Ketotic hypoglycemia. This condition usually develops in boys between 18 months and 5 years of age. Attacks typically arise from caloric deprivation. These attacks may be episodic and are more frequent in the morning and during periods of illness.

○ **What are the neurologic signs and symptoms associated with hypoglycemia?**

Hypoglycemia may produce mental and neurologic dysfunction. Neurologic manifestations can include paresthesias, cranial nerve palsies, transient hemiplegia, diplopia, decerebrate posturing, and clonus.

○ **What lab findings are expected with diabetic ketoacidosis?**

Elevated ß-hydroxybutyrate, acetoacetate, acetone, and glucose. Ketonuria and glucosuria are present. Serum bicarbonate levels, pCO_2, and pH are decreased. Potassium levels may be elevated but will fall when the acidosis is corrected.

○ **Outline the basic treatment for DKA.**

Administer fluids. Start with normal saline (the total deficit may be 5 to 10 L), followed by potassium, 100 to 200 mEq in the first 12 to 24 hours. Prescribe insulin, 5 - 10 unit bolus followed by 5 to 10 units/hour. (Editors' note: Many physicians no longer give bolus.) Add glucose to the IV fluid when the glucose level falls below 250 mg/dL and give the patient a phosphate supplement when the levels drop below 1.0 mg/dL.

For pediatric patients, administer NS, 20 mL/kg/hour for 1 to 2 hours, and insulin, 0.1 units/kg bolus, followed by 0.1 units/kg/hour drip.

○ **What are the complications of bicarbonate therapy in DKA?**

Paradoxical CSF acidosis, cardiac arrhythmias, decreased oxygen delivery to tissue, and fluid and sodium overload.

○ **A 42-year-old female presents with a history of palpitations, sweating, diplopia, blurred vision, and weakness. Her husband states she has been confused, most notably before breakfast. What is a probable diagnosis?**

Islet cell tumor of the pancreas which can result from fasting hypoglycemia.

❍   **What are the key features of nonketotic hyperosmolar coma?**

Hyperosmolality, hyperglycemia, and dehydration. Blood sugar levels should be > 800 mg/dL, serum osmolality should be > 350 mOsm/kg, and serum ketones should be negative.

❍   **What is the treatment for nonketotic hyperosmolar coma?**

Normal saline, potassium, 10 to 20 mEq/hour, and insulin, 5 to 10 units/hour. Glucose should be added to the IV if the blood sugar level drops below 250 mg/dL.

❍   **What is the overall mortality rate of nonketotic hyperosmolar coma?**

Approximately 50%.

❍   **Distinguish between lactic acidosis type A and B.**

Type A is associated with inadequate tissue perfusion, the resultant anoxia, and subsequent lactate and hydrogen ion accumulation. This condition usually occurs because of shock and is often seen in the ED. Type B includes all forms of acidosis in which there is no evidence of tissue anoxia.

❍   **What is the most common precipitant of thyroid storm?**

Pulmonary infections.

❍   **What signs and symptoms are helpful for diagnosing thyroid storm?**

Eye signs of Graves' disease, a history of hyperthyroidism, widened pulse pressure, hypertension, a palpable goiter, tachycardia, fever, diaphoresis, increased CNS activity, emotional lability, heart failure, and coma.

❍   **What pH decrease is expected with an increase of pCO_2 of 10 mm Hg?**

0.08.

❍   **What pH increase is expected with a decrease of pCO_2 of 10 mm Hg?**

0.13.

❍   **What pH increase is expected with a rise in HCO_{23} of 5.0 mEq/L?**

0.08.

❍   **What decrease in pH is expected with a decrease in HCO_3 of 5.0 mEq/L?**

0.10.

❍   **How is the anion gap calculated from electrolyte values?**

Anion gap = Na - (Cl - HCO_3)
The normal gap is 12 ± 4 mEq/L.

❍   **Acidosis is closely related to anion gap measurement. Name the causes of increased anion gap acidosis.**

A MUD PILE CAT
Alcohol

Methanol
Uremia
DKA

Paraldehyde
Iron and isoniazid
Lactic acidosis
Ethylene glycol

Carbon monoxide
Aspirin
Toluene

○   **How can the magnitude of the anion gap be useful in narrowing the differential of an anion gap acidosis?**

An anion gap > 35 mEq/L is usually caused by ethylene glycol, methanol, or lactic acidosis. An anion gap 23 to 30 mEq/L may be due to an increase in organic acids, and an anion gap 16 to 22 mEq/L may be a result of advanced uremia.

○   **How is the osmolar gap determined?**

Osmolality is a measure of the concentration of particles in a solution with units of osmoles per kg water. Osmolarity is a measure of osmoles per liter of solution. For dilute solutions, like body fluids, these two measures are roughly equivalent. An osmolar gap is the difference between the measured osmolality and the calculated osmolarity; normally 275 to 285 mOsm/L.

○   **How much do different substances contribute to the osmolar gap?**

	mg/dL to increase serum osmol 1 mOsm/L	mOsm/L increase per mg/dL
Methanol	2.6	0.38
Ethanol	4.3	0.23
Ethylene glycol	5.0	0.20
Acetone	5.5	0.18
Isopropyl alcohol	5.9	0.17
Salicylate	14.0	0.07

Small amounts of methanol cause greater increases in osmolality. Large amounts of salicylate will eventually increase the osmolar gap. Note also that the contribution to an osmolar gap due to ethanol may be calculated; this can be useful when a mixed alcohol ingestion is suspected.

○   **What clinical findings can narrow the differential of an anion gap acidosis?**

Methanol:	Visual disturbances and headache are common; can produce wide gaps
Uremia:	Must be advanced to contribute to gap
Diabetic ketoacidosis:	Usually occurs with both hyperglycemia and glucosuria
Alcoholic ketoacidosis:	Often has lower blood sugar and mild or absent glucosuria
Salicylates:	High levels required to contribute to gap
Lactic acidosis:	Can check serum level and has a broad differential
Ethylene glycol:	Causes calcium oxalate or hippurate crystals in urine

○   **What causes an oxygen saturation curve to shift to the right?**

A shift to the right delivers more O2 to the tissue. Remember:

CADET! Right face!

Hyper	**C**arbia
	Acidemia
2,3	**D**PG
	Exercise
Increased	**T**emperature
	Release to tissues

○ **When body waste materials, urine, and stool are internally recycled, they can cause a normal anion gap metabolic acidosis. Remember: USED CRAP.**

USED CRAP

Ureteroenterostomy
Small bowel fistula
Extra chloride (NH4Cl or amino acid chlorides 2° TPN)
Diarrhea

Carbonic anhydrase inhibitors
Renal tubular acidosis
Adrenal insufficiency
Pancreatic fistula

○ **Name the two primary causes of metabolic alkalosis.**

Loss of hydrogen and chloride from the stomach and overzealous diuresis with loss of hydrogen, potassium, and chloride.

○ **Which types of nodules are more likely to be malignant on a thyroid scan, hot or cold?**

Cold. This procedure should not be considered confirmatory. Cysts and benign adenomas can also read as cold. Some types of thyroid cancers will read as "warm" and thus be dismissed. Use caution when interpreting results.

○ **What test should be performed to distinguish a benign cystic nodule from a malignant nodule?**

Fine needle aspiration biopsy and cytological evaluation.

○ **What is a solitary thyroid nodule most likely to be?**

A nodular goiter (50%). Other possibilities to consider include cancer (20%), adenoma (20%), cyst (5%), or thyroiditis (5%).

○ **What are the key predisposing factors to hypoglycemia in diabetic patients on insulin?**

Exercise, poor oral intake, worsening renal function, and medications are the key predisposing factors to consider.

○ **What is the major mechanism of hyponatremia in DKA patients?**

Dilution of sodium due to shifting of water out of the cells into the vascular space.

○ **What will orthostatic drops in blood pressure in a diabetic patient usually reflect?**

Autonomic dysfunction.

○ **What major insults are likely to lead to DKA in an otherwise controlled diabetic?**

Always look for infection (even a minor one), cardiac ischemia, medications, lack of compliance with insulin and diet.

○ **Which medications are likely to worsen glucose control in a diabetic patient?**

The list is long, but includes thiazide diuretics, beta-blockers, steroids, estrogens, dilantin, cyclosporine, diazoxide.

○ **What are the key factors leading to hypernatremia in a patient with non-ketogenic hyperosmolar coma?**

Profound dehydration with greater losses of water than salt as well as impaired thirst.

○ **What are some complications of hypophosphatemia seen in treated DKA?**

Rhabdomyolysis, cardiac dysfunction, arrhythmias, hemolysis, poor neutrophil function.

○ **What are the key factors predisposing diabetics to soft tissue infections?**

Microvascular disease, poor wound healing and trauma often masked by neuropathy.

○ **What are some agents used to treat severe diabetic gastroparesis?**

Cisapride and metoclopramide are the key agents. Erythromycin has also been tried in very severe cases.

○ **Diffuse abdominal pain with bloody stools and a high serum lactate in a diabetic might suggest what gastrointestinal disease?**

Ischemic or necrotic bowel.

○ **What medications are likely to lead to acute hyperkalemia in a diabetic patient?**

NSAID's, ACE inhibitors, beta-blockers, potassium sparing diuretics and salt substitutes (these are usually potassium salts).

○ **What are some common causes of abdominal pain, nausea and vomiting in a diabetic patient?**

Diabetic gastroparesis, gallbladder disease, pancreatitis, and perhaps, ischemia bowel.

○ **Atypical chest pain in an elderly diabetic individual should always suggest what syndrome?**

Cardiac ischemia. Diabetic patients have high a high risk of cardiac ischemia and this must always be strongly considered even if the pain is somewhat atypical.

○ **What is the most desirable agent used to treat severe hyperglycemia in pregnancy?**

These patients must have tight control achieved by multiple injections of insulin.

○ **Increasing quantities of acetone seen during treatment of DKA are due to what phenomenon?**

The conversion of beta-hydroxybutyrate into acetone.

○   **What do profound polyuria and dehydration in DKA reflect?**

Severe osmotic diuresis caused by glycosuria.

○   **What is the possible adverse effect seen during very rapid correction of severe hyperglycemia?**

Cerebral edema.

○   **What are the major adverse effects of intravenous radiocontrast dye given to diabetic patients?**

Acute tubular necrosis is well known. One should also watch for worsening of CHF, precipitation of angina pectoris and hemodynamic compromise.

○   **If autoimmune adrenal disease is the underlying disorder, which zone of the adrenal gland is spared?**

Medulla.

○   **What characteristic lab findings are associated with primary adrenal insufficiency?**

Hyperkalemia, hyponatremia, hypoglycemia, azotemia (if volume depletion is present), and a mild metabolic acidosis.

○   **What are the main causes of death during an adrenal crisis?**

Circulatory collapse and hyperkalemia induced arrhythmias.

○   **What are the causes of acute adrenal crisis?**

Major stress, such as surgery, severe injury, myocardial infarction, or any other acute illness in a patient with primary or secondary adrenal insufficiency.

○   **Secretion of which adrenal hormone is not impaired by secondary adrenal insufficiency?**

Aldosterone. Aldosterone secretion is more dependent upon angiotensin II than corticotropin, and aldosterone deficiency is not a problem in hypopituitarism. Selective aldosterone hypersecretion can manifest as a result of increased renin and angiotensin II formation.

○   **What are the causes of acute abrupt primary adrenal insufficiency?**

Adrenal hemorrhage, necrosis, thrombosis in meningococcal disease, sepsis, anticoagulation therapy or the antiphospholipid syndrome.

○   **What are the causes of acute abrupt secondary adrenal insufficiency?**

Sheehan's Syndrome (postpartum pituitary necrosis), bleeding into a pituitary macroadenoma, and head trauma.

○   **What diseases produce slow insidious progression to primary adrenal insufficiency?**

Autoimmune diseases, tuberculosis, systemic fungal infections (histoplasmosis, blastomycosis, cryptococcosis), AIDS, (CMV, Kaposi's sarcoma), metastatic carcinoma (lung, breast, kidney), and lymphoma.

○ **What are the common clinical manifestations of adrenal insufficiency?**

Fatigue, lethargy, anorexia, weight loss, hyperpigmentation, hyponatremia, and hyperkalemia are common. Depression, dizziness, orthostatic hypotension, nausea and vomiting, diarrhea, lymphocytosis, eosinophils and normocytic, normochromic anemia are also significant manifestations.

○ **In a critical care setting, patients refractory to which type of medications suggest adrenal insufficiency?**

Catecholamines/Vasopressors.

○ **Are orthostatic hypotension and electrolyte abnormalities more common in primary or secondary adrenal insufficiency?**

Primary, because of the aldosterone deficiency and hypovolemia.

○ **What are the most specific signs of primary adrenal insufficiency?**

Hyperpigmentation of the skin and mucosal membranes due to high ACTH levels as a consequence of cortisol feedback and salt craving.

○ **Does a normal cortisol level in a critically ill patient rule out adrenal insufficiency?**

No. With critical illness, one should expect a cortisol level greater than normal and a normal level could be considered relatively insufficient. An absolute level of 25 ug/dl probably rules out adrenal insufficiency, although the lower cutoff is unknown.

○ **After an endocrinologic diagnosis has been established by hormonal studies, the radiologic study of choice to assess for pituitary or hypothalamic tumor would be?**

MRI with analysis of the sagittal and coronal sections. A CT scan can be helpful if bony invasion is suspected.

○ **Are imaging studies of the adrenal glands necessary in primary adrenal insufficiency?**

Yes. In cases other than autoimmune or adrenal myeloneuropathy, a CT scan of the adrenal should be performed to aid in the differential diagnosis. Enlarged glands with/without calcifications in patients with TB are a sign of active disease and warrant anti-infective therapy. Enlargement also occurs in other fungal infections, lymphoma, cancer and AIDS. A biopsy by CT guidance may also be helpful.

○ **What is the emergent steroid replacement in adrenal insufficiency?**

Hydrocortisone 50-100 mg IV every eight hours initially.

○ **What is the daily replacement of hydrocortisone once the patient is stabilized?**

Hydrocortisone 15 mg in the a.m. and 10 mg in the p.m. The dose should be the smallest possible to alleviate clinical symptoms yet prevent weight gain and osteoporosis. Measurements of urinary cortisol may help determine the appropriate dosing.

○ **Which patients should receive fludrocortisone?**

Patients with primary adrenal insufficiency should receive 50-200 ug/day of fludrocortisone as a substitute for aldosterone, guided by measurements of blood pressure, potassium and plasma renin activity.

○   **What added precautions should be taken by all patients with adrenal insufficiency?**

They should wear a medic alert bracelet, carry a card detailing their medications and the recommendations for treatment in emergencies, and to double or triple their dose of hydrocortisone when they sustain injury or illness. They should secure ampules of glucocorticoids for self injection or suppositories when vomiting or unable to take oral steroids.

○   **What accounts for the almost immediate effect of cortisol on blood pressure in patients with adrenal insufficiency?**

Cortisol exerts a permissive effect on catecholamine vascular responsivity and a vital role in the maintenance of vascular tone, vascular permeability and distribution of body water within the vascular compartment.

○   **What is the characteristic hemodynamic pattern of adrenal insufficiency?**

Predominantly, decreased systemic vascular resistance to a lesser degree, decreased cardiac contractility depending upon the volume status.

○   **The use of which sedating agent has been shown to increase mortality in critically ill patients by inducing primary adrenal insufficiency?**

Etomidate. This sedating agent is a selective inhibitor of adrenal 11-hydroxylase, the enzyme that converts deoxycortisol to cortisol. Mortality reportedly increased in a trauma unit that began using etomidate by continuous infusion for sedation and for this reason, etomidate is not used for continuous sedation in the critically ill.

○   **Is there any evidence to support the use of corticosteroids in septic shock?**

No beneficial effects of corticosteroids have been shown in sepsis or septic shock. In fact, they may be harmful, according to several studies.

○   **Randomized propspective trials have shown benefit from corticosteroids in which disease states?**

Bacterial meningitis, acute spinal injury, typhoid fever, *Pneumocystis carinii* pneumonia, and possibly treatment of the fibroproliferative phase of acute respiratory distress syndrome.

○   **What symptoms should increase the suspicion of adrenal insufficiency in the critically ill?**

Unexplained circulatory instability, high fever without cause, unresponsive to antibiotics, hypoglycemia, hyponatremia, hyperkalemia, neutropenia, eosinophilia, unexplained mental status changes, disparate anticipated severity of disease and the actual state of the patient.

○   **What are the adverse effects of using excessive dosing when covering for stress?**

Catabolic effects on muscle, impaired wound healing, antagonizing insulin and the effects on glucose metabolism and the anti-inflammatory effect on active infection.

○   **What are the current dosing recommendations for stress doses in patients with suspected adrenal insufficiency?**

Minor stress	25 mg/day
Moderate stress	50-75 mg/day
Major stress	100-150 mg/day

○ **How is the etiology of type 1 DM different from type II DM?**

Type I DM is associated with Human Leukocyte Antigens (HLA), autoimmunity, and or islet cell antibodies. Type II DM usually involves a genetic mutation resulting in inactive pancreatic and liver enzymes as well as insulin receptor defects.

○ **What etiologies are responsible for secondary DM?**

Exocrine pancreatic diseases like cystic fibrosis, pancreatic cancer and Cushing's disease.

○ **What condition should be suspected in a patient with a serum glucose of 942 mg/dl, mild ketonuria, depressed sensorium and positive Babinski sign?**

Non-ketotic hyperosmolar coma (NKHC).

○ **What is the appropriate mixture of regular and intermediate acting insulin in a daily insulin injection regimen?**

2/3 of the total dose should be intermediate acting with 1/3 being regular insulin. The single injection should be given 30 minutes prior to breakfast.

○ **What is the appropriate mixture of regular and intermediate acting insulin in a twice daily insulin injection regimen?**

2/3 of the dose should be given 30 minutes prior to breakfast; the remaining 1/3 given 30 minutes prior to dinner. Both injections should be 2/3 intermediate acting and 1/3 short acting insulin.

○ **What is the significance of the Hgb A1C?**

It represents the fraction of hemoglobin that has been nonenzymatically glycosylated. It provides an accurate estimation of the relative blood glucose level over the preceding 6-8 weeks.

○ **What is the Somogyi phenomenon?**

A hyperglycemic event that results from an over zealous response by counter regulatory hormones during a period of hypoglycemia.

○ **What happens to a patient with hyperthyroidism when exogenous TRH is administered?**

The TRH receptors are blocked thus preventing a rise in TSH levels. In a patient with a normal thyroid a concomitant rise in TSH would occur.

○ **What are the causes for elevated TBG levels?**

Pregnancy, newborn state, estrogens, and heroin.

○ **What is the most common cause of acquired hypothyroidism?**

Lymphocytic thyroiditis.

○ **What are the clinical manifestations of acquired hypothyroidism?**

Myxedema of the skin, cold intolerance, constipation, low pitched voice, menorrhagia, mental and physical slowing, dry skin, coarse brittle hair, and decreased energy level with increased need for sleep.

○ **What is the most common clinical manifestation of Lymphocytic thyroiditis?**

The appearance of a goiter.

○   **Patients with lymphocytic thyroiditis are usually hypothyroid, euthyroid, or hyperthyroid?**

The majority will be euthyroid. However , many will eventually become hypothyroid, while only a few will manifest the symptoms of hyperthyroidism.

○   **What is de Quervain's disease?**

A subacute, nonsupparative thyroiditis. Clinical manifestations involve a tender thyroid, fever and chills usually remitting within several months.

○   **What is the etiology of de Quervain's thyroiditis?**

Most likely due to a viral infection such as mumps or Coxsackievirus.

○   **Which medications are commonly found to result in sporadic goiters?**

Lithium, amiodarone and iodide containing asthma inhalers.

○   **What is a thyrotropin receptor stimulating antibody?**

An antibody commonly found in Graves' disease, which binds to the TSH receptor leading to thyroid stimulation and goiter production.

○   **Is Graves' disease more common in boys or girls?**

Girls are affected five times more than boys.

○   **What are the classical signs and symptoms of Graves' disease?**

Emotional lability, autonomic hyperactivity, exophthalmos, tremor, increased appetite with no weight gain or weight loss, diarrhea, and a goiter in nearly all affected individuals.

○   **How is Graves' disease confirmed by laboratory testing?**

Increased bound and free T3 and T4 with decreased TSH. Frequently, the presence of thyroid peroxidase and TSH receptor stimulating antibodies are present.

○   **What treatment options exist for patients with Graves' disease? What treatment is recommended?**

Patients can be managed medically with propylthiouracil (PTU) or methimazole, surgically with a subtotal thyroidectomy or with radioiodine therapy. Medical management is the treatment of choice.

○   **What are the three largest concerns with surgical management of Graves' disease?**

Hyper- or hypothyroidism depending on the amount of tissue removed, vocal cord paralysis and hypoparathyroidism.

○   **If fine needle aspiration of a thyroid nodule reveals parafollicular cells, what type of carcinoma should be suspected?**

Medullary carcinoma of the thyroid.

○   **What combination of disorders account for multiple endocrine neoplasia type IIA?**

Medullary carcinoma of the thyroid, adrenal medullary hyperplasia or pheochromocytoma, and parathyroid hyperplasia.

○   **What is the mode of inheritance of MEN Type IIA?**

Autosomal dominant.

○   **How is MEN Type-IIA different from MEN Type IIB?**

Men Type IIB is associated with multiple neuromas. It, too, is autosomal dominant.

○   **What are the hallmarks of polyglandular autoimmune disease type I?**

Autoimmune hypoparathyroidism, Addison's disease, and chronic mucocutaneous candidiasis.

○   **What are the symptoms of a thyroid storm?**

Tachycardia, systolic hypertension, tremulousness, delirium and hyperthermia.

○   **How do you manage acute thyrotoxicosis?**

Propranolol at 10 mg/kg IV over 10-15 minutes for hypertension and increased metabolic rate. Lugol's iodide, 5 drops PO every eight hours or sodium iodide 125-250 mg/dl IV over 24 hours will stop thyroxine production.

○   **What measures can be taken to further reduce peripheral conversion of T4 to T3?**

Oral dexamethasone at .2 mg/kg or oral hydrocortisone 5 mg/kg.

○   **What is the Waterhouse-Friderichsen Syndrome?**

Adrenal insufficiency due to adrenal hemorrhage. It is often secondary to meningococcemia- induced shock.

○   **Name four conditions that can be attributed to hyperadrenocortical stimulation.**

Cushing's syndrome, hyperaldosteronism, adrenogenital syndrome, and feminization.

○   **What is a pheochromocytoma?**

An uncommon tumor derived from neural crest cells found in the adrenal medulla.

○   **What two autosomal dominant diseases have a high prevalence of pheochromocytomas?**

Neurofibromatosis and Von Hippel-Lindau disease.

○   **What laboratory tests help make the diagnosis of pheochromocytoma?**

An increased total 24 hour urinary catecholamines and their metabolites (i.e., epinephrine, norepinephrine, metanephrine and VMA).

○   **What are the classic signs and symptoms of pheochromocytomas?**

Paroxysmal hypertension, autonomic hyperactivity, headache, visual changes and weight loss.

❍   **Which class of antihypertensive drugs are recommended for the temporary treatment of pheochromocytoma associated hypertension?**

Alpha adrenergic blocking agents like phenoxybenzamine and prazosin.

❍   **How do you manage a hypertensive crisis in a patient with a pheochromocytoma?**

1 mg of IV phentolamine or .5-.8mg/kg/min of sodium nitroprusside.

❍   **What specific disease process should be considered in a child who presents with dehydration, hypernatremia, decreased urine osmolarity and a high level of circulating ADH?**

Nephrogenic diabetes insipidus.

❍   **What is central diabetes insipidus?**

A lack of ADH secretion which results in an inability to concentrate the urine despite functioning kidneys.

❍   **What is the danger of rigorously hydrating a patient who has hypernatremia due to diabetes insipidus?**

Cerebral edema, seizures and death.

❍   **What should the physician consider if the patient with diabetes insipidus continues to diurese despite repeated doses of DDAVP?**

The patient most probably has nephrogenic diabetes insipidus, due to unresponsive kidney receptors for ADH, whether the ADH is endogenous or exogenous.

❍   **If nephrogenic diabetes insipidus is assumed, what further pharmacological treatment may be helpful?**

Thiazide diuretics have a paradoxical effect and may work in decreasing fluid losses.

❍   **What are the clinical manifestations of acromegaly?**

Coarse facial features, enlarged tongue, enlargement of the distal extremities and hypogonadism.

❍   **What pituitary tumor is the most common?**

Prolactinoma.

❍   **What are the common presenting signs of a prolactinoma?**

Headache, amenorrhea and galactorrhea.

❍   **What two options exist for the treatment of prolactinomas?**

Bromocriptine and surgery via a transphenoidal approach.

❍   **What is Cushing's disease?**

Pituitary adenomas leading to increased ACTH secretion with resultant bilateral adrenal hyperplasia and elevated cortisol levels.

O **Is Cushing's disease different than Cushing's syndrome?**

Cushing's disease results from pituitary adenomas, while Cushing's syndrome is elevated cortisol levels from various causes, including paraneoplastic syndromes, primary adrenal tumors, and exogenous use of cortisol.

O **What clinical manifestations are common to all patients with Cushing's syndrome?**

Moon facies, buffalo hump, obesity, hypertrichosis, hypertension, growth retardation, easy bruising, purple striae on the hips and abdomen, and amenorrhea in girls.

O **How is Cushing's syndrome diagnosed?**

Using the dexamethasone suppression test. Patients with ACTH dependent Cushing's demonstrate suppression with the larger doses of dexamethasone while those with ectopic tumors cannot be suppressed at any level.

O **What is Conn's syndrome?**

Primary hyperproduction of adrenal mineralcorticoids usually resulting from an aldosteronoma.

O **What are the clinical manifestations of primary aldosteronism?**

Hyperplasia of the zona glomerulosa leading to hypertension, sodium and water retention, hypokalemia and decreased serum renin levels.

O **What are the clinical manifestations of primary hypogonadism?**

Failure of development of the secondary sexual characteristics with abnormally small penis and testes.

O **What is hypogonadotropic hypogonadism?**

A delayed onset of puberty, due to decreased levels of FSH and LH, with functioning ovaries or testes.

O **How is the diagnosis of primary hypogonadism made?**

The levels of FSH and LH are abnormally elevated for the corresponding age. Testosterone levels remain low and show little response to the administration of hCG.

O **What is the deficient hormone in secondary hypogonadism?**

FSH or LH. The defect is in the pituitary rather than in the testes or ovaries.

O **What is Kallmann's syndrome?**

Hypogonadotropic hypogonadism with anosmia.

O **Is the pituitary gland responsible for parathyroid regulation?**

No. Unlike the thyroid gland, the parathyroids are not regulated by the pituitary gland, but rather, by circulating calcium levels.

O **What is the difference between primary and secondary hyperparathyroidism?**

In primary hyperparathyroidism, the defect is in the parathyroid gland, (i.e., an adenoma or hyperplasia), while in secondary hyperparathyroidism, the elevated PTH is a physiologic response to a low calcium level, usually a result of renal disease.

○ **What are the diagnostic laboratory findings seen in hyperparathyroidism?**

Elevated serum calcium and PTH with concomitant decreased phosphorous levels.

○ **What is von Recklinghausen's disease?**

Hyperparathyroidism, leading to cystic changes in bone, due to osteoclastic resorption with fibrous replacement, forming non neoplastic "brown tumors".

○ **What is pseudohypoparathyroidism?**

An autosomal recessive disorder characterized by kidneys unresponsiveness to PTH, shortened fourth and fifth metacarpals and metatarsals, and short stature, all occurring without evidence of parathyroid dysfunction.

○ **What other mineral must be considered in the patient who appears hypocalcemic?**

Magnesium. Giving calcium will not correct the problem, however the administration of magnesium will correct both the calcium level and the magnesium level.

○ **What are the clinical manifestations of polycystic ovarian disease (PCO)?**

Obesity, hirsutism, secondary amenorrhea and bilaterally enlarged polycystic ovaries.

○ **How are patients with PCO treated?**

Contraceptive pills for menstrual regulation and ovarian suppression.

○ **What laboratory findings are seen in PCO?**

Most patients have increased ratio of LH to FSH and an increased amount of LH due to an exaggerated response to GnRH.

○ **What are the sodium concentrations of the most common commercially available IV fluids?**

0.9 normal saline = 154 mEq/l
0.45 normal saline = 77 mEq/l
0.3 normal saline = 54 mEq/l
0.2 normal saline = 33 mEq/l

○ **What disorder has autosomal dominant inheritance and is associated with episodic weakness or paralysis along with transient alterations in serum potassium?**

Periodic paralysis, most commonly associated with episodes of hypokalemia, but may occur with hyperkalemia as well. Patients are normal between attacks. The condition becomes progressively worse in adulthood.

○ **What is the predominant energy source used during starvation by a healthy subject?**

Lipids.

○ **How long does the body's reserve of carbohydrates last during starvation?**

Glycogen stores are consumed within 24 hours.

O   **How much protein is required for balance in a healthy stable adult?**

Approximately 0.6 g/kg ideal body weight/day.

NEUROLOGY

○ **A 50 year old female with hearing loss over the last six months presents at 2 a.m. with vertigo that has progressively become worse over the last two months. Upon examination, she is mildly ataxic. What is the diagnosis?**

Eighth nerve lesion, possibly an acoustic schwannoma or meningioma.

○ **What is a vestibular schwannoma?**

An acoustic neuroma or a tumor of the eighth cranial nerve. In addition to hearing loss and vertigo, patients also present with tinnitus. Surgical removal is the treatment of choice because this tumor may spread to the cerebellum and the brainstem.

○ **Where are congenital berry aneurysms located?**

In the circle of Willis.

○ **What is the prognosis for a patient recently diagnosed with amyotrophic lateral sclerosis (ALS)?**

Death 3 to 10 years after the onset of symptoms. ALS, also known as Lou Gehrig's disease, involves a progressive loss of the anterior horn cell function of the motor neurons. No sensory abnormalities are involved, just gradual weakness and atrophy of the muscles.

○ **Which three bacterial illnesses present with peripheral neurologic findings?**

Botulism, tetanus, and diphtheria.

○ **Which type of bacteria are most commonly cultured from brain abscesses, aerobic or anaerobic?**

Anaerobic.

○ **What are the most common neurologic findings in adult botulism cases?**

Eye and bulbar muscle deficit.

○ **What is an Argyll Robertson pupil?**

A small and irregular pupil that can narrow to focus but not in response to light. This can be a sign of neurosyphilis. Other symptoms include headache, dizziness, diplopia, nuchal rigidity, weakness, paralysis, tabes dorsalis, memory loss, dementia, lethargy, and delusions.

○ **What is the legal definition of blindness?**

Visual acuity of 20/400 at best, with external correction such as glasses or contacts.

○ **A child with blurry vision has an abnormal pupillary reflex and a white reflex upon funduscopic examination. What is the treatment?**

125

Surgical removal of the eye. This is a retinoblastoma that can grow to other sites in the brain or body. This condition is inheritable and thus the parents should be counseled about the risks.

○   **A patient presents with facial droop on the left and weakness of the right leg. Where is the most likely site of the lesion?**

The brainstem, specifically the left pons.

○   **What area of the brain is dysfunctional when a patient has Cheyne-Stokes respirations?**

The cortex. The nervous system is relying on diencephalic control.

○   **What are the most common brain tumors in children?**

Cerebellar astrocytomas and medulloblastomas.

○   **What are the most common origins of metastatic brain lesions in adults?**

Breast adenocarcinoma, bronchogenic carcinoma, and malignant melanoma. Twenty percent of adult brain tumors are metastatic.

○   **What causes cerebral palsy?**

70% of cases are idiopathic. Other causes include utero infection, chromosomal abnormality, or stroke. Cerebral palsy is a defect of the central nervous system that occurs prenatally, perinatally, or before age three.

○   **Which subtypes of cerebral palsy are associated with mental retardation?**

Spastic and sometimes athetotic. Mental retardation occurs in 25% of patients with cerebral palsy.

○   **A 25-year-old was knocked unconscious for ten seconds while playing touch football one week ago. Since then, he has had intermittent vertigo, nausea, vomiting, blurred vision, a headache, and malaise. His neurological examination and CT are normal. What is the diagnosis?**

Post concussive syndrome. Most individuals recover fully over a 2 to 6 week time span. A small percentage of patients with post concussive syndrome will have persistent deficits.

○   **Differentiate between decerebrate and decorticate posturing.**

Decerebrate posturing: elbows and legs extended (indicative of a midbrain lesion).

Decorticate posturing: elbows flexed and legs extended (suggesting a thalamic lesion).

Remember: De**COR**ticate = hands by the heart.

○   **When does the onset of epilepsy usually occur?**

Before age 20.

○   **How long must a generalized tonic-clonic seizure last without a period of consciousness to be considered status epilepticus?**

30 minutes. Status epilepticus may result from grand mal seizures or anticonvulsant therapy withdrawal.

○ **Recurrent seizures in patients with a history of a febrile seizure generally occur in what time frame?**

About 85% occur within the first two years. The younger the child, the more likely recurrence. If a patient has a febrile seizure in the first year of life, the recurrence rate is 50%. If it occurs in the second year, the recurrence rate is only 25%.

○ **What is the most common malignant brain tumor in adults?**

Glioblastoma.

○ **What is the most common benign brain tumor in adults?**

Meningioma.

○ **What happens if light is directed into the eyes of a patient who is in a diabetic coma?**

The pupils will constrict.

○ **Distinguish between the gait of a patient with a cerebellar lesion and that of a patient with an extrapyramidal lesion.**

A patient with a cerebellar lesion will have truncal ataxia, an unsteady, irregular gait with broad steps. A patient with an extrapyramidal lesion will have a festinating gait, several small, shuffling steps taken without swinging the arms.

○ **The Weber's test is performed on a patient complaining of hearing loss. The patient hears sounds more loudly in his right ear. Which types of hearing loss may this patient have?**

Conductive hearing loss on the right or sensory hearing loss on the left.

○ **Describe Rinne's test and explain the normal findings.**

Rinne's test is performed by placing the tip of the tuning fork on the mastoid process until the patient can no longer hear the tone. The fork is then relocated to just in front of the pinna until the patient can no longer hear the tone. In normal patients, the ratio is 1:2 of the duration of time the patient can hear the fork.

○ **What is the most common cause of subarachnoid hemorrhage?**

Saccular aneurysm.

○ **What are other common causes of a subarachnoid hemorrhage?**

Rupture of cerebral artery aneurysm and arteriovenous malformation. These patients present with an abrupt, severe headache that can progress to syncope, nausea, vomiting, nuchal rigidity, and non-focal neurological changes.

○ **Damage to the middle meningeal artery results in what kind of hematoma?**

Epidural.

○ **A 29 year old drunken male presents after having his head pounded into the concrete. The patient had a brief episode of LOC but was then ambulatory and alert. Now he appears drowsy and just threw up on you. What is the probable diagnosis?**

Epidural hematoma.

○   **Which is more common, subdural or epidural hemorrhaging?**

Subdural. Subdural hemorrhaging can result from the tearing of the bridging veins. Bleeding occurs less rapidly because the veins, not arteries, are damaged.

○   **A 26 year old woman complains of a throbbing, dull, unilateral headache that lasts for hours then goes away with sleep. She also has been nauseated and has vomited twice. She reports small areas of visual loss plus strange zig-zag lines in her vision. What is the most likely diagnosis?**

Classic migraine headache. Classic migraine accounts for only 1% of migraines. It can be differentiated from the common migraine because it involves visual disturbances of scotomata and fortification spectra, in addition to all the other migraine symptoms.

○   **What factors may precipitate migraine headaches?**

Bright lights, cheese, hot dogs and other foods containing tyramine or nitrates, menstruation, monosodium glutamate, and stress.

○   **A 30 year old man with severe orbital and temporal pain on the right side has tearing out of the right eye but not the left. The patient's pain tends to occur when he arrives home from work. Also, he knows he will get a headache if he comes home and grabs a beer. The headaches last only about an hour. What syndrome can be associated with this man's headache?**

Horner's syndrome (anhidrosis, mitosis, and ptosis). This man has a cluster headache, which typically occurs in men ranging from ages 20 to 50. A cluster headache can recur at the same time and location each day, and is exacerbated by alcohol and vasodilators. Relief is achieved with 100% O_2, ergots, lithium, or prednisone. Intranasal viscous lidocaine can also be effective.

○   **Which type of headache usually afflicts adults?**

Tension headaches. This is a bilateral "bandlike" fronto-occipital headache accompanied by constant pain. Tension headaches are generally muscular in nature therefore a patient may also have tense neck and scalp muscles.

○   **Describe the key signs and symptoms of classic, common, ophthalmoplegic, and hemiplegic migraine headaches.**

Common:	This headache is indeed the most common. It is a slowly evolving headache that lasts for hours to days. A positive family history as well as two of the following are prevalent: nausea or vomiting, throbbing quality, photophobia, unilateral pain, and increase with menses. A lack of visual symptoms distinguishes common migraine from classic migraine.
Classic:	The prodrome lasts up to 60 minutes. The most common symptom is visual disturbance (homonymous hemianopsia, scintillating scotoma, fortification spectra, and photophobia). Lip, face, and hand tingling, aphasia, extremity weakness, nausea and vomiting may occur.
Ophthalmoplegic:	These headaches are most common in young adults. The patient has an outwardly deviated, dilated eye with ptosis. The third, fourth, and sixth nerves are usually involved.
Hemiplegic:	Unilateral motor and sensory symptoms and mild hemiparesis to hemiplegia are exhibited.

O   **How can you tell if a headache is caused by an intracranial tumor?**

Through a CT or MRI. However, everyone who walks into the office complaining of a headache cannot be subjected to these procedures.   Patients complaining of the "worst headache of their life" have written a ticket for a scan and LP. Other signs that may suggest a serious underlying disease are headaches that (1) wake patients from their sleep (although cluster headaches may do this), (2) are worse in the morning, (3) increase in severity with postural changes or Valsalva maneuvers, (4) are associated with nausea and vomiting (though migraines have similar symptoms), (5) are associated with focal defects or mental status changes, and (6) occur with a new onset of seizures.

O   **A man developed Huntington's chorea at the age of 44. What are the chances of his daughter developing the same disease?**

50%. Huntington's chorea is an autosomal dominant disorder that first manifests itself between ages 30 to 50. Symptoms include dementia, amnesia, delusions, emotional instability, depression, paranoia, antisocial behavior, and irritability. If the daughter inherits the disease, she will also develop chorea, bradykinesia, hypertonia, hyperkinesia, clonus, schizophrenia, intellectual impairment, and bowel incontinence. She will eventually die a premature death about 15 years after the onset of her symptoms.

O   **What chromosome carries the genetic defect for Huntington's chorea?**

The short arm of chromosome 4.

O   **Differentiate between Korsakoff's psychosis and Wernicke's encephalopathy.**

Korsakoff's psychosis: Inability to process new information, i.e., to form new memories. This is a reversible condition resulting from brain damage induced by a thiamine deficiency that is generally secondary to chronic alcoholism.

Wernicke's encephalopathy: Also due to an alcohol-induced thiamine deficiency. This is an irreversible disease in which the brain tissues break down, become inflamed, and bleed. Patients experience decreased muscle coordination, ophthalmoplegia, and confusion.

O   **A 35 year old woman with a history of flu-like symptoms (URI) one week ago presents with vertigo, nausea, and vomiting. No auditory impairment or focal deficits are noted. What is the likely diagnosis?**

Labyrinthitis or vestibular neuronitis.

O   **A 50 year old female with acute vertigo, nausea, and vomiting reports similar episodes over the last 20 years that are sometimes associated with hearing change, hearing loss, and tinnitus. She has permanent right > left sensorineural hearing loss. What is the diagnosis?**

Menière's disease.

O   **At what age is bacterial meningitis most common?**

Infants under 1 year old.

O   **What bacteria is the most common cause of meningitis in infants under 1 year old?**

Group B Streptococci and *E. coli*.

O   **What organism is frequently responsible for bacterial meningitis in adults?**

Neisseria meningitides.

❍   **How does bacterial meningitis differ from viral meningitis in terms of the corresponding CSF lab values?**

Bacterial meningitis is associated with low glucose and high protein levels, while viral meningitis will have normal glucose and normal protein levels.

❍   **On LP, opening pressure is markedly elevated. What should be done?**

Close the 3-way stopcock, remove only a small amount of fluid from the manometer, abort the LP, and initiate measures to decrease the intracranial pressure.

❍   **A patient presents with acute meningitis. When should antibiotics be initiated?**

Immediately. Do not wait for results of LP. Patients should receive a CT prior to LP only if papilledema or a focal deficit is present.

❍   **What is the most worrisome diagnosis of a purpuric, petechial rash in an infant?**

Meningococcemia.

❍   **Mononeuropathies are most commonly induced by what?**

Trauma that results in compression or entrapment of the involved nerve.

❍   **A 28 year old woman complains of a two-day history of weakness and tingling in her right arm and leg. She reports a previous episode of right eye pain and blurred vision that resolved over one month, but that occurred two years ago. She also recalls a two week episode of intermittent blurred vision the previous year. What is the diagnosis?**

Presumptive multiple sclerosis. Confirm with MRI and CSF (look for oligoclonal bands).

❍   **What is the most common presenting symptom of multiple sclerosis (MS)?**

Optic neuritis (about 25%).

❍   **A patient with MS presents with a fever. The nurse asks, "Should I give the patient Tylenol?" What is your response?**

Yes! Reducing a fever is important for MS patients. Existing signs and symptoms can worsen with small increases in temperature.

❍   **Which is the most common type of muscular dystrophy?**

Duchenne's muscular dystrophy.

❍   **A 32 year old female who complains of periods of weakness, especially when she chews her food, presents with ptosis, diplopia and dysarthria. Her muscles weaken with repetitive exercise. What test confirms the diagnosis of myasthenia gravis?**

Administration of exogenous anticholinesterase. Myasthenia gravis produces autoimmune antibodies against the acetylcholine receptors in the neuromuscular junction. Therefore, giving exogenous anticholinesterase will lead to an increase of acetylcholine and thereby relieve the symptoms.

○   **What neoplastic process is most commonly associated with myasthenia gravis?**

Thymoma.

○   **What is the most common medication associated with Neuroleptic Malignant Syndrome?**

Haloperidol. Other drugs, especially antipsychotic medications, are also causative.

○   **What is the hallmark motor finding in neuroleptic malignant syndrome?**

"Lead pipe" rigidity.

○   **A resting tremor is usually related to what disease?**

Parkinson's disease. Parkinson's tremors are generally asymmetrical and have the characteristic "pill rolling" appearance.

○   **What ECG finding makes phenytoin relatively contraindicated?**

Second or third degree heart block. If the patient is in status epilepticus, there may be no other choice. Phenytoin is relatively ineffective for seizures due to cyclic antidepressant overdose.

○   **Polio most frequently affects which age group?**

Polio is now extremely rare in the US, i.e., two cases per year. When it does infect, it afflicts the pediatric age group three months to 16 years.

○   **In the US, what animals are most likely to be infected with the rabies virus?**

Bats, skunks, and raccoons. Dogs are the usual carriers in developing countries.

○   **Can rabies be transmitted via a rat bite?**

No, rodents do not carry the virus. And no, bats are not rodents.

○   **Do individuals infected with the rabies virus really foam at the mouth?**

Yes, hypersalivation is one of the symptoms of furious rabies, along with hyperactivity, fear of water, hyperventilation, aerophobia, and autonomic instability. Patients with paralytic rabies develop either ascending paralysis or paralysis that affects one or more limbs individually. Rabies is 100% fatal once symptoms are exhibited.

○   **What is the classic EEG finding associated with petite mal seizures?**

A three second spike and wave pattern.

○   **What is Shy-Drager syndrome?**

A rare, gradually progressive nerve disorder characterized by very low blood pressure, lack of coordination, muscle wasting, stiffness, and lack of bladder and/or bowel control. This syndrome occurs most often in young people.

○   **What artery is most commonly involved in stroke?**

The middle cerebral artery.

❍   **Unilateral occlusion of the vertebrobasilar arterial distribution results in what kind of symptoms?**

Ipsilateral cranial nerve abnormalities and contralateral motor and sensory deficits.

❍   **A patient with aphasia most likely had a stroke involving which hemisphere?**

The dominant hemisphere. Patients who stroke in the nondominant hemisphere have apraxia and sensory neglect.

❍   **What is the most common cause of syncope?**

Vasovagal or simple fainting (50%).

❍   **What is tabes dorsalis?**

Progressive loss of all or part of the body's reflexes. The large joints of affected limbs are destroyed. Patients experience severe, stabbing pains in their legs, sensory deficits, and difficulty walking. Forty percent of patients with neurosyphilis are afflicted with tabes dorsalis.

❍   **A 9 month old child is having frequent convulsions and cannot control his muscles enough to hold up his head. You noted a developmental road block at the age of 6 months, and now it seems the child is regressing in both motor and cognitive skills. Upon examination, the patient has a cherry red macula. What is the patient's prognosis?**

This patient probably has Tay-Sachs disease. As the disease progresses the child will loose his sight, suffer dementia and become paralyzed. Death will occur before age 4.

❍   **What is the probable ethnic background of the patient described in the above case?**

Eastern European, Jewish, or French Canadian.

❍   **What body parts are most commonly affected in an essential tremor?**

Head and upper extremities. Essential tremors are sporadic and slowly progressive. These tremors are rare at rest but become worse when the limbs are used.

❍   **A 74 year old male presents with a unilateral burning headache that is worse around his temples and his eye. He also complains of visual disturbances and pain in his jaw after heavy use. Upon examination, you palpate a prominent temporal artery that is very tender. What tests should be run to make a diagnosis?**

Biopsy of the temporal artery. This patient most likely has temporal arteritis or giant cell arteritis. A sed rate of over 50 mm/hr suggests this diagnosis.

❍   **Why is the above case a medical emergency?**

Giant cell arteritis affects the large blood vessels. It usually involves the arteries branching off of the carotids. Therefore, involvement of the temporal artery may also indicate involvement of the central retinal artery. Twenty-five percent of patients with temporal arteritis have thromboses in the central retinal artery which leads to blindness. An immediate course of high dose prednisone should be started to decrease the inflammation in all patients.

❍   **A 67 year old woman complains of severe episodes of pain in her nose, cheek, and upper lip. She says it feels like a "lightning bolt hitting my face." What is the diagnosis?**

Tic douloureux or trigeminal neuralgia. This is a nerve condition of unknown etiology, possibly a microvascular compression causing a neuronal breakdown. It involves the trigeminal nerve and is most common in the V1 and V2 branches, although it may affect all three.

O   **How is the above patient treated?**

Perform an MRI to rule out a brainstem process, such as a tumor. Carbamazepine treats trigeminal neuralgia.

O   **For the following clinical presentations, identify which are associated with peripheral vertigo or with central vertigo.**

1) Intense spinning, nausea, hearing loss, diaphoresis
2) Swaying or impulsion, worse with movement, tinnitus, acute onset
3) Unidirectional nystagmus inhibited by ocular fixation, fatigable
4) Mild vertigo, diplopia, and ataxia
5) Multidirectional nystagmus not inhibited by ocular fixation, non-fatigable

Answers: peripheral vertigo: (1), (2), and (3); central vertigo: (4) and (5).

O   **A patient has an irritative lesion in the left hemisphere. What way do the eyes deviate?**

To the right.

O   **What motor deficit occurs with an anterior cerebral artery infarct?**

Leg weakness greater than arm weakness on the contralateral side.

O   **What two signs are displayed in a middle cerebral artery stroke?**

1) Contralateral sensory/motor deficits
2) Arm and face weakness greater than leg weakness

O   **What is the significance of bilateral nystagmus with cold caloric testing?**

It signifies that an intact cortex, midbrain, and brainstem are present.

O   **How are upper motor neuron (UMN) lesions of CN VII (facial nerve) distinguished from peripheral lesions?**

UMN: A unilateral weakness of the lower half of the face
Peripheral: Involves the entire half of the face, as seen in Bell's Palsy.

O   **What are the two main forms of neurofibromatosis?**

Type 1 (NF1), von Recklinghausen's disease or peripheral neurofibromatosis : consists of cafe-au-lait spots, neurofibromas, plexiform neuromas, iris hamartomas (Lisch nodules), optic gliomas, and osseous lesions. Type 1 Neurofibromatosis is caused by a mutation in the gene on chromosome 17, and accounts for 85% of all neurofibromatosis. Type 2 (NF2), central neurofibromatosis : involves tumors of cranial nerve VIII and the gene is linked to chromosome 18.

O   **Heterozygotes for homocystinuria can present with what problem in adulthood?**

Adults who are heterozygotes for homocystinuria can present with a history of stroke at a younger age than expected. Deficiency of cystathionine beta-synthetase is the most common cause of homocystinuria. Homozygotes present early in life with ectopia lentis, mental retardation and early strokes.

○   **What is the enzyme defect in Lesch-Nyhan disease?**

Hypoxanthine-guanine phosphoribosyltransferase (HGPRT).

○   **What are the two most common organisms that cause meningitis in patients with ventriculo-peritoneal (VP) shunts?**

Staphylococcus epidermidis and *Staphylococcus aureus*.

○   **Which vitamin should be given routinely during the treatment of tuberculous meningitis?**

B6. Isoniazid can induce a peripheral neuropathy, which can be prevented by the co-administration of vitamin B6 (pyridoxine).

○   **What is the most common cranial neuropathy seen in Borreliosis (Lyme disease)?**

Unilateral or bilateral facial palsy. Less frequently, the VIII cranial nerve can also be affected.

○   **Which is the cranial nerve most affected in pseudotumor cerebri?**

Cranial nerve IV can be involved with clinical signs of diplopia. Other findings include decreased visual acuity and restricted peripheral fields with enlargement of the blind spot.

○   **When should steroids be used in the treatment of increased intracranial pressure (ICP)?**

Steroids are beneficial in the treatment of vasogenic edema, so they should be used to treat increased ICP associated with tumors, abscesses and brain trauma.

○   **What cutaneous manifestation is seen in patients with Sturge-Weber disease?**

A Port wine stain, or angiomatous nevus, is seen in the distribution of cranial nerve V. This may be associated with pial angiomas. Seizures are the main clinical manifestation, but hemiparesis can also be seen.

○   **What are the clinical findings of Klein-Levin syndrome?**

This syndrome occurs in adolescent males and presents with episodes of hypersomnia, hyperphagia and frontal lobe type personality changes.

○   **A 63 year old previously healthy man awakens at 6 AM with weakness of the left arm and leg and difficulty walking. He arrives at the hospital at 7 AM and a CT scan is immediately performed, the results of which are normal. What dose of t-PA should he receive?**

None. It must be assumed that the stroke onset was the time the patient was last known to be normal, i.e., when he went to sleep. Thrombolysis is contraindicated beyond 3 hours, and controversial prior to that.

○   **What is the risk of symptomatic intracranial hemorrhage in patients who receive t-PA?**

Six percent. The risk of fatal intracranial hemorrhage is 3 percent.

○   **Carotid endarterectomy is indicated for symptomatic patients with what degree of stenosis?**

70% or greater.

○   **What is the single most important modifiable risk factor for stroke?**

Hypertension.

O   **When is maximum cerebrospinal fluid xanthochromia observed after subarachnoid hemorrhage?**

48 hours.

O   **Which of the following signs is not part of the classic Wallenberg syndrome: nystagmus, Horner's syndrome, contralateral hemiparesis, ipsilateral ataxia, contralateral loss of pain and temperature sense.**

Hemiparesis.

O   **What is the usual localization of the pure sensory stroke?**

Thalamus.

O   **Rank the following vascular malformations in order of risk of hemorrhage: arteriovenous malformation, capillary telangiectasia, cavernous malformation, and venous angioma.**

1) Arteriovenous malformation, 2) cavernous malformation, 3) capillary telangiectasia, 4) venous angioma.

O   **What stroke type is increased most in the postpartum period?**

Cerebral venous thrombosis.

O   **Bilateral cortical hemorrhagic infarcts associated with increased intracranial pressure are observed in what stroke syndrome?**

Superior sagittal sinus syndrome.

O   **What disorder presents with chemosis, proptosis, and an ocular bruit?**

Carotid cavernous fistula.

O   **What are the antiplatelet mechanisms of action of aspirin and ticlopidine?**

Aspirin interferes with platelet function by inhibiting the enzyme cyclooxygenase. Ticlodipine inhibits ADP-induced platelet aggregation.

O   **What potential adverse effect requires monitoring in patients treated with ticlopidine?**

Neutropenia.

O   **What is the CSF volume in a typical adult?**

150 ml.

O   **How is SIADH distinguished from cerebral salt wasting syndrome?**

In cerebral salt wasting syndrome, urinary sodium loss persists, despite fluid restriction, and there is a normal or reduced extracellular fluid volume.

O   **Rapid correction of chronic hyponatremia will cause which neurologic disorder?**

Central pontine myelinolysis may be caused by rapid correction of serum sodium level (> 0.5 mEq/L/hr).

O   **What are the clinical features of epidural abscess?**

Spinal tenderness, fever, radicular pain, myelopathy, elevated CSF protein and CSF pleocytosis.

O   **What is the treatment of an epidural abscess?**

Immediate laminectomy, drainage of the abscess, and antibiotic therapy. A delay may result in permanent disability.

O   **What are the causes of subdural empyema?**

Sinusitis, meningitis, head trauma, otitis, and osteomyelitis.

O   **What is the drug treatment for acute traumatic spinal cord injury?**

The treatment for acute (<8 hours) spinal cord injury is Methylprednisolone 30 mg/kg bolus followed by 5.4 mg/kg-hour for the next 23 hours.

O   **What are the complications that occur following subarachnoid hemorrhage?**

Vasospasm, recurrent hemorrhage, hydrocephalus, seizures, cardiac arrhythmias, hypertension, neurogenic pulmonary edema, stress ulcers and SIADH.

O   **What drug will reduce the risk of vasospasm following subarachnoid hemorrhage?**

Nimodipine.

O   **What are the causes of cerebral hemorrhage?**

Trauma, hypertension, ruptured aneurysms, cerebral amyloid angiopathy, vascular malformations, hemorrhage into a tumor (e.g. melanoma, choriocarcinoma, renal cell carcinoma), anticoagulant use, hemophilia, thrombocytopenia, stimulant drugs (amphetamines, cocaine, phenylpropanolamine) and vasculitis (e.g. Wegener's granulomatosis).

O   **What is the drug treatment for convulsive status epilepticus?**

Lorazepam (0.1 mg/kg) administered at 2 mg/minute, followed by intravenous fosphenytoin (18 mg of phenytoin equivalent/kg).

O   **What are the clinical features of spinal cord compression from metastatic cancer?**

Localized spinal tenderness, radicular pain, sensory level, paraparesis or quadriparesis, bowel and bladder incontinence, brisk deep tendon reflexes, upgoing plantar reflexes, and spasticity.

O   **What is the treatment for acute spinal cord compression from metastatic cancer?**

Usually high dose corticosteroids and radiation therapy. Surgical therapy is used instead of radiation therapy if the primary cancer type is unknown, the tumor is radioresistant, spinal instability makes surgery necessary or the patient has received the maximum radiation dose.

O   **What is myasthenic crisis?**

A myasthenia gravis patient with significant impairment in respiratory function. Myasthenic crisis may require emergency intubation and assisted ventilation.

○ **What is the treatment for neuroleptic malignant syndrome?**

Rapid cooling methods. Immediate withdrawal of the neuroleptic drug. Sinemet, bromocriptine or dantrolene may be used as needed.

○ **What are the features of botulism infection?**

A history of recent ingestion of home canned or prepared foods, followed by sudden onset of diplopia, dysphagia, muscle weakness, dry mouth, fixed dilated pupils and respiratory paralysis. Treatment is with botulism antitoxin.

○ **What are the earliest clinical features of uncal herniation?**

Uncal herniation begins with a unilateral enlarged pupil and a sluggish pupillary light reaction.

○ **How is a subarachnoid hemorrhage diagnosed?**

CT scan may show blood in the suprasellar cistern, interhemispheric fissure, sylvian fissure, or surface of the brain. If the CT scan is normal, a spinal tap may show xanthochromia, or blood.

○ **What is the Cushing reflex?**

The elevation in blood pressure and reduction in pulse that follows a increase in intracranial pressure. It is a brainstem mediated reflex.

○ **What is the treatment for cerebral metastatic brain tumors?**

High dose corticosteroids to reduce the mass effect from cerebral edema, and usually radiation therapy. Surgery replaces radiation if a biopsy for the diagnosis of a metastatic lesion is needed, or if a single metastatic lesion is present.

○ **Are there any psychiatric symptoms seen in MS?**

In about 50% of cases, depression, irritability, low mood, anxiety, and poor concentration occur. Less common is confusion and psychosis.

○ **Does multiple sclerosis affect cognition?**

Yes, in 50% of cases manifesting mostly as deficits in short term memory, attention and speed of processing with frank dementia in only < 5%.

○ **What is a Marcus-Gunn pupil?**

An afferent papillary defect (APD). Shining a light into the affected eye causes sluggish constriction. Swinging the light from the normal eye to the affected one dilates both pupils because the brain perceives less light via the abnormal eye.

○ **What percent of MS patients will never experience a relapse?**

15%.

○ **What is the pathology of MS?**

Demyelination of CNS (white matter) with relative axonal preservation, although there is evidence of a moderate degree of axonal loss as well as some plaques encroaching upon the cortex with sparing of neuronal cell bodies and axis cylinders.

○   **What are good prognostic indicators for MS?**

Female sex, younger age at onset, relapsing-remitting form, less rate of relapses early in the course, long first inter-attack interval, and, if an initial symptom is sensory or cranial nerve dysfunction.

○   **What other conditions can produce MRI findings similar to MS?**

Ischemia, SLE, Behcet's disease, other vasculitides, HTLV-1 and sarcoidosis.

○   **What is the preferred therapy for acute MS?**

High dose IV methylprednisolone (6-15 mg/kg) for 3-5 days with or without a taper of oral prednisone, will induce objective improvement in >85% of cases.

○   **What are the symptomatic therapies commonly used in MS?**

Fatigue: Amantadine, Pemoline, and Fluoxetine.
Pain: Tegretol, Misoprostol (Prostaglandin E analog), TCA, Dilantin, Baclofen, and Depakote
Spasticity: Baclofen, Benzodiazepines, and Dantrolene.
Intention tremor: Clonazepam, Inderal, and Artane.

○   **What are some predisposing factors to Guillain-Barre Syndrome (GBS)?**

Viral infection, gastrointestinal infection, immunization or surgery often precede the neurological symptoms by 5 days to 3 weeks.

○   **Does early treatment with IVIG or plasmapheresis accelerate recovery in GBS?**

Yes. It also diminishes the incidence of long term neurologic disability.

○   **How would you differentiate acute anterior poliomyelitis from GBS?**

The former shows asymmetry of paralysis, signs of meningeal irritation, fever and CSF pleocytosis.

○   **What are the other differential diagnoses of GBS?**

1- porphyria
2- AIDS
3- hypophosphatemia
4- toxic neuropathies (hexane, thallium, arsenic)
5- botulism

○   **What types of memory are impaired earliest in Alzheimer's disease?**

Episodic, explicit, declarative, and short term memory.

○   **What is the difference between dysarthria and aphasia?**

Dysarthria is a disorder of speech, a motor function. Aphasia is a disorder of language, a higher cortical function.

○   **What are the typical features of transient global amnesia?**

Abrupt onset of amnesia that spares personal identity, resolves within 24 hours, has no other neurologic deficits, and occurs typically between ages 50 and 70.

○   **What is the characteristic triad of normal pressure hydrocephalus?**

Dementia, incontinence, and a gait ataxia (often described as a "magnetic" gait due to difficulty picking up the feet).

○   **The post concussive syndrome includes what symptoms?**

Headaches, dizziness, impaired memory and concentration, irritability, and depression.

○   **What is the Wernicke-Korsakoff syndrome?**

Chronic, severe impairment in anterograde memory (Korsakoff's syndrome) with acute confusion, ataxia, ophthalmoplegia, and nystagmus (Wernicke's encephalopathy). This syndrome results from lesions of the dorsomedial nuclei of the thalamus and mamillary bodies.

○   **How should Wernicke's encephalopathy be treated?**

Immediate intravenous thiamine replacement.

○   **What are the major risk factors for Alzheimer's disease?**

Age, Down's syndrome (Trisomy 21), and family history.

○   **How do donepezil (Aricept) and tacrine (Cognex) treat Alzheimer's disease?**

Both are acetylcholinesterase inhibitors and help compensate for the cholinergic deficits in Alzheimer's disease.

○   **What is Tourette's syndrome?**

A tic disorder with motor and vocal tics developing before age 18. Vocal tics may be unformed or formed (words). Coprolalia (cursing) and echolalia may occur. Tourette's syndrome may be accompanied by Attention Deficit Disorder and Obsessive Compulsive Disorder.

○   **What are symptoms of Attention Deficit Disorder?**

Impulsivity, distractibility, and often hyperactivity.

○   **What are some disorders of myelination in the CNS?**

Multiple sclerosis is an autoimmune disorder of central myelin.
Pelizaeus-Merzbacher is a hereditary CNS demyelinating disorder caused by a mutation in myelin proteolipid protein. Metabolic demyelinating diseases include metachromatic leukodystrophy (deficiency of arylsulfatase A), adrenoleukodystrophy (faulty metabolism of very long chain fatty acids) and Krabbe's globoid cell leukodystrophy. Central pontine myelinolysis, a catastrophic disruption of corticospinal pathways in the brainstem resulting in a "locked-in" syndrome, occurs with overrapid correction of hypo- or hypernatremia. Progressive multifocal leukoencephalopathy (PML) is a viral patchy white matter encephalopathy (due to JC virus, but associated with HIV infection).

○   **What are some disorders of peripheral nervous system myelin.**

Guillain-Barre Syndrome (GBS, a.k.a. acute inflammatory demyelinating polyradiculoneuropathy, AIDP) is an autoimmune attack on peripheral myelin, often after a viral or bacterial illness, resulting in sudden rapidly progressive weakness and areflexia. EMG shows slowing of nerve conduction and conduction block. Prognosis is worse if *Campylobacter jejuni* is involved. Treatment options include plasma exchanges or intravenous IgG. CIDP (chronic immune demyelinating polyradiculoneuropathy) is a chronic or relapsing form of GBS. CIDP responds to steroids; GBS doesn't. Charcot-Marie-Tooth is an autosomal recessive (usually) or X-linked (rarely) distal peripheral neuropathy; mutations in myelin membrane binding proteins (Po) or connexin gap junction proteins result in progressive demyelination, distal weakness and atrophy with foot drop and a "stork-like" gait. There is also an axonal form (HSMN2).

○   **What is the main excitatory neurotransmitter in brain?**

Glutamate.

○   **What is the main inhibitory neurotransmitter in the brain?**

Gamma-aminobutyric acid

○   **What drugs act at GABA receptors?**

Benzodiazepines (e.g. diazepam), barbiturates (phenobarbital), neurosteroids, and the novel anticonvulsant loreclezole enhance GABA receptors. They are inhibited by convulsants including bicuculline, picrotoxin, penicillin, and Zn^{++}.

○   **What are the major monoamine neurotransmitters in the CNS?**

Acetylcholine, epinephrine, norepinephrine, serotonin, dopamine, and histamine.

○   **What drugs act at CNS muscarinic acetylcholine receptors?**

Antimuscarinic agents (atropine, scopolamine, etc.) and antimuscarinic side effects of other agents (e.g. tricyclic antidepressants) result in initial CNS excitation, irritability, hallucinations or delirium, progressing to coma and respiratory paralysis. Clinical uses include decreasing secretions or GI motility, paralyzing the iris, reversing bradycardia or bronchospasm, preventing motion sickness, and inducing sleep. Anticholinergics are sometimes helpful in treating early Parkinson's disease, especially for tremor, but can cause confusion, dry mouth, and urinary retention.
Anticholinesterases (physostigmine, neostigmine) are used to treat hypotonic bladder, glaucoma, and myasthenia gravis (see above). Tacrine (Cognex) and donepezil (Aricept) cause modest symptomatic improvement of Alzheimer's disease.
Organophosphate insecticides irreversibly inhibit AChE resulting in sweating, salivation, lacrimation, urination, defecation (SLUD), bradycardia, hypotension and death.

○   **What is the role of acetylcholine in CNS disease?**

Loss of cholinergic neurons may be responsible for some of the symptoms of Alzheimer's Disease, and has led to use of AChE inhibitors in treatment (see above). A mutation in the membrane spanning region of the a4 subunit of the nicotinic AChR is likely responsible for autosomal dominant frontal lobe epilepsy; the disease mechanism is unknown.

○   **What pathologies are associated with dopamine?**

Parkinson's disease (PD) results from loss of SNc dopaminergic neurons. Schizophrenia is undoubtedly related to dopamine receptor function, but the etiology remains elusive. Long-term treatment with neuroleptics can result in dopamine receptor upregulation and tardive dyskinesia/dystonia.

○   **What drugs act at CNS dopamine receptors?**

Sinemet is a preparation of L-DOPA and carbidopa, which prevents peripheral metabolism of L-DOPA and reduces side effects (nausea). Bromocriptine is a direct dopamine agonist, used occasionally in PD, for suppression of pituitary prolactinomas, and formerly used to stop lactation (parlodel), but is now restricted due to incidence of hypertension, seizure and stroke. Antidopaminergics (neuroleptics) are used to treat psychosis/schizophrenia and other problems. Clozapine is an antipsychotic D4 receptor antagonist that does not exacerbate Parkinson's disease. Deprenyl, an MAO-type B inhibitor, provides minimal symptomatic benefit in early PD; latest analyses of the DATATOP study data no longer support a protective effect on SNc neurons.

❍   **What drugs act as adrenergic receptors?**

Alpha-2 agonist agents (clonidine) suppress sympathetic outflow in hypertension. Beta-1 receptors are found in the cerebral cortex and beta-2 in the cerebellum. Isoproterenol is a relatively pure beta-agonist. Deprenyl and pargyline are antidepressants that inhibit catabolism of epinephrine and NE by blocking MAO. Desipramine and other tricyclic antidepressants (TCA's) block NE reuptake. Amphetamine blocks reuptake and facilitates increased release of NE. Beta-blockers (propranolol, nadolol, atenolol, etc.) are used in hypertension, to prevent arrhythmias, and in migraine prophylaxis.

❍   **What are the major peptide neurotransmitters in the CNS?**

Opioid peptides, substances P and Y, and "gut peptides" including somatostatin, colecystokinin, neurotensin, VIP, calcitonin gene-related peptide, corticotropin releasing factor, etc., are present in neurons, and may act as neurotransmitters or neuromodulators. Substance P is one of several tachykinin peptides, which is present in dorsal root ganglion neurons that project to the substantia gelatinosa of dorsal spinal cord (pain modulation), also in projection neurons from striatum back to substantia nigra.

❍   **Below what value of cerebral perfusion pressure (CPP) is autoregulation of cerebral blood flow impaired?**

40 - 50 mm Hg: CPP = MAP - ICP, where MAP is mean arterial pressure and ICP is intracranial pressure.

❍   **What is the recommended duration of antibiotic therapy for brain abscess?**

Six to eight weeks of intravenous antibiotics.

❍   **What are common electrocardiographic changes seen with brain injuries?**

Sinus tachycardia, QT-interval prolongation, and pan precordial T-wave inversion. More severe findings include QRS widening and ventricular tachycardia.

❍   **Are fixed and dilated pupils only found with structural dysfunction?**

No. Metabolic dysfunction (e.g., hepatic encephalopathy) or toxins (e.g., atropine) can give enlarged unreactive pupils.

❍   **What are "pontine pupils"?**

"Pinpoint", but reactive, pupils secondary to injury of the sympathetic fibers descending through the tegmentum. It results from intrinsic pontine tegmental injury or from cerebellar or other posterior fossa mass effect causing compression of the tegmentum: Narcotic administration causes similar pupillary findings.

❍   **What is meant by the term "communicating" (or 'non-obstructive") hydrocephalus?**

All of the ventricles are dilated, including the cerebral aqueduct and basal cisterns. Obstructive hydrocephalus is either secondary to aqueductal stenosis or CSF outflow blocked by a mass.

❍   **Lesions containing what substances are of high attenuation on unenhanced CT scan?**

Blood, calcium, or melanin. High attenuation with blood results from the protein fraction of hemoglobin (92 - 93%), rather than the iron, which only contributes 7 - 8% to the brightness.

❍   **What diagnosis must be investigated in the patient presenting with pulsating exophthalmos?**

Carotid cavernous fistula. Patients without a history of trauma, usually women, over forty years of age, often present with orbito-fronto-temporal headache, dilated conjunctival veins, and may have a sixth nerve palsy.

❍   **What is the most common symptom of a glioblastoma multiforme?**

Headache, in 3/4 of patients.

❍   **Carotid bifurcation aneurysms may cause intracerebral hemorrhage into what areas of the brain?**

Frontal lobe, temporal lobe, and basal ganglia.

❍   **What is the risk of cerebral infarction in the first 5 years following posterior circulation transient ischemic attacks?**

35%.

❍   **What is the most common tumor of the sellar and parasellar region?**

Pituitary adenoma.

❍   **What is the most common endocrine disorder associated with suprasellar extension of pineal tumors?**

Diabetes insipidus.

❍   **What are the most common initial symptoms of an acoustic neuroma?**

Tinnitus, hearing loss, and unsteadiness.

❍   **What symptoms, related to lumbar disc herniation, are indications for emergency surgery?**

Urinary retention, perineal numbness, and motor weakness of more than a single nerve root. These are findings suggestive of cauda equina compression.

❍   **What are the most common clinical problems seen at the initial presentation of an intracranial arteriovenous malformation?**

Seizures and hemorrhage.

O   **A 62 year old patient presents with right shoulder pain. What is the diagnosis?**

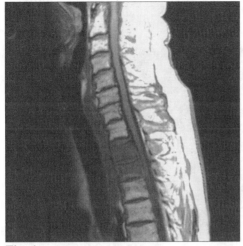

Fig. A

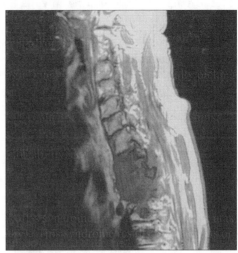

Fig. B

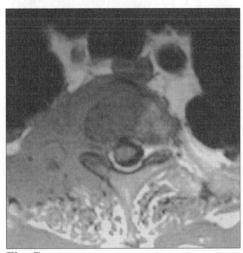

Fig. C

Sagittal (Fig. A and B) and axial T1 (Fig. C) noncontrast sections through the upper thoracic spine demonstrate a mass lesion involving both vertebral bodies and the nearby lung pleura with some extension into the epidural space on the right. This patient was subsequently shown to have a Pancoast tumor at biopsy.

○   **A 36 year old presents with altered mental status and history of a fall with severe headache. What is the diagnosis after viewing only the CT? (Fig. A)**

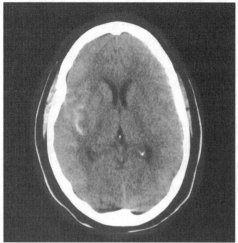

Fig. A

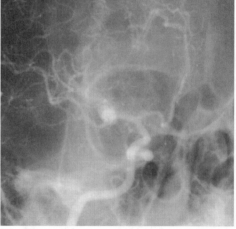

Fig. B

Acute right sided subarachnoid hemorrhage confined mostly to the sylvian fissure. The differential diagnosis is between trauma and ruptured intracerebral aneurysm. In this patient, a large right middle cerebral artery trifurcation aneurysm is confirmed by contrast angiography. (Fig. B)

○   **This is a 68 year old with new onset right homonomous hemianopsia. Based on the images shown, what is the diagnosis? (Fig. A)**

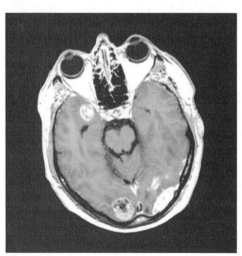

Fig. A

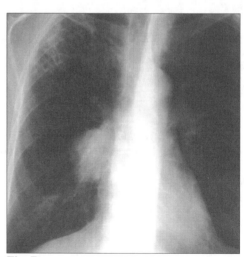

Fig. B

Multiple inhomogeneously enhancing lesions are present throughout the brain, several of which are shown here. The left occipital lesion would explain the patient's visual symptoms. The chest x-ray demonstrates a large mass in the right hilum (Fig. B) in this patient with lung carcinoma and multiple brain metastases.

○   **A 69 year old presents with confusion of new onset. What is the diagnosis?**

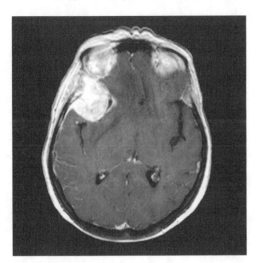

A large dural based enhancing mass with a dural tail arises near the greater wing of the sphenoid at the junction of the right frontal and temporal lobes. The mass has characteristics of an extra-axial lesion and is consistent with a meningioma. Note that the finding of a small dural tail of enhancement along the edge of the mass is quite characteristic of meningioma along with its broad-based dural attachment.

CLINICAL PHARMACOLOGY AND TOXICOLOGY

○ **What is the clinical presentation of anticholinergic poisoning?**

Mydriasis, tachycardia, hypoactive bowel sounds, urinary retention, dry axilla, hyperthermia, and mental status changes. Remember:

Dry as a bone,
Red as a beet,
Mad as a hatter,
Hot as hades,
Blind as a bat.

○ **Name 7 primary actions of cyclic antidepressant overdose.**

1) Inhibition of amine reuptake
2) Sodium channel blockade, which causes negative inotropy
3) Anticholinergic effects, primarily antimuscarinic
4) CNS depression
5) α-Adrenergic antagonism, which contributes further to hypotension
6) GABA antagonism
7) Q-T prolongation

○ **What is the appropriate treatment for TCA induced seizures?**

Benzodiazepines (clorazepam or diazepam) and barbiturates (phenobarbital) are the agents of choice. Phenytoin is not generally effective but may be tried for recurrent seizures or those unresponsive to treatment. Bicarbonate and alkalosis are the main stays of treatment..

○ **What is the treatment for TCA induced hypotension?**

Isotonic saline and pepid alkalinization. If the patient is resistant to fluid resuscitation, a directly acting α-agonist, such as norepinephrine, should be started. Dopamine acts in part by releasing norepinephrine. This agent may already be depleted by the reuptake inhibition of the cyclic antidepressant and by stress.

○ **What period of observation is required prior to medically clearing a TCA overdose?**

6 hours.

○ **A 32 year old female is prescribed meperidine (Demerol) for an open fracture. The patient is chronically on fluoxetine (Prozac). What is a potential complication?**

The serotonin syndrome.

○ **What signs and symptoms are typical of the serotonin syndrome?**

Agitation, anxiety, altered mental status, ataxia, diaphoresis, incoordination, sinus tachycardia, hyperthermia, shivering, tremor, hyperreflexia, myoclonus, muscular rigidity, and diarrhea.

○   **What are potential pharmacological treatments for the serotonin syndrome?**

Serotonin antagonists, such as methysergide and cyproheptadine. Benzodiazepines and propranolol have also been successfully employed.

○   **What are the major pharmacological effects of neuroleptics?**

Blockade of dopamine, α-adrenergic, muscarinic, and histamine receptors.

○   **What findings occur with neuroleptic malignant syndrome?**

Altered mental status, muscular rigidity, autonomic instability, hyperthermia, and rhabdomyolysis.

○   **What level of lithium is generally considered toxic?**

2.0 mEq/L.

○   **Will charcoal bind lithium?**

No.

○   **What are the signs and symptoms of lithium toxicity?**

Neurological signs and symptoms include tremor, hyperreflexia, clonus, fasciculations, seizures, coma. GI signs and symptoms consist of nausea, vomiting, and diarrhea. Cardiovascular effects include ST-T wave changes, bradycardia, conduction defects, and arrhythmias.

○   **What is the treatment for lithium toxicity?**

Supportive care, normal saline diuresis, hemodialysis for patients with clinical signs of severe poisoning, i.e., seizures and arrhythmias, renal failure, or decreasing urine output.

○   **What is the pharmacological effect of barbiturates and benzodiazepines?**

Both enhance chloride influx through the GABA receptor associated chloride channel. Benzodiazepines increase the frequency of channel opening, whereas barbiturates increase the duration of channel opening.

○   **What is a "Mickey Finn"?**

A mixture of alcohol and chloral hydrate.

○   **At what rate is alcohol metabolized in an acutely intoxicated person?**

About 20 mg/dL/hour.

○   **What is the pharmacological treatment for alcohol withdrawal?**

Benzodiazepines or barbiturates.

○   **Isopropanol is metabolized by what enzyme to what metabolite?**

Isopropanol is metabolized by alcohol dehydrogenase to acetone in the liver.

○   **What is a normal osmolar gap?**

< 10 mOsm.

○ **What cofactor is required to convert formic acid to carbon dioxide and water?**

Folate. Leucovorin, folinic acid, the active form of folate, is preferentially administered at 1 mg/kg. Folate may be substituted at the same dose if leucovorin is not available.

○ **Is NaHCO₃ beneficial in the management of methanol poisoning?**

Yes. In animal models, maintenance of a normal pH through bicarbonate administration decreased toxicity, including visual impairment.

○ **What methanol level mandates dialysis?**

50 mg/dL. Other indications include visual impairment, severe metabolic acidosis, and ingestion of greater than 30 cc.

○ **What cofactors are administered to a patient with ethylene glycol poisoning?**

Thiamine and pyridoxine. These cofactors will aid in transforming glyoxylic acid to nontoxic metabolites. Both are administered intravenously in 100 mg increments.

○ **Name the three clinical phases of ethylene glycol poisoning?**

Stage I: Neurological symptomatology (i.e., inebriation)
Stage II: Metabolic acidosis and cardiovascular instability
Stage III: Renal failure

○ **When should dialysis be initiated for an ethylene glycol poisoning case?**

When the serum level is > 25 mg/dL, or when renal insufficiency or severe metabolic acidosis occurs.

○ **What is the toxic dose of naloxone?**

None. Narcan is a safe drug and may be given in large quantities. The usual adult dosage is 2 mg IV; the usual pediatric dose is 0.01 mg/kg. Narcan may precipitate acute withdrawal and may therefore be titrated to effect.

○ **How does treatment for a cocaine induced MI differ from a typical MI?**

Both are treated the same except that ß-blockers are **not** used for a cocaine-induced MI secondary to potential unopposed α-adrenergic activity. The tachycardia of a cocaine associated MI is first treated with benzodiazepine sedation.

○ **What syndrome is associated with Jimson Weed?**

Anticholinergic poisoning.

○ **What is the mechanism of salicylate toxicity?**

Salicylates uncouple oxidative phosphorylation and thereby halt cellular ATP production.

○ **Which acid-base disturbance is typical for salicylate poisoning?**

Mixed respiratory alkalosis, secondary to central respiratory center stimulation, and metabolic acidosis, secondary to uncoupling of oxidative phosphorylation.

O   **What order are the kinetics of elimination for an ASA overdose?**

Zero order elimination with hepatic enzymatic clearance saturated and renal clearance becoming important.

O   **What is the "magic number" for the dose of a nonenteric coated ASA that must be exceeded to cause toxicity (mg/kg)?**

150 mg/kg.

O   **What is the "magic number" for the dose of an enteric coated ASA that must be exceeded to require admission for observation and for the determination of serial salicylate levels?**

150 mg/kg.

O   **Is hemodialysis used to treat salicylate toxicity?**

Yes. For severely poisoned patients, i.e., coma, ARDS, cardiac toxicity, serum levels > 100 mg/dL, and for patients who are unresponsive to maximal therapy.

O   **Can a patient present with salicylate poisoning and a therapeutic level?**

Yes. Patients with chronic salicylate poisoning have a large Vd (volume of distribution) and thus may present with mental status changes and a therapeutic level.

O   **What are the 4 stages of acetaminophen (APAP) poisoning?**

Stage I: 30 minutes to 24 hours, nausea and vomiting
Stage II: 24 to 48 hours, abdominal pain and elevated LFTs
Stage III: 72 to 96 hours, LFTs peak, nausea and vomiting
Stage IV: 4 days to 2 weeks, resolution or fulminant hepatic failure

O   **APAP poisoning produces which type of hepatic necrosis?**

Centrilobular necrosis. The toxic metabolite of APAP is generated in the liver via the P-450 system, which is located in the centrilobular region.

O   **How is APAP usually metabolized in non-overdose conditions?**

Most APAP is metabolized is by glucuronidation. However, some APAP metabolism occurs in conjugation with sulfate. This percentage increases with decreasing age. Four percent or less APAP is transformed into an extremely toxic intermediary compound by P-450 MFOs. It is theorized that this toxic intermediary immediately conjugates with glutathione and is harmlessly excreted in the urine.

O   **How does N-acetylcysteine (NAC, Mucomyst) work?**

The precise mechanism is still not well understood. However, it is known that NAC enters cells and is metabolized to cysteine, which serves as a glutathione precursor.

O   **Which measure of hepatic function is a better prognostic indicator in APAP overdose :liver enzyme levels or bilirubin level and prothrombin time?**

Bilirubin level and prothrombin time.

○   **An acutely intoxicated, nonalcoholic, otherwise healthy patient ingests APAP. Is this patient more or less likely to develop hepatotoxicity?**

Less likely. An acute ingestion of alcohol will tie up the P-450 system thereby inhibiting the formation of NAPQI. A chronic alcoholic has an induced P-450 system and will suffer greater APAP hepatic toxicity through increased NAPQI formation.

○   **What is the minimum dose of APAP that can cause hepatotoxicity in the child? In the adult?**

Child: 140 mg/kg. Adult: 140mg/kg (or about 7.5 g).

○   **According to the Rumack-Matthew nomogram, at what four hour APAP level should treatment be initiated?**

150 mg/mL.

○   **What is the proposed mechanism of theophylline induced seizures?**

Adenosine antagonism. Adenosine is released into the synaptic cleft from presynaptic terminals along with excitatory neurotransmitters. Adenosine binds to presynaptic adenosine receptors, inhibiting the release of more excitatory neurotransmitters or additionally increasing concentrations of cAMP or inhibition of phosphodiasterase PDE III,PDE IV.

○   **What is the appropriate initial treatment of theophylline induced seizures?**

Benzodiazepines and barbiturates. Theophylline induced seizures warrant hemodialysis or charcoal hemoperfusion.

○   **What is the treatment of theophylline induced hypotension?**

Fluid administration and ß-blockers. Theophylline induced cardiovascular instability is secondary to ß-agonist effects. Therefore, ß-blockers can be beneficial in the treatment of arrhythmias and hypotension.

○   **What are absolute indications for hemodialysis or hemoperfusion in theophylline toxicity?**

Seizures or arrhythmias that are unresponsive to conventional therapy, a theophylline level >100ug/mg in an acute overdose or 50 ug/MG in a chronic overdose

○   **What abnormal laboratory parameters are typical in a patient with acute theophylline poisoning?**

Hypokalemia, hyperglycemia, and leukocytosis. The ß-agonist properties of theophylline produce these abnormalities.

○   **What are the absolute indications for Digibind administration in digoxin poisoning?**

Ventricular arrhythmias, hemodynamically significant bradyarrhythmias that are unresponsive to standard therapy, and a potassium level greater than 5.0 mEq/L.

○   **Why is calcium chloride administration contraindicated in digoxin poisoning?**

Digoxin inhibit the Na+/K+/Na/K+ATPase. This mechanism increases the intracellular concentration of sodium. The sodium calcium exchange pump is then activated, which leads to high intracellular concentrations of calcium. Calcium chloride administration would further increase intracellular calcium, which would cause myocardial irritability.

O   **A patient on Digoxin is bradycardic and hypotensive with significantly peaked T waves. What is the initial line of treatment?**

Administer 10 vials of Digibind intravenously while simultaneously treating the presumed hyperkalemia with insulin and glucose, sodium bicarbonate, and Kayexalate. After the Digibind is administered, hyperkalemic induced arrhythmias may safely be treated with calcium chloride.

O   **What is the antidote for ß-blocker poisoning?**

Glucagon. Glucagon receptors, located on myocardial cells, are G protein coupled receptors that activate adenylate cyclase, leading to increased levels of intracellular cAMP. Thus, glucagon administration causes the same intracellular effect as ß-agonist.

O   **What are potential treatment modalities for a calcium channel blocker poisoning?**

Therapeutic interventions include IV calcium, isoproterenol, glucagon, transvenous pacer, atropine, and vasopressors, such as norepinephrine, epinephrine, or dopamine.

O   **What is the mechanism and treatment for clonidine induced hypotension?**

Treatment: Includes IV fluid administration and dopamine.
Mechanism: Decreased cardiac output secondary to a decreased sympathetic outflow from the CNS.

O   **What typical eye response is related to clonidine poisoning?**

Pinpoint pupils.

O   **At what adrenergic receptor is clonidine active?**

Clonidine is an α-2 agonist.

O   **What is the pharmacological basis of the anticonvulsant effect of phenytoin?**

Sodium channel blockade. Phenotoin causes an increasing efflux or a decreasing influx of sodium ions across cell membranes in the motor cortex durring generation of a nerve impulse

O   **Why does IV phenytoin administration lead to cardiovascular toxicity?**

The propylene glycol diluent is a myocardial depressant and vasodilator.

O   **What are the four stages of iron poisoning?**

Stage I: 0-6 hours : Abdominal pain, nausea, vomiting, and diarrhea secondary to the corrosive effects of iron. In more severe cases hematemasis, hypotension and altered mental status.

Stage II: 6 to 24 hours : quiescent period during which iron is absorbed (in severe poisoning a latent period may be absent).

Stage III: 12-24 hours : GI hemmorhage, shock, metabolic acidosis, heart failure, CV collapse, coma, seizures, coagulopathy, hepatic and renal failure

Stage IV: 4-6 weeks postingestion: gastric outlet or small bowel obstruction secondary to scarring

O   **What dose of iron is expected to produce clinical toxicity?**

20 mg/kg of <u>elemental</u> iron. For example, a toddler ingests 10 tablets of 324 mg ferrous sulfate, i.e., 20% <u>elemental</u> iron; this equals 648 mg of elemental iron. The dose would be toxic to a 20 kg child at 32.4 mg/kg.

○   **What 4 hour iron level is generally considered toxic?**

300 to 350 ug/dL.

○   **What are indications for deferoxamine therapy?**

1. All symptomatic patients exhibiting more than merely transient symptomatology
2. Patients with lethargy, significant abdominal pain, hypotension, mental status changes, hypovolemia or metabolic acidosis
3. Patients with a positive KUB
4. Any symptomatic patient with a level greater than 300 mg/dL

○   **What oral chelator reduces iron absorption in animal model studies?**

Magnesium hydroxide or milk of magnesia.

○   **What historical disclosure warrants an evaluation after a hydrocarbon ingestion?**

Coughing. Any patient who coughs after ingesting a hydrocarbon has the potential for developing chemical pneumonitis.

○   **At what point can a patient who has ingested a hydrocarbon be safely discharged?**

After six hours asymptomatic patients, with a normal chest x-ray and pulse oxygen, may be discharged to home.

○   **Chronic solvent abusers develop what metabolic complication?**

Renal tubular acidosis.

○   **A 2 year old child is asymptomatic after ingestion of a button battery. A KUB reveals the foreign body in his stomach. What is the disposition for this patient?**

Discharge to home. If the battery is lodged in the esophagus, an endoscopy must be performed immediately. Otherwise, reassure the patient's parents and instruct them to check their son's stools.

○   **What is the potent ingredient in Sarin?**

An organophosphate

○   **What enzyme is inhibited by organophosphates?**

Acetylcholinesterase.

○   **How do organophosphates enter the body?**

They can be inhaled, ingested or absorbed through the skin.

○   **What are the signs and symptoms of organophosphate poisoning?**

1 – 2 hours after poisoning patients may have GI upset, bronchospasm, miosis, bradycardia, excessive salivation and sweating, tremor, respiratory muscle paralysis, muscle fasciculations, agitation, seizures, coma and death. Remember SLUDGE (salivation, lacrimation, urinary incontinence, diarrhea, gastric upset and emesis).

○   **What antihypertensive agent may induce cyanide poisoning?**

Nitroprusside. One molecule of sodium nitroprusside contains five molecules of cyanide. To prevent toxicity with long duration infusions, sodium thiosulfate should be infused with sodium nitroprusside at a ratio of 10:1, thiosulfate to nitroprusside. Beware of thiocyanate toxicity!

○   **What is the antidote for isoniazid induced seizures?**

Pyridoxine.

○   **What regions of the liver lobules contain the greatest amount of P-450 related mixedfunction oxidases (P-450 MFOs)?**

The centrilobular regions, accounting for primarily centrilobular necrosis.

○   **Clonidine is a centrally acting presynaptic α-2 adrenergic agonist that decreases the central sympathetic outflow.   Although its primary use is to treat hypertension, clonidine has additional emergency value in blunting withdrawal symptoms from opiates and ethanol. A clonidine overdose closely resembles an overdose with which other class of drugs?**

Opiates.

○   **Toxicity from clonidine (Catapres) usually occurs within what time period?**

Within 4 hours.

○   **Which agent is a useful "antidote" for clonidine overdose?**

Naloxone (Narcan)

○   **Name a few substances that have anticholinergic properties.**

Antihistamines, cyclic antidepressants, phenothiazine, atropine, and, Jimson weed.

○   **What ECG abnormality is most common in patients who suffer from anticholinergic toxicity?**

Sinus tachycardia. Other dangerous arrhythmias include conduction problems and V-Tach.

○   **What is cornpicker's pupil?**

Mydriasis from contact of the eye with Jimson weed. Jimson weed contains atropine, scopolamine, and hyoscyamine. It is a common plant and is available through health food stores.

○   **ß-adrenergic antagonists have three main effects on the heart. Name these effects.**

1) Negative chronotropy
2) Negative inotropy
3) Decrease AV nodal conduction velocity (negative dromotropy)

○   **T/F: ß-adrenergic antagonists can cause mental status changes and seizures.**

True.

○   **What is the treatment for an opiate overdose?**

Naloxone, 0.4 to 2.0 mg in an adult and 0.01 mg/kg in a child. Naloxone's duration of action is about 1 hour. Higher doses and continuous infusion may be required.

○   **Which types of nystagmus are expected with a PCP overdose?**
Vertical, horizontal, and rotary. Vertical nystagmus is not common with other conditions/ingestions. The most common findings of a PCP overdose are hypertension, tachycardia, and nystagmus.

○   **How can the pesticide PCP enter the body?**

Through inhalation, skin and ingestion

○   **What is the clinical presentation of PCP intoxication?**

Irritation of skin, eyes and upper respiratory tract, headache, vomiting, weakness, sweating, hyperthermia, tachycardia, tachypnea, convulsions, coma, pulmonary edema, cardiovascular collapse and death.

○   **What is the most common cause of chronic heavy metal poisoning?**

Lead.

○   **Organophosphates are found in what kinds of compounds?**

Pesticides, flame retardants and plasticizers.

○   **What is the most common arrhythmia induced by chronic, heavy ethanol bingeing ?**

Atrial fibrillation.

○   **In a non-drinker what blood ethanol level will cause confusion or stupor?**

180mg/dl to 300mg/dl. The minimum blood alchohol level that can cause coma in a nondrinker is 300mg/dl.

○   **In chronic alcohol users, alcohol withdrawal seizures occur approximately how many hours after cessation of heavy alcohol consumption?**

6-48 hours from the time of the last drink.

○   **Delirium tremens occur how long after the cessation of alcohol consumption?**

On average 3-5 days.

○   **T/F: Status epilepticus is commonly seen in alcohol withdrawal seizures.**

False. Status epilepticus is rare in alcohol withdrawal seizures and should suggest the need to find other causative pathology.

○   **What is the classic triad of Wernicke's encephalopathy?**

Global confusion, oculomotor disturbances and ataxia.

156   USMLE STEP 2 AND STEP 3 REVIEW

○   **What constellation of findings should prompt consideration of ethylene glycol toxicity?**

Ethanol-like intoxication (with no odor), large anion gap acidosis, increased osmolal gap, altered mental status leading to coma, and calcium oxalate crystals in the urine

○   **In life threatening theophylline overdose, what is definitive management?**

Charcoal hemoperfusion.

○   **T/F: Lithium has a narrow therapeutic toxic range.**

True. Therapeutic lithium levels are between .5 - 1.5 mEq/L, and must be monitored closely.

○   **How is lithium eliminated after metabolism?**

By renal excretion.

○   **What are the typical CNS findings in mild lithium toxicity?**

Rigidity, tremor, hyperreflexia.

○   **What are the typical CNS findings in severe lithium toxicity?**

Seizures, coma, myoclonic jerking.

○   **What are the indications for hemodialysis in lithium toxicity?**

Serum lithium level above 4.0 mEq/l, renal failure and severe clinical symptoms (stupor, seizures etc.).

○   **T/F: Permanent neurologic sequelae (encephalopathy) can develop from lithium toxicity.**

True.

○   **A 30 year old man presents to the ED 20 minutes after ingesting 30 tablets of Amitriptyline. What is the preferred method of gastric emptying?**

Immediate gastric lavage using a large (34-36 French) orogastric tube. Ipecac should not be used due to the potential for a rapid deterioration in mental status and seizures.

○   **What class of antidysrthythmics are contraindicated in cyclic antidepressant overdoses?**

The type 1A and 1C antidysrthythmics. They have quinidine-like effects on the sodium channels and will enhance the cardiotoxcity of the cyclic antidepressants.

○   **What is the initial treatment for hypotension in antidepressant overdose?**

Intravenous fluids - normal saline or Ringer's lactate

○   **What vasopressor should be used to treat hypotension not responsive to IV fluids in antidepressant overdose?**

Norepinephrine should be used because it is a direct acting alpha-adrenergic agonist.

❍   **The onset of toxicity of monoamine oxidase inhibitors (MAOI) can occur up to what period of time after ingestion?**

12 to 24 hours.

❍   **What over-the-counter cold medications should not be used by people taking MAOI's?**

Decongestants, antihistamines and products containing dextromethorphan.

❍   **Name 5 hebal remedies associates with bleeding**

Ginger, garlic, ginkgo, ginseng, and feverfew.

❍   **What herbal remedies as are associated with CNS stimulation?**

Guarance, ma huang, St. John's wart, yohimbe and ginseng.

❍   **If a patient has a sulfa or ASA allergy can they be prescribed a COX II inhibitor?**

No.

❍   **Ingestion of benzene (an ingredient in pesticides, detergent, and paint remover) causes dermatitis, leukemia, and aplastic anemia. How can it be identified as a causative agent in such illnesses?**

Phenol, the metabolite, can be found in the urine.

INFECTIOUS DISEASES

○ **Describe the pathophysiologic features of HIV.**

HIV attacks the T4 helper cells. The genetic material of HIV consists of single stranded RNA. HIV has been found in semen, vaginal secretions, blood and blood products, saliva, urine, cerebrospinal fluid, tears, alveolar fluid, synovial fluid, breast milk, transplanted tissue, and amniotic fluid. There has been no documentation of infection from casual contact.

○ **How quickly do patients infected with HIV become symptomatic?**

5 to 10% develop symptoms within three years of seroconversion. Predictive characteristics include a low CD4 count and a hematocrit less than 40. The mean incubation time is about 8.23 years for adults and 1.97 years for children less than 5 years old.

○ **An HIV positive patient presents with a history of weight loss, diarrhea, fever, anorexia, and malaise. She is also dyspneic. Lab studies reveal abnormal LFTs and anemia. What is the most likely diagnosis?**

Mycobacterium avium intracellulare. Lab confirmation is made by an acid fast stain of body fluids or by a blood culture.

○ **What is the most common cause of focal encephalitis in AIDS patients?**

Toxoplasmosis. Symptoms include focal neurologic deficits, headache, fever, altered mental status, and seizures. Ring enhancing lesions are evident on CT.

○ **The differential diagnosis of ring enhancing lesions in AIDS patients includes:**

Lymphoma, cerebral tuberculosis, fungal infection, CMV, Kaposi's sarcoma, toxoplasmosis, and hemorrhage.

○ **What are the signs and symptoms of CNS cryptococcal infection in an AIDS patient?**

Headache, depression, lightheadedness, seizures, and cranial nerve palsies. A diagnosis is confirmed by an India ink prep, a fungal culture, or by a testing for the presence of cryptococcal antigens in the CSF.

○ **What is the most common eye finding in AIDS patients?**

Cotton wool spots. It has been proposed that the cotton wool spots are associated with PCP. These finding may be hard to differentiate from the fluffy, white, often perivascular retinal lesions that are associated with CMV.

○ **What is the most common cause of retinitis in AIDS patients?**

Cytomegalovirus. Findings include photophobia, redness, scotoma, pain, or a change in visual acuity. On examination, fluffy white retinal lesions may be evident.

○ **What is the most common opportunistic infection in AIDS patients?**

Pneumocystis carinii (PCP). Symptoms may include a non-productive cough and dyspnea. A chest x-ray may reveal diffuse interstitial infiltrates, or it may be negative. Although Gallium scanning is more sensitive, false positives occur. Initial treatment includes TMP-SMX. Pentamidine is an alternative.

O   **How is candidiasis of the esophagus diagnosed?**

An air contrast barium swallow shows ulcerations with plaques. In contrast, herpes esophagitis produces punched out ulcerations with no plaques. Definitive diagnosis is made by upper GI endoscopy and fungal and viral cultures.

O   **What is the most common gastrointestinal complaint in AIDS patients?**

Diarrhea. Many of the medications used to treat HIV have GI side effects. Hepatomegaly and hepatitis are also typical. Conversely, jaundice is an uncommon finding. *Cryptosporidium* and *Isospora* are the common causes of prolonged watery diarrhea.

O   **A patient is infected with *Treponema pallidum*. What is the treatment?**

The type of treatment depends upon the stage of the infection. Primary and secondary syphilis are treated with benzathine penicillin G (2.4 million units IM X 1 dose) or doxycycline (100 mg bid po for 14 day). Tertiary syphilis is treated with benzathine penicillin G, 2.4 million units IM X 3 doses 3 weeks apart.

O   **Describe the lesions associated with lymphogranuloma venereum (LV).**

LV caused by *Chlamydia* presents as painless skin lesions with lymphadenopathy. Lesions may be papular, nodular, or herpetiform vesicles. Sinus formation, involving the vagina and rectum, are common in women.

O   **What is the cause of chancroid?**

Haemophilus ducreyi. Patients with this condition present with 1 or more painful necrotic lesions. Suppurating inguinal lymphadenopathy may also be present.

O   **What is the cause of granuloma inguinale?**

Calymmatobacterium granulomatis. Onset occurs with small papular, nodular, or vesicular lesions that develop slowly into ulcerative or granulomatous lesions. Lesions are painless and are located on mucous membranes of the genital, inguinal, and anal areas.

O   **What causes tetanus?**

Clostridium tetani. This organism is a Gram positive rod; it is vegetative and a spore former. It produces tetanospasmin, an endotoxin, which induces the disinhibition of the motor and autonomic nervous systems and thus the exhibition of tetanus clinical symptoms.

O   **What is the incubation period of tetanus?**

Hours to over 1 month. The shorter the incubation period, the more severe the disease. Most patients who contract tetanus in the US are over 50 years old.

O   **What is the most common presentation of tetanus?**

"Generalized tetanus" with pain and stiffness in the trunk and jaw muscles. Trismus develops and results in risus sardonicus ("The Devil's Smile").

O   **Outline the treatment for tetanus.**

Respiratory: Administer succinylcholine for immediate intubation if required.

Immunotherapy: Human tetanus immune globulin will neutralize circulating tetanospasmin and the toxin in the wound. However, it will not neutralize toxin fixed in the nervous system. Dose TIG 3000 to 5000 units. Prescribe tetanus toxoid, 0.6 mL IM, at 1 week and 6 weeks and 6 months.

Antibiotics: *Clostridium tetani* is sensitive to cephalosporins, tetracycline, erythromycin, and penicillin, but penicillin G is the drug of choice.

Muscle relaxants: Administer diazepam or dantrolene.

Neuromuscular block: Prescribe pancuronium bromide, 2 mg plus sedation.

Autonomic dysfunction: Prescribe labetalol, 0.25 to 1.0 mg/minute IV, or magnesium sulfate, 70 mg/kg IV load, then 1 to 4 g/hour continuous infusion is used to treat autonomic dysfunction. Administer MS, 5 to 30 mg IV infusion every 2 to 8 hours, and clonidine, .1-.3 mg every 8 hour per NG.

Note: Fatal cardiovascular complications have occurred in patients treated with ß-adrenergic blocking agents alone. Adrenergic blocking agents used to treat autonomic dysfunction may precipitate myocardial depression.

○ **Where is the hookworm *Necator americanus* infection acquired?**

In areas where human fertilizer is used and people don't wear shoes. Patients present with chronic anemia, cough, low grade fever, diarrhea, abdominal pain, weakness, weight loss, eosinophilia, and guaiac positive stools. A diagnosis is confirmed if ova are present in the stool. Treatment includes mebendazole or pyrantel pamoate.

○ **What are the signs and symptoms of *Trichuris trichiura*?**

This hookworm lives in the cecum. Complaints include anorexia, abdominal pain especially RUQ, insomnia, fever, diarrhea, flatulence, weight loss, pruritus, eosinophilia, and microcytic hypochromic anemia. A diagnosis is made by examining for ova in the stool. Mebendazole is the treatment of choice.

○ **List three common protozoa that can cause diarrhea.**

Entamoeba histolytica: Found worldwide. Although half of the infected patients are asymptomatic, the usual symptoms consist of N/V/D/F, anorexia, abdominal pain, and leukocytosis. Determine the presence of this organism by ordering stool tests and performing an ELISA for extraintestinal infections. Treatment is with metronidazole or tinidazole followed by chloroquine phosphate.

Giardia lamblia: Found worldwide. This organism is one of the most common intestinal parasites in the US. Symptoms include explosive watery diarrhea, flatus, abdominal distention, fatigue, and fever. The diagnosis is confirmed via a stool examination. Treatment is with metronidazole.

Cryptosporidium parvum: Found worldwide. Symptoms are profuse watery diarrhea, cramps, N/V/F, and weight loss. Treatment is supportive care. Medications may be needed for immunocompromised patients.

○ **Explain the pathophysiology of rabies.**

Infection occurs within the myocytes for the first 48 to 96 hours. It then spreads across the motor endplate and ascends and replicates along the peripheral nervous system, axoplasm, and into the dor-sal root ganglia, spinal cord, and CNS. From the gray matter, the virus spreads by peripheral nerves to tissues and organ systems.

○ **What are the signs and symptoms of rabies?**

Incubation period of 12 to 700 days with an average of 20 to 90 days. Initial signs and systems are fever, headache, malaise, anorexia, sore throat, nausea, cough, and pain or paresthesias at the bite site.

In the CNS stage, agitation, restlessness, altered mental status, painful bulbar and peripheral muscular spasms, bulbar or focal motor paresis, and opisthotonos are exhibited. As in the Landry-Guillain-Barré syndrome, 20% develop ascending, symmetric flaccid and areflexic paralysis. In addition, hypersensitivity to water and sensory stimuli to light, touch, and noise may occur.

The progressive stage includes lucid and confused intervals with hyperpyrexia, lacrimation, salivation, and mydriasis along with brainstem dysfunction, hyperreflexia, and extensor planter response.

Final stages include coma, convulsions, and apnea, followed by death between the fourth and seventh day for the untreated patient.

O   **What is the diagnostic procedure of choice in rabies?**

Fluorescent antibody testing (FAT).

O   **How is rabies treated?**

Wound care includes debridement and irrigation. The wound must not be sutured; it should remain open. This will decrease the rabies infection by 90%.

RIG 20 IU/kg, half at wound site and half in the deltoid muscle, should be administered along with HDCV, 1 mL doses IM on days 0, 3, 7, 14, and 28, also in the deltoid muscle.

O   **A patient presents has a 40°C fever and a erythematous, macular, and blanching rash which becomes deep red, dusky, papular, and petechial. The patient is vomiting and has a headache, myalgias, and cough. Where did the rash begin?**

Rocky Mountain Spotted Fever (RMSF) rash typically begins on the flexor surfaces of the ankles and wrists and spreads centripetally and centrifugally.

O   **Which test confirms RMSF?**

Immunofluorescent antibody staining of a skin biopsy or serologic fluorescent antibody titer. The Weil-Felix reaction and complement fixation tests are no longer recommended.

O   **Which antibiotics are prescribed for the treatment of RMSF?**

Tetracycline or chloramphenicol. Antibiotic therapy should not be withheld pending serologic confirmation.

O   **What is the most deadly form of malaria?**

Plasmodium falciparum.

O   **What lab findings are expected for a patient with malaria?**

Normochromic normocytic anemia, a normal or depressed leukocyte count, thrombocytopenia, an elevated sed rate, abnormal kidney and LFTs, hyponatremia, hypoglycemia, and a false positive VDRL.

O   **How is malaria diagnosed?**

Visualization of parasites on Giemsa stained blood smears. In early infection, especially with *P. falciparum*, parasitized erythrocytes may be sequestered and undetectable.

O **What is the drug of choice for treating *P. vivax*, *P. ovale*, and *P. malariae*?**

Chloroquine.

O **How is uncomplicated chloroquine resistant *P. falciparum* treated?**

Quinine plus pyrimethamine-sulfadoxine plus doxycycline or mefloquine.

O **What are the adverse effects of chloroquine?**

N/V/D/F, pruritus, headache, dizziness, rash, and hypotension.

O **Name the most common intestinal parasite in the US.**

Giardia. Cysts are obtained from contaminated water or by hand-to-mouth transmission. Symptoms include explosive foul smelling diarrhea, abdominal distention, fever, fatigue, and weight loss. Cysts reside in the duodenum and upper jejunum.

O **How is Chagas' disease transmitted?**

By the blood sucking Reduviid "kissing" bug, blood transfusion, or breast feeding. A nodule or chagoma develops at the site. Symptoms include fever, headache, conjunctivitis, anorexia, and myocarditis. CHF and ventricular aneurysms can occur. The myenteric plexus is involved and may result in megacolon. Lab findings include anemia, leukocytosis, elevated sed rate, and ECG changes, such as PR interval, heart block, T wave changes, and arrhythmias.

O **Which 2 diseases are transmitted by the deer tick, *Ixodes dammini*?**

Lyme disease and Babesiosis.

O **How do patients present with *Babesia* infection?**

Intermittent fever, splenomegaly, jaundice, and hemolysis. The disease may be fatal in patients without spleens. Treatment is with clindamycin and quinine.

O **What is the most frequently transmitted tick-borne disease?**

Lyme disease. The causative agent is a spirochete (*Borrelia burgdorferi*), the vectors are *Ixodes dammini*, *I. pacificus*, *Amblyomma americanum*, and *Dermacentor variabilis*.

O **What areas of the United States report the highest incidence of Lyme disease?**

New England, the middle Atlantic and upper Midwestern states

O **What are the signs and symptoms of Lyme disease?**

Stage I: In the first month after the tick bite, patients can present with fever, fatigue, malaise, myalgia, headache, and a circular macule or papule lesion with a central clearing at the site of the tick bite that gradually enlarges (erythema chronicum migrans).

Stage II: (Weeks to months later) This stage involves neurological abnormalities such as meningoencephalitis, cranial neuropathies, peripheral neuropathies, myocarditis, and conjunctivitis to blindness.

Stage III: (Months to years) Migratory oligoarthritis of the large joints, neurological symptoms such as subtle encephalopathy (mood, memory and sleep disturbances) polyneuropathy, cognitive dysfunction and incapacitating fatigue.

○ **How is Lyme disease diagnosed?**

Immunofluorescent and immunoabsorbent assays identify the antibodies to the spirochete. Treatment includes doxycycline or tetracycline, amoxicillin, IV penicillin (V in pregnant patients), or erythromycin.

○ **What tick-borne disease is also harbored in wild rabbits?**

Tularemia

○ **What are the signs and symptoms of tularemia?**

Indurated skin ulcers at the site of inoculation, regional lymphadenopathy, fever, shaking chills, cough, hemoptysis, SOB, rales or pleural rub, hepatosplenomegaly and a maculopapular rash.

○ **What is the treatment for tularemia?**

Streptomycin. Mortality rate is 5 – 30% without antibiotic treatment.

○ **A patient presents a with sudden onset of fever, lethargy, a retro-orbital headache, myalgias, anorexia, nausea, and vomiting. She is extremely photophobic. The patient has been on a camping trip in Wyoming. What tick-borne disease might cause these symptoms?**

Colorado tick fever. This is caused by a virus of the genus *Orbivirus* and the family *Reoviridae*. The vector is the tick *D. andersoni*. The disease is self-limited; treatment is supportive.

○ **What is the most common cause of cellulitis?**

Streptococcus pyogenes. Staphylococcus aureus can also cause cellulitis though it is generally less severe and more often associated with an open wound.

○ **What is the most common cause of cutaneous abscesses?**

Staphylococcus aureus.

○ **What percentage of dog and cat bites become infected?**

About 10% of dog bites and 50% of cat bites become infected. *Pasteurella multocida* are the causative agents for 30% of dog bites and 50% of cat bites.

○ **A 6 year old child presents with headache, fever, malaise, and tender regional lymphadenopathy about a week after a cat bite. A tender papule develops at the site. What is the diagnosis?**

Catscratch disease. This condition usually develops 3 days to 6 weeks following a cat bite or scratch. The papule typically blisters and heals with eschar formation. A transient macular or vesicular rash may also develop.

○ **What is the probable cause of an animal bite infection arising that develops in less than 24 hours? More than 48 hours?**

Less than 24 hours*: Pasteurella multocida* or streptococci. More than 48 hours: *Staphylococcus aureus*.

○ **What is the most common cause of gas gangrene?**

Clostridium perfringens.

○   What is the most common site of a herpes simplex I infection?

The lower lip. These lesions are painful and can frequently recur since the virus remains in the sensory ganglia. Recurrences are generally triggered by stress, sun, and illness.

○   What is the recommended treatment for neurosyphilis?

Intravenous penicillin G. Follow up CSF examinations are mandatory.

○   What complication may arise from aggressive treatment of neurosyphilis with penicillin?

Jarisch-Herxheimer reaction. It is due to a release of endotoxin when large numbers of spirochete are lysed during the penicillin treatment, and consists of mild fever, malaise, headache, arthralgia, and may produce a temporary worsening of the neurological status.

○   At which stage of Lyme disease does neurological involvement occur?

The second and third stages. 2nd stage cranial neuropathies, meningitis and radiculoneuritis. 3rd stage-encephalitis, and a variety of CNS manifestations including stroke like syndromes, extrapyramidal and cerebellar involvement.

○   What is Weil's disease?

Weil's syndrome is the less common variety of leptospirosis, with icterus, marked hepatic and renal involvement along with a bleeding diasthesis being the main features, and hence the name leptospirosis-ictero-hemorrhagica.

○   What clinical feature of leptospirosis sets it apart from other infections of the nervous system and hints at the diagnosis?

Hemorrhagic complications. These are not uncommon, and intraparenchymal and subarachnoid hemorrhages have been reported.

○   What are the neurological features of brucellosis?

Mainly a chronic meningitis and the vascular complications thereof. However, cranial neuropathies, demyelination and mycotic aneurysms have all been described.

○   How is brucellosis spread?

By ingestion of contaminated milk and milk products. It may also be spread by contact with an infected animal (usually cattle). *Brucella melitensis* is the culprit.

○   What are the characteristic features of cerebral amebiasis, and what is the pathogenic organism?

Cerebral amebiasis is usually a secondary infection, and patients often have intestinal or hepatic amebiasis. The causative organism is Entamoeba Histolytica. The clinical features are that of intracerebral abscesses causing focal neurological signs. Frontal lobes and basal nuclei are common sites of abscess formation.

○   What is the current recommended treatment for intracranial toxoplasmosis in HIV disease?

This is usually a combination therapy with sulfadiazine, pyrimethamine, and folinic acid.

○ **What is the nature of CNS lymphoma in AIDS?**

They are almost all tumors of B cell origin. They may be large cell immunoblastic, or small non-cleaved cell lymphoma.

○ **Which virus is considered responsible for AIDS associated CNS lymphoma?**

Epstein-Barr virus

○ **How is botulism contracted, and what are the principle clinical features?**

It is contracted by consumption of contaminated foods, by injury from non-sterile objects (wound botulism) and in infants from intestinal colonization by *Clostridium botulinum* (lack of normal intestinal flora permit this colonization). The clinical features are that of a descending paralysis with complete ophthalmoplegia, bulbar and somatic palsy.

○ **Is the motor paralysis induced by botulinum toxin reversible?**

It's an irreversible paralysis, and recovery is from axonal sprouting from old sarcolemmal area to a new locus.

○ **Which condition resembles Guillain-Barre syndrome, the appropriate treatment of which results in miraculous complete improvements often within a day?**

Tick paralysis, which results in an ascending paralysis within a few days of attack by the tick *Dermacentor* (hard tick). This releases a toxin in its saliva, which is responsible for the neuromuscular blockade. Removal of the tick results in resolution of the weakness that begins within hours.

○ **What is the cause of Sydenham's chorea, and what are the principal clinical features?**

This is caused by an immunological cross-reaction after group A streptococcus infections. The chorea often occurs several months after the acute infection. It is characterized by development of involuntary choreiform movements that may be unilateral, and remits spontaneously after a while. There are also associated behavioral changes that may reach the severity of obsessive compulsive disorder.

○ **To which group of viruses does the Poliovirus belong?**

Poliovirus is an enterovirus that belongs to the picornavirus group.

○ **What is the meaning of the term reverse transcriptase in the description of HIV?**

Under normal circumstances, the transcription of a protein in a human cell occurs in a forward direction going from DNA to RNA. In reverse transcriptase, the transcription proceeds from RNA to DNA. HIV is a reverse transcriptase or a 'retrovirus' that needs to be incorporated into the human genome by the reverse transcription before replicating.

○ **Is AIDS dementia a cortical or subcortical dementia?**

Cortical. There is no evidence of myelin breakdown in AIDS dementia. The white matter pallor is probably secondary to blood brain barrier breakdown

○ **A 31 year old stepped on a nail at his job. The nail pierced through his sneaker and into his foot. His tetanus status is up to date. What is your main concern?**

Infection with *Pseudomonas* that can lead to osteomyelitis. Pseudomonal infection is most commonly associated with hot, moist environments, such as sneakers.

○   **How do viral meningitis and bacterial meningitis differ with regards to CSF pressure? CSF leukocytes? CSF glucose?**

The pressure in bacterial infection is increased, whereas it is normal or slightly increased in viral meningitis. The leukocytosis is greater than 1000 (up to 60K) in bacterial, and rarely over 1000 in viral meningitis. The glucose concentration is decreased in bacterial meningitis and is generally normal in viral meningitis.

○   **What is the sine-quo-non of botulism poisoning presentation?**

Bulbar palsy.

○   **What is thought to be the mode of inoculation in cat-scratch disease?**

Rubbing the eye after contact with a cat.

○   **A patient is diagnosed with impetigo from group A streptococcus. What sequelae do you have to keep an eye out for?**

Acute post-streptococcal glomerulonephritis. It will not, however, lead to rheumatic fever, for reasons that are not fully understood. (Possibly the strains for pharyngitis and impetigo are different).

○   **What are the major Jones criteria used to diagnose rheumatic fever?**

Carditis, chorea (Sydenham's), erythema marginatum, migratory polyarthritis, and subcutaneous nodules. The diagnosis requires either 2 major or 1 major and 2 minor with evidence of previous strep. infection.

○   **What is the drug of choice for meningococcal disease?**

Aqueous penicillin G (250k-300k units/kg/day IV in 6 doses) is the ideal, though patients can be started effectively on empiric cefotaxime or ceftriaxone for suspected cases and in patients with penicillin allergy.

○   **Should people who have had contact with patients with meningococcal meningitis be given prophylactic antibiotics?**

Yes. Rifampin or ceftriaxone are recommended.

○   **What is the most common cause of aseptic meningitis?**

Enteroviruses.

○   **What is the recommended initial treatment for cases of gonorrhea?**

Third generation cephalosporins (especially ceftriaxone) plus either doxycycline (100 mg BID for seven days) or azithromycin (1 gram PO x 1 dose) for presumptive coinfection with chlamydia.

○   **What is the cause of epidemic keratoconjunctivitis?**

Adenovirus.

○   **After finishing the prescribed dosage of penicillin for pharyngitis, your patient's repeat culture still grows streptococcus. What do you do?**

Nothing. Most people are asymptomatic carriers and in most cases it is inconsequential.

○   **What are the most common causes of herpangina?**

Coxsackie A and B viruses, and Echovirus.

○   **Why does therapy for TB take several months, when other infections usually clear in a matter of days?**

Because the mycobacterium divide very slowly and have a long dormant phase, during which time they are not responsive to medications.

○   **What is the most common side effect of rifampin?**

Orange discoloration of urine and tears.

○   **What are the organisms most commonly thought to be associated with Guillain-Barre Disease?**

CMV, EBV, Coxsackievirus, *Campylobacter jejuni*, and *Mycoplasma pneumoniae*.

○   **In what disease is cerebrospinal fluid albuminocytologic dissociation seen and what does it mean?**

Guillain-Barré Disease. An increase in cerebrospinal fluid protein without a corresponding increase in cerebrospinal fluid white cells is referred to as albuminocytologic dissociation.

○   **What are five infectious agents associated with erythema nodosum?**

Erythema nodosum has been associated with many infectious and some non-infectious processes. Some of its better known associates are Group A streptococcus, meningococcus, syphilis, *Mycobacterium tuberculosis*, and *M. leprae*, as well as histoplasmosis, coccidioidomycosis, blastomycosis and herpes simplex virus. Some of the less common associates of erythema nodosum include *Chlamydia trachomatis*, *C. psitacci*, *Corynebacterium diphtheriae*, *Campylobacter*, *Haemophilus ducreyi*, *Yersinia*, *Rochalimea henselae*, *Trichophyton*, filariasis, sarcoidosis, and various drugs.

○   **What is the risk of transmission of HIV from an HIV infected person following a needle stick exposure?**

0.3%-0.5% on average. (Though this varies depending on needle gauge and depth and site of insertion).

○   **What two common urinary pathogens do not give a positive urine nitrate test?**

Enterococcus and *Staphylococcus saprophyticus*. *Acinobacter* also fails to give a positive urine nitrate test.

○   **What are the features of typhoid fever?**

Braydcardia, **I**nsidious onset, **R**ose spots, **D**icrotic pulse, **S**plenomegaly, **F**ever, **L**eukopenia, **E**pidemic, **W**idal reaction. (BIRDS FLEW).

○   **In a patient who presents with diarrhea, high fever, headache, lethargy, confusion, a normal lumbar puncture, 45% band forms on the differential of his white blood count, and a blood culture that is positive for Escherichia coli, what is the most likely cause of the diarrhea?**

Shigella. Blood cultures in *Shigella* diarrhea are virtually never positive for *Shigella*. When they are positive, they are more likely to be positive for *Escherichia coli*. Perhaps this is due to the fact that while *Shigella* is locally quite invasive at the mucosal level, it is very poorly invasive at the systemic level. Resident *Escherichia coli* in the gut, however, take advantage of the disrupted mucosa and invade the blood stream.

O   **Which hemoglobin provides the greatest innate resistance to falciparum malaria?**

Erythrocytes of patients that are heterozygous for sickle cell hemoglobin (sickle cell trait) are resistant to malaria.

O   **What is the most common infectious disease complication of both measles and influenza?**

Pneumococcal pneumonia.

O   **On Tuesday you are driving home from work in rural California and pass 3 dead squirrels. On Wednesday, taking a different route, you pass two more dead squirrels. The following morning you see a twenty six year old male with enlarged tender lymphadenitis and a 105° F fever. What illness might you suspect?**

Cases of human plague (*Yersinia pestis*) are sometimes heralded by squirrel die-offs. A squirrelly die-off occurs when the organism is introduced into a highly susceptible mammalian population, causing a high mortality rate among infected animals. This is referred to as epizootic plague.

O   **One day after a previously healthy adult has been admitted to the hospital after an accidental overdose of oral iron, she appears to become septic. What is the most likely organism causing her sepsis?**

Yersinia enterocolitica. The growth of *Y. enterocolitica* appears to be enhanced after exposure to excess iron. This combined with intestinal damage to the mucosa by the iron may play a role in pathogenesis.

O   **If the result of a patient's PPD is read as 3 mm of induration and then 15 mm of induration following the placement of the second PPD two weeks later, which study should be considered the more reliable?**

The second study with an induration of 15 mm. With time, the body's memory of the tuberculosis infection may want. The placement of a PPD may stimulate that memory. This is what is referred to as the "booster phenomenon". The boosted result is considered to be the reliable result.

O   **A patient from the Philippines has a hypopigmented patch that is lacking in sensation. What is the most likely cause of his problem?**

Leprosy (*Mycobacterium leprae*).

O   **Which intestinal parasites are known to cause anemia as their major manifestation?**

Hookworms. Three species of hookworms affect humans. These include *Ancylostoma duodenale*, *Necator americanus*, and *A. ceylanicum*.

O   **What is the most common symptom of tularemia?**

Skin sores at the site of inoculation and lymphadenopathy (75%). Other symptoms include pneumonia, lesions in the GI system, infection of the eyes, fever, and headache.

O   **How is tularemia most commonly transmitted?**

Ticks and rabbits. Tularemia is caused by *F. tularensis*.

O   **Which has a longer incubation period, staphylococci or *Salmonella*?**

Salmonella; it is generally ingested in small doses and then multiplies in the GI tract. Symptoms occur 6 to 48 hours after ingestion. *Staphylococcus aureus* has an incubation period of just 3 hours.

RHEUMATOLOGY, IMMUNOLOGY AND ALLERGY

○ **Which class of immunoglobulins is responsible for urticaria (hives) and angioedema?**

IgE.

○ **Which class of immunoglobulins is responsible for food allergies?**

IgE.

○ **What are the most common food allergies?**

Dairy products, eggs, and nuts.

○ **When do the clinical manifestations of a new drug allergy usually become apparent?**

One to two weeks after starting the drug.

○ **Which class of drugs is commonly associated with angioedema?**

Angiotensin converting enzyme (ACE) inhibitors. A patient who has suffered angioedema from one ACE inhibitor should not be prescribed another one. Complication can result from any member of this class of antihypertensive agents. ACE triggered angioedema can occur at any time during the course of therapy.

○ **What drug is the most common pharmaceutical cause of true allergic reactions?**

Penicillin. It accounts for approximately 90% of true allergic drug reactions and more than 95% of fatal anaphylactic drug reactions. Parenterally administered penicillin is more than twice as likely to cause a fatal anaphylactic reaction as compared to orally administered penicillin.

○ **How long after exposure to an allergen does anaphylaxis occur?**

Seconds to 1 hour.

○ **After penicillin, what is the most common cause of anaphylaxis-related deaths?**

Insect stings. Approximately 100 deaths occur in the US annually because of anaphylaxis induced by insect stings.

○ **A patient on ß-blockers who develops anaphylactic cardiovascular collapse may not respond to epinephrine or dopamine infusions. What drug can be used in this setting?**

Glucagon, 5 to 15 mg/minute IV.

○ **What percentage of patients with Kawasaki's disease also develop acute carditis?**

50%, usually myocarditis with mild to moderate congestive heart failure. Pericarditis, conduction abnormalities, and valvular disturbances may occur but are less common.

○   **Are the nodules of erythema nodosum more often symmetrical or asymmetrical in distribution?**

Symmetrical. These nodules are distinctive, bilateral, tender nodules with underlying red or purple shiny patches of skin that develop in a symmetric distribution along the shins, arms, thighs, calves, and buttocks.

○   **Is there an effective treatment for erythema nodosum?**

No. The disease usually lasts several weeks, but the pain associated with the tender lesions can be relieved with non-steroidal antiinflammatory agents.

○   **A patient presents with fever, acute polyarthritis, or migratory arthritis a few weeks after a bout of streptococcal pharyngitis. What disease should be suspected?**

Acute rheumatic fever. Although the early symptoms may be nonspecific, a physical examination eventually reveals signs of arthritis (60 to 75%), carditis (30%), choreiform movements (10%), erythema marginatum, or subcutaneous nodules.

○   **What treatment should be started when acute rheumatic fever has been diagnosed?**

Penicillin or erythromycin. This treatment should be started even if cultures for group A streptococci are negative. High dose aspirin therapy is used at an initial dose of 75 to 100 mg/kg/day. Carditis or congestive heart failure is treated with prednisone, 1 to 2 mg/kg/day.

○   **What is Lhermitte sign in ankylosing spondylitis?**

A sensation of electric shock that radiates down the back when the neck is flexed. This is a sign that atlantoaxial subluxation and C-spine instability may be present. Lhermitte sign may also be present in patients with rheumatoid arthritis and multiple sclerosis.

○   **What rheumatic syndrome may lead to corneal irritation, ulceration, and infection?**

Sjogren's syndrome. This syndrome involves the lymphocytic infiltration of the lacrimal and salivary glands and may occur as an independent entity or as an accompaniment to other rheumatologic diseases. Patients with Sjogren's syndrome present with a dry mouth and eyes.

○   **What organisms are typically responsible for septic arthritis and osteomyelitis of the foot in an immunocompetent adult?**

Staphylococcus and *Pseudomonas*.

○   **How is gout distinguished from pseudogout by using a microscope with a polarizing filter?**

When the plane of polarization is perpendicular to the crystal, pseudogout (calcium pyrophosphate) crystals appear yellow and rhomboidal, while gout (uric acid) crystals appear blue and needle shaped. The mnemonic CUB, or "crossed urate blue" is a reminder.

○   **Is the onset of pain more rapid in gout or in pseudogout?**

Gout. The onset of pain in acute gouty arthritis occurs over a few hours, whereas the pain associated with pseudogout usually evolves over a day or more.

○   **Cite an example for each of the four major types of allergic reactions: Type I (immediate hypersensitivity); type II (cytotoxic); type III (Arthus reaction); and type IV (delayed hypersensitivity).**

Type I: Asthma, food allergies (IgE)
Type II: Transfusion reaction (IgG and IgM)
Type III: Serum sickness, post streptococcal glomerulonephritis (complex activates complement)
Type IV: Skin testing (activated T-lymphocytes)

○   **What is the common name for granulomatous arteritis of the thoracic aorta and its branches? What are its common symptoms?**

Temporal arteritis. Symptoms include tender scalp, headache, fluctuating vision, reduced brachial pulse, and jaw or tongue pain.

○   **Myocardial infarction can occur with which two rheumatic diseases?**

Kawasaki disease and polyarteritis nodosa (PAN).

○   **What is the most common cause of anaphylactoid reactions?**

Radiographic contrast media. Other causes include ASA , NSAIDS and codeine.

○   **What is the difference between anaphylactoid and anaphylaxis reactions?**

Anaphylactoid reactions resemble anaphylaxis reactions in symptomatology but do not require prior exposure and are not immunologically mediated.

○   **A bacterial infection and an allergic phenomenon can both cause a generalized confluent exfoliation of the skin. What are the two diseases and what test should be performed to distinguish between them?**

Bacterial infection: Ritter's disease. This disorder is caused by *Staphylococcus* and thus is also known as staphylococcal scalded skin syndrome. Ritter's disease causes exfoliation at the superficial granular layer of the epidermis.

Allergic phenomenon: Toxic epidermal necrolysis (TEN).

A skin biopsy distinguishes between the two conditions because the exfoliative cleavage plane is deeper at the dermal-epidermal junction or lower with TEN.

○   **How is mucocutaneous lymph node syndrome (Kawasaki disease) diagnosed in a young patient with prolonged fever?**

Diagnosis requires four of the following findings:

1) Conjunctival inflammation
2) Rash
3) Adenopathy
4) Strawberry tongue and injection of the lips and pharynx
5) Erythema and edema of extremities

Desquamation of the fingers and the toes may be striking, but it is a late finding and is not one of the key clinical features of the disease.

○   **What is the treatment of choice for a patient in anaphylactic shock?**

Epinephrine.
Mild anaphylaxis (uticaria, rhinitis, mild bronchospasm) : 0.3 – 0.5cc 1 :1,000 SQ
Moderate (generalized uticaria, angioedema, hypotension) : 1 – 5 cc 1 :10,000 IM q 5 – 20 min x 3
Severe (laryngeal edema, repiratory failure, shock) : 1 – 5cc IV over 10 minutes. If no improvement start an epi drip.

○   **How long should a patient with a generalized anaphylactic reaction be observed?**

24 hours. Recurrence of hemodynamic collapse and airway compromise is common within this period of time. Treat with antihistamines and steroids for 72 hours.

○   **What is the diagnostic approach for SLE with a pleural effusion?**

All pleural effusions in patients with rheumatic disease require thoracentesis to distinguish inflammatory effusions from infectious effusions. Pulmonary embolisms are common in patients with SLE; thus, a nuclear ventilation-perfusion (V/Q) scan is also indicated.

○   **What percentage of patients with Kawasaki disease will develop coronary artery aneurysms if not treated?**

Approximately 20%. 1 to 2% of these patients will die from acute myocardial infarction during the resolution phase of the illness.

○   **What cardiac complication commonly occurs with SLE, juvenile rheumatoid arthritis, and rheumatoid arthritis?**

Pericarditis.

○   **What are the symptoms of atlantoaxial subluxation?**

Changes in bowel or bladder function, limb paresthesias, or new weakness.

○   **What vascular disease is accompanied by polymyalgia rheumatica in 10 to 30% of the cases?**

Temporal arteritis.

○   **A patient is suspected of having a new onset of acute gouty arthritis. What must be determined?**

The exclusion of a septic arthritis must assume top priority because the signs and symptoms of the two diseases may be indistinguishable.

○   **What complication of rheumatoid arthritis may produce signs and symptoms that mimic those of deep vein thrombosis (DVT)?**

A Baker's cyst. This cyst can occasionally be distinguished clinically from DVT when deep hemorrhage from the ruptured cyst produces bruising or staining in a purple crescent below the malleoli, or when localized swelling at the site of the ruptured popliteal cyst spares the more distal parts of the leg and the foot.

○   **Arthritis of the elbow joint causes limitation of all motion at the joint. In what way does olecranon bursitis differ?**

Pain from olecranon bursitis may limit flexion and extension at the elbow, but it usually does not affect pronation and supination.

O **How should a potentially septic olecranon bursitis be treated?**

Aspirate as much fluid as possible from the bursa via a large-bore needle. Antibiotics should be started immediately.

O **How should a new monarthritis be approached in a patient with rheumatoid arthritis?**

Assume it is septic until proven otherwise. The risk for infection is higher in a joint that has been previously injured or affected by arthritis.

O **A 10 year old child is limping; he complains of several weeks of groin, hip, and knee pain that worsens with activity. What diseases should be considered?**

Transient tenosynovitis of the hip, slipped capital femoral epiphysis, Legg-Calvé-Perthes, suppurative arthritis, rheumatic fever, juvenile rheumatoid arthritis, and tuberculosis of the hip.

O **What is Legg-Calvé-Perthes disease? How does it present? Who is affected?**

Legg-Calvé-Perthes disease is avascular necrosis of the femoral head, presenting in children between 2 and 13 years of age as subacute groin, hip, and knee pain that worsens with activity. The disease is also known as Coxa Plana. The cause is unknown.

O **What is the diagnosis for a preadolescent child with activity related knee pain and a thickened and tender patellar tendon?**

Osgood-Schlatter. This disease is an inflammatory repetitive injury process in which cartilaginous fragments are pulled loose from the tibial tuberosity by the ligamentum patellae of the quadriceps tendon. Treatment involves several months of restriction from excessive physical activity.

O **What disease is suspected in an adolescent with a tender, purpuric dependent rash on the lower extremities, colicky abdominal pain, migratory polyarthritis, and microscopic hematuria?**

Henoch-Schonlein purpura, a leukoblastic vasculitis. Intestinal or pulmonary hemorrhage may occur, and 7 to 9% of the cases will develop chronic renal sequelae. Salicylates are effective for the arthritis. Other treatments are directed at the symptoms. Steroids are not particularly effective.

O **A child has painful swollen joints along with a spiking high fever, shaking chills, signs of pericarditis, and a pale erythematous coalescing rash on the trunk, palms, and soles. Hepatosplenomegaly is found. What is your diagnosis?**

Systemic juvenile rheumatoid arthritis. Arthrocentesis is necessary to eliminate the possibility of septic arthritis. The rheumatoid factor and the antinuclear antibody usually are negative; one-fourth of patients will proceed to have joint destruction. This is the least common of the three types of JRA.

O **What treatment, besides aspirin, prevents the complications of Kawasaki disease?**

IV immunoglobulins can reduce the incidence of coronary artery aneurysms to less than 5%. Corticosteroids are thought to increase the likelihood of development of coronary artery disease.

O **What are the cardiovascular manifestations of Rheumatic Arthritis?**

Pericarditis and aortitis.

O **Which patients are more likely to get recurrences of rheumatic fever?**

Recurrences are most common in children and patients who have had carditis during their initial episode. 20% of these patients will have a second episode within 5 years.

○   **A 70 year old patient has had progressive pain and motion restriction of the shoulder for several months. There is minimal tenderness to palpation, but active and passive range of motion are limited in abduction and rotation. What is the probable diagnosis?**

Adhesive capsulitis. The pain is usually a poorly localized diffuse ache that is often worse at night. The etiology is unclear but the condition commonly follows injury or chronic inflammation, particularly after immobilization.

○   **What is the treatment for adhesive capsulitis?**

An intensive physical therapy program with range of motion exercises. Intraarticular steroids and oral prednisone.

○   **What disease produces erythematous plaques with dusky centers and red borders resembling bull's eye targets?**

Erythema multiforme. This disease can also produce non-pruritic urticarial lesions, petechiae, vesicles, and bullae.

○   **What is the appropriate management for toxic epidermal necrolysis (TEN)?**

Admit the patient for management similar to that required for extensive second degree burns. The mortality rate of TEN can be as high as 50% because of fluid loss and secondary infections.

○   **What drugs are most commonly implicated in toxic epidermal necrolysis?**

Sulfonamides and sulfones, phenylbutazone and related drugs, barbiturates, antiepileptic drugs, and antibiotics.

○   **What can cause erythema multiforme?**

Viral or bacterial infections, drugs of nearly all classes, and malignancy.

○   **What is the most common cause of allergic contact dermatitis?**

Toxicodendron species, such as poison oak, poison ivy, and poison sumac. These allergens are responsible for more cases than all the other allergens combined.

○   **Why does scratching spread poison oak and poison ivy?**

The antigenic resin contaminates hands and fingernails. A single contaminated finger can produce more than 500 reactive groups of lesions.

○   **How is the antigen of poison oak or poison ivy inactivated?**

Careful washing with soap and water destroys the antigen. Special attention must be paid to the fingernails, otherwise the antigenic resin can be carried for weeks.

○   **What underlying illnesses should be considered in a patient with nontraumatic uveitis?**

Collagen vascular diseases, sarcoid, ankylosing spondylitis, Reiter's syndrome, tuberculosis, syphilis, toxoplasmosis, juvenile rheumatoid arthritis, and Lyme disease.

○ **In what way does trochanteric bursitis mimic lumbar radiculopathy?**

Both conditions produce pain that involves the hip and radiates along the iliotibial band to the lateral knee.

○ **A patient has myalgias, arthralgias, headache, and an annular erythematous lesion accompanied by central clearing. What is your diagnosis?**

Stage I Lyme disease with the classic lesion of erythema chronicum migrans (ECM). The primary lesion occurs at the site of the tick bite.

○ **What rheumatologic ailments produce pulmonary hemorrhage?**

Goodpasture's disease, systemic lupus erythematosus, Wegener's granulomatosis, and nonspecific vasculitides.

○ **What rheumatologic ailments can produce acute airway obstruction?**

Relapsing polychondritis and rheumatoid arthritis.

○ **How is septic bursitis contracted?**

A puncture wound or an overlying cellulitis are the typical sources for septic bursitis.

○ **What lymphocyte surface molecule is responsible for HLA class II antigens?**

CD4.

○ **Which are the only complement fixing immunoglobulins?**

IgG and IgM..

○ **Which immunoglobulin is the major host defense against parasites?**

IgE.

○ **What are the two main functions of T cells?**

To signal B cells to make antibody, and to kill virally infected or tumor cells.

○ **What causes fatality in hereditary angioedema?**

Edema of the larynx.

○ **Reactive leukocytosis, resembling a leukemia-like picture, can occur in what clinical scenarios?**

Sepsis, hepatic failure, diabetic acidosis, and azotemia

○ **What is the definition of neutropenia?**

Absolute Neutrophil Count (ANC) < 1500 cell/ml.

○ **Aside from chemotherapeutics, which suppress bone marrow, what other agents are most commonly implicated in neutropenia?**

Phenothiazines, semisynthetic penicillin, NSAIDs, aminopyrine derivatives, and antithyroid medications

O   **What is the most common cause of transient neutropenia?**

Viral infections which most commonly include Hepatitis A, Hepatitis B, Influenza A and B, measles, rubella, and varicella.

O   **How long would you expect the neutropenia to persist?**

It may persist for the first three to six days of the acute viral syndrome.

O   **What nutritional deficiencies may precipitate neutropenia?**

Vitamin B12, folic acid, and copper.

O   **Neutropenia and bacterial infection may herald the onset of what?**

Overwhelming sepsis.

O   **Briefly explain the cellular basis for the Type I hypersensitivity reaction (wheal and flare). Give a clinical example.**

This immediate type or anaphylactic hypersensitivity is mediated by circulating basophils and mast cells, which become activated by crosslinking of IgE on their membrane surface. The prototypic IgE mediated disease is ragweed hay fever. Other, sometimes fatal, anaphylactic reactions are the classic insect venom or food induced allergies.

O   **Briefly explain the cellular basis for the Type II hypersensitivity reaction (cytotoxic). Give a clinical example.**

These immune interactions involve integral cellular antigen components and IgG and IgM antibody formation to these foreign antigen determinants. The classic example is immune mediated hemolysis such as that seen in transfusion reaction, or hemolytic disease of the newborn.

O   **Briefly explain the cellular basis for the Type III hypersensitivity reaction (Arthus or immune complex). Give a clinical example.**

Tissue injury is caused by immune complex deposition in various tissues, which are toxic to that tissue, by mechanisms, such as complement activation or proteolytic enzyme release. Examples include immune complex pericarditis, and arthritis following meningococcal, or H. influenzae infection.

O   **In Type IV hypersensitivity reaction (cell-mediated or delayed type), pathologic changes follow interaction of antigen with what cellular component of the immune system?**

Antigen specific sensitized T cells.

O   **What features of the physical exam which should be highlighted when examining an atopic individual?**

Height, weight, pulsus paradoxus, Alae nasi flaring, mouth breathing, allergic 'shiner', allergic 'salute' (transverse nasal creasing from habitual nose wiping), and Dennie lines (wrinkles beneath lower eyelids).

O   **What other conditions would you see eosinophilia?**

Neoplasm (Hodgkin's lymphoma), immunodeficiency, parasitic infestation, Addison's disease, Collagen vascular disease, Cystic fibrosis, Infections (CMV, EBV, Leprosy, systemic Candidiasis, Coccidioidomycosis), Guillain-Barré, hemosiderosis, interstitial nephritis, and Kawasaki disease.

○ **What are some possible adverse effects of chronic steroid use?**

Posterior subcapsular cataract, Osteoporosis, Hypertension, Diabetes mellitus, Cushingoid body habitus, Infections, Pancreatitis, Gastritis, and Myopathy.

○ **What is the basis of antigen desensitization?**

Injection of antigenic extract into patients blunts the anamnestic rise of IgE via production of IgG, which effectively sequesters antigen by binding it.

○ **What are the likely causative agents implicated in perennial allergic rhinitis?**

Components of house dust, feathers, allergens, dander of household pets, and mold spores are the most common inciting agents.

○ **What constitutes triad asthma?**

The syndrome of nasal polyps, asthma, and aspirin intolerance comprise triad asthma (also called Sampter's Triad).

○ **What is the most effective treatment of allergic rhinitis?**

Topical use of corticosteroids, such as beclomethasone nasal spray.

○ **What is extrinsic asthma?**

Asthmatic exacerbation following environmental exposure to allergens such as dust, pollens, and dander.

○ **What is intrinsic asthma?**

Asthmatic exacerbation not associated with an increase in IgE or a positive skin.

○ **What is atopic dermatitis?**

An inflammatory skin disorder characterized by erythema, edema, pruritus, exudation, crusting, and scaling. 80% have elevated serum IgE levels.

○ **What is the most effective treatment for control of urticaria?**

0.5 mg/kg Hydroxyzine (Atarax) is the most effective therapy, but diphenhydramine (Benadryl) is also useful.

○ **What are typical initial symptoms of an anaphylactic reaction?**

Initially patients usually report a tingling sensation around the mouth followed by a warm feeling and tightness in chest or throat.

○ **Patients with severe allergic reaction to eggs should avoid receipt of which vaccines?**

Influenza and yellow fever vaccines.

○ **What is the most serious complication of serum sickness?**

The most serious complications are Guillain-Barre syndrome, and peripheral neuritis, most commonly of the brachial plexus.

○   **What is the major cause of serum sickness?**

Drug allergy, particularly penicillin.

○   **In what post-operative time period is acute rejection the greatest?**

3 months status post transplantation.

○   **What commonly used immunosuppressive agent would be contraindicated in heart-lung transplant patients?**

Steroids. Their use may affect airway healing.

○   **What is the most sensitive and specific sign of an infectious disease in an immunocompromised host?**

Fever.

○   **At what CD4 cell count is prophylaxis indicated in these patients and what antimicrobial is used?**

Just as with immunodeficiency virus, a CD4 count of <200cells/mm^3 is indication for prophylaxis with TMP-SMX (Bactrim).

○   **A renal transplant patient, 30 days posttransplant, presents with fever, oliguria, hypertension, and elevated serum creatinine. What two diagnostic tests would you perform next?**

Renal ultrasound and renal scan to evaluate renal blood flow.

○   **What diagnostic study is necessary to differentiate between rejection reaction, acute tubular necrosis, cyclosporine toxicity, or recurrence of renal disease?**

Renal biopsy.

○   **What is the major cause of death in renal transplant recipients one year following transplant?**

Infection.

○   **In transplant patients receiving immunosuppressive therapy, how does one evaluate abdominal pain?**

Chronic steroid use often masks abdominal catastrophes. Therefore, abdominal pain in a transplant patient is a surgical EMERGENCY until otherwise proven.

○   **Following an acute episode of CMV, patients with renal or liver transplants are at an increased risk for?**

Graft Rejection. CMV has been shown to upregulate MHC II D/DR in allografts, which may precipitate rejection reaction.

○   **A liver transplant patient presents with increased liver aminotransferase and direct bilirubin without pain or fever. Which diagnostic test would be most useful?**

Doppler flow study to rule out arterial thrombosis.

○   **What would you suspect if a liver transplant patient presented with rapidly increasing ascites and liver dysfunction?**

Portal vein thrombosis.

○ **What is the mechanism of immunosuppression with hydroxychloroquine?**

Alkalinization of proteolytic vesicles.

○ **Anti-dsDNA antibodies are most indicative of what disease?**

Systemic lupus erythematosus.

○ **The presence of antineutrophil cytoplasmic antibodies (c-ANCA) with a diffuse staining pattern in serum immunofluorescence is most commonly associated with what disease?**

Wegener's granulomatosus. It can also be seen in HIV and Kawasaki disease.

○ **What is the overall prognosis of JRA patients?**

At least 75% of patients with JRA will have long term remissions without significant residual deformity or loss of function.

○ **How does ankylosing spondylitis differ from rheumatoid arthritis?**

Involvement of the sacroiliac joints and lumbodorsal spine, predilection for males, occurrence of aortitis, familial incidence, a negative RF, and lack of rheumatoid nodules or incidence of acute iridocyclitis characterize ankylosing spondylitis.

○ **Reiter's disease may occur following infection with which microbial agents?**

Shigella, *Yersinia*, *Enterocolitica*, *Campylobacter*, and *Chlamydia*.

○ **What percent of patients with inflammatory bowel disease have articular manifestations of the disease?**

10%.

○ **What are the most frequent early symptoms of SLE?**

The most frequent early symptoms in children are fever, malaise, arthritis or arthralgia, and rash.

○ **What is the most sensitive seum marker in SLE?**

ANA is positive in 95 – 100% of patients with SLE but it is not very specific. ANA will also be positive in RA, hepatitis and interstitial lung disease.

○ **What hematologic conditions are seen in patients with SLE?**

Anemia, thrombocytopenia, and leukopenia occur frequently.

○ **What pharmacologic agents are most commonly associated with drug induced lupus?**

Anticonvulsants, hydralazine and isoniazid.

○ **What are the major causes of SLE mortality?**

Nephritis, with resultant renal failure
Central nervous system complications
Infection
Pulmonary lupus
Myocardial infarction

○ When is anticoagulation therapy indicated in SLE?

In patients with the persistent presence of antiphospholipid antibodies (because of the risk of venous or arterial thrombosis), migraine, recurrent fetal loss, TIA, stroke, avascular necrosis, transverse myelitis, pulmonary hypertension or embolus, livedo reticularis, leg ulcers, or thrombocytopenia.

○ What are the diagnostic criteria for Kawasaki disease?

Fever lasting at least 5 days, plus:
Presence of four of the following five conditions:
   1. Bilateral nonpurulent conjunctival injection.
   2. Changes in the mucosa of the oropharynx, including infected pharynx, dry fissured lips, strawberry tongue.
   3. Changes in peripheral extremities, such as edema and/or erythema of the hands or feet desquamation.
           4. Primarily truncal rash.
           5. Cervical lymphadenopathy.
Illness not explained by any other known disease process

○ A 30 year old patient presents with progressive destruction and ulcerations of upper respiratory tract and associated arthritis and acute glomerulitis. The presumptive diagnosis of Wegener's granulomatosis is made. What are the therapeutic options?

Corticosteroids, cyclosporine, or trimethoprim-sulfamethoxazole (Bactrim)

○ What clinical manifestations differentiate SYSTEMIC from FOCAL scleroderma?

In focal scleroderma, one sees cutaneous fibrosis and no systemic involvement, such as diffuse fibrosis or Raynaud's phenomenon, both of which are components of systemic scleroderma.

○ A 18 year old female presents with complains of fever and malaise one week prior to the development of 1-3 cm painful, red, ovoid nodules on her shins bilaterally. The patient's mom states she had an episode of severe sore throat the previous week also. Hilar lymphadenopathy is demonstrated on chest x-ray. What is the diagnosis?

Erythema nodosum.

○ The combination of pain, tenderness, and swelling of the costosternal junction is referred to as what syndrome?

Tietze's syndrome or costochondritis.

○ What is the clinical scenario of Familial Mediterranean Fever and what is the attributed cause?

Amyloid deposition is the cause of this condition, which manifests with proteinuria that progresses to nephrotic syndrome and renal failure. Colchicine may greatly lessen the occurrence of the amyloid deposition.

O   **What connective tissue disease is characterized by sicca complex and anti-SSA and SSB autoantibodies?**

Sjogren's syndrome.

O   **Which vasculitis affects predominantly the extracranial vessels?**

Takayasu's arteritis.

O   **A patient presents with pain along the radial aspect of the wrist extending into the forearm. What is the diagnostic test of choice?**

Finkelstein's test. This test confirms the diagnosis of deQuervain's tenosynovitis, an overuse inflammation of the extensor pollicis brevis and the abductor pollicis where they pass along the groove of the radial styloid. Finkelstein's test is performed by instructing the patient to make a fist with his thumb tucked inside the other fingers. The test is positive if pain is reproduced when the examiner gently deviates the fist in the ulnar direction.

O   **In carpal tunnel syndrome, Tinel's sign is produced by tapping the volar wrist over the median nerve. If the test is positive, what does the patient experience?**

Paresthesias extending into the index and long fingers.

O   **What are the three most common cervical problems that produce pain radiating to the shoulder?**

Degenerative disease of the C-spine, degenerative disc disease, and herniated nucleus pulposus.

O   **What herniated cervical disc causes pain that mimics the pain of a rotator cuff injury?**

C5–C6.

GENITOURINARY

○ **What is the most common cause of acute renal failure?**

Acute tubular necrosis. This occurs after toxic or ischemic renal injuries caused by shock, surgery, or rhabdomyolysis.

○ **What percentage of men with BPH are afflicted with occult prostate cancer?**

10 to 30%.

○ **How well does the size of the prostate in BPH correlate with the symptoms?**

Not well. Symptoms can arise because of a small fibrous prostate as well as a large one. Additional symptoms can also develop as a result of median bar hypertrophy of the posterior vesicle neck, detrusor muscle decompensation, or instability.

○ **Which is the most common type of bladder cancer?**

Transitional cell carcinoma. Schistosomiasis infection, aniline dyes, smoking, and the male gender are all risk factors.

○ **Why is surgical correction of cryptorchidism important?**

Surgical correction is required to preserve fertility, but the procedure has no bearing on the future development of testicular cancer. Surgery must be performed before age 5 to preserve fertility.

○ **How is testicular torsion distinguished from epididymitis?**

By the rate of the pain onset. Torsional pain typically begins instantaneously at maximum intensity, whereas epididymal pain grows steadily over hours or days. In torsion you classically have a loss of the cremasteric reflex and a swollen firm high riding testical. Clinically, elevation of the scrotum may relieve pain related to epididymitis but is not effective with torsional pain (Prehn's sign). This test is not, however, considered diagnostic.

○ **How is testicular torsion diagnosed?**

By emergency surgical exploration. A doppler exam is also very sensative but should not delay treatment.

○ **What is the testicular viability after 6 hours, 10 hours and 24 hours of ischemia?**

6 – 80%
10 – 20%
24 – near 0%

○ **A 75 year old diabetic man presents with a fever, appearing toxic, complaining of acute onset of pain and swelling in his scrotum. He denies urinary symptoms and has a painful, erythematous, edematous scrotum with crepitus. What is the diagnosis and treatment?**

Fournier's gangrene. This usually presents in immunocompromised elderly patients and is due to infection or trauma of the perianal area. *Bacteriodes fragilis* and *E. coli* predominate. Treatment is supportive plus broad-spectrum parenteral antibiotics against anaerobes and gram negative enteric organisms. Urological consult for surgical debridement is necessary.

❍   **What is the most common cause of epididymitis in the following age groups: prepubertal boys, men under 35 and men over 35?**

Prepubertal boys: Coliform bacteria
Men younger than 35:   *Chlamydia* or *Neisseria* gonorrhea
Men older than 35:   Coliform bacteria

Epididymitis is also frequently caused by urinary reflux, prostatitis, or urethral instrumentation.

❍   **What does epididymitis in childhood suggest?**

Obstructive or fistulous urinary defects. Epididymitis is rare in children.

❍   **What does a blue dot sign suggest?**

Torsion of the epididymis or appendix testis. With transillumination of the testis, a blue reflection occurs. When detected early, a patient with torsion of the appendix testis will experience intense pain near the head of the epididymis or testis, which is frequently associated with a palpable tender nodule. If normal flow to the affected testis can be confirmed by a testicular ultrasound, immediate surgery can be avoided. Most appendages will calcify or degenerate within 10 to 14 day without harm to the patient.

❍   **How does the pain associated with epididymitis differ from that produced by prostatitis?**

Epididymitis: Pain begins in the scrotum or groin and radiates along the spermatic cord. It intensifies rapidly, is associated with dysuria, and is relieved with scrotal elevation (Prehn's sign).

Prostatitis: Patients have frequency, dysuria, urgency, bladder outlet obstruction, and retention. They may have low back pain and perineal pain associated with fever, chills, arthralgias, and myalgias.

❍   **What percentage of patients with epididymitis will also have pyuria?**

25%.

❍   **What four clinical findings are indicative of acute glomerulonephritis (GM)?**

1) Oliguria.
2) Hypertension.
3) Pulmonary edema.
4) Urine sediment containing RBCs, WBCs, protein, and RBC casts.

❍   **What is the most common cause of post-infectious glomerulonephritis?**

Poststreptococcal Group A ß-hemolytic. However, other infections may also produce GN-related infections. GN is caused by an immune complex deposition in glomeruli. Most patients recover renal function spontaneously within a few weeks.

❍   **What syndrome is characterized by a rapidly progressive, antiglomerular basement membrane antibody induced GN that is preceded by pulmonary hemorrhage and hemoptysis?**

Goodpasture's syndrome.

○   **What are some causes of false positive hematuria?**

Food coloring, beets, paprika, rifampin, phenothiazine, Dilantin, myoglobin, or menstruation.

○   **A urinalysis reveals RBC casts and dysmorphic RBCs. What is the probable origin of hematuria?**

Glomerulus.

○   **A 4 year old boy presents with a painless mass in his scrotum that fluctuates in size with palpation. The mass transilluminates. What is the probable diagnosis?**

A communicating hydrocele. An inguinal scrotal ultrasound should distinguish hydrocele from bowel, and a testicular nuclear scan should rule out testicular torsion.

○   **What percentage of urinary calculi are radiopaque?**

90%.

○   **What are the admission criteria for patients with renal calculi?**

Infection with concurrent obstruction, a solitary kidney and complete obstruction, uncontrolled pain, intractable emesis, or large stones. Only 10% of stones > 6 mm pass spontaneously. Other indications include renal insufficiency and complete obstruction or urinary extravasation, as demonstrated by the IVP.

○   **What percentage of patients with urinary calculi do not have hematuria?**

10%.

○   **A urinary pH of 7.3 is conducive to the formation of what kind of stones?**

Struvite and phosphate stones. Alkalotic urine actually inhibits the formation of uric acid and cysteine stones. Conversely, struvite and phosphate stones are inhibited by a more acidic urine.

○   **Which type of stone formation is caused by a genetic error?**

Cysteine stones. These stones are produced because there is an error in the transport of amino acids that results in cystinuria.

○   **Where is kidney stone formation most likely to occur?**

In the proximal portion of the collecting system.

○   **What is the 5 year recurrence rate for kidney stones?**

50%. The 10 year recurrence rate is 70%.

○   **What percentage of patients spontaneously pass kidney stones?**

80%. This is largely dependent on size. Seventy-five percent of stones less than 4 mm pass spontaneously, while only 10% of those larger than 6 mm pass spontaneously. Analgesics and increased fluid intake aid in outpatient management of kidney stones.

○   **What is the most common systemic cause of impotence?**

Diabetes.

O   **What is the postvoid residual volume that suggests urinary retention?**

A volume greater than 60 cc.

O   **What is the most common cause of nephrotic syndrome in children? In adults?**

Children: Minimal change disease. Adults: Idiopathic glomerulonephritis.

O   **Name some common nephrotoxic agents.**

Aminoglycosides, NSAIDs, contrast dye, and myoglobin.

O   **What is the definition of oliguria? Of anuria?**

Oliguria: Urine output < 500 mL/day
Anuria: Urine output < 100 mL/day

O   **When is a retrograde urethrogram necessary to evaluate a patient with a penile fracture?**

Patients with hematuria, blood at the urethral meatus, or the inability to void should undergo this procedure to rule out a urethral injury. A penile fracture is rupture of the corpus cavernosum with tearing of the tunica albuginea. It occurs as a result of a blunt trauma to the erect penis. Urethral injury occurs in approximately 10% of patients with a penile fracture.

O   **What is the initial treatment for priapism?**

Terbutaline, 0.25 to 0.5 mg subcutaneously.

O   **What are the causative organisms of prostatitis?**

E. coli (80%), *Klebsiella*, *Enterobacter*, *Proteus*, and *Pseudomonas*.

O   **What is the outpatient treatment for prostatitis?**

TMP-SMX, double strength po bid for 30 days; or ciprofloxacin, 500 mg po bid for 30 days; or norfloxacin, 400 mg po bid for 30 days.

O   **Which is the most common type of prostate cancer?**

Acinar adenocarcinoma (95%).

O   **Where is prostate cancer most commonly found?**

In the peripheral regions of the prostate.

O   **What is the most common cause of proteinuria?**

Pathology of the glomerulus. Other causes include tubular pathology or overproduction of protein.

O   **Outpatient management of pyelonephritis should be reserved for what patients?**

Young, otherwise healthy patients who are not vomiting, are hemodynamically stable, are defervesing with antipyretics, and are able to drink fluids. These patients should be treated with IV fluids, antipyretics, and a dose of IV antibiotics, such as gentamycin, a third-generation cephalosporin, or TMP-SMX.

○ **The rule of 2's is a wonderful pearl, described by Dr. David S. Howes of the University of Illinois, that explains the appropriate outpatient management for women who present at that institution with uncomplicated pyelonephritis. Outline the rule of 2's.**

1) Give 2 L of IV fluid.
2) Give 2 tablets of Tylenol 3.
3) Give 2 g of ceftriaxone.
4) If the patient can tolerate 2 glasses of water and his or her fever decreases by 2 degrees, give TMP-SMX double strength bid for 2 weeks and plan a follow-up in 2 days.

Editors' note: We provide 1 g of ceftriaxone or use other IV antibiotics.

○ **What are the risk factors for subclinical pyelonephritis?**

Multiple prior UTIs, longer duration of symptoms, recent pyelonephritis, diabetes, anatomic abnormalities, immunocompromised patients, and indigents.

○ **What is the most common cause of chronic renal failure?**

NIDDM.

○ **When are renal insufficiency symptoms displayed?**

When 90% of the nephrons have been destroyed. Hypertension, diabetes mellitus, glomerulonephritis, polycystic kidney disease, tubulointerstitial disease, and obstructive uropathy are all causes of chronic renal failure.

○ **What is the most common cause of intrinsic renal failure?**

Acute tubular necrosis (80 to 90%), resulting from an ischemic injury (the most common cause of ATN) or from a nephrotoxic agent. Less frequent causes of intrinsic renal failure (10 to 20%) include vasculitis, malignant hypertension, acute GN, or allergic interstitial nephritis.

○ **Name an abnormal ultrasound finding that suggests chronic renal failure?**

Kidneys < 9 cm in length are abnormal. A difference in length between the two kidneys of > 1.5 cm suggests unilateral kidney disease. Kidneys with a small or absent renal cortex are also indicative of chronic renal failure.

○ **What is the life expectancy of chronic renal patients after the disease has progressed to dialysis?**

Patients younger than 60 have a 4 to 5 year life expectancy. Patients over 60 have a 2 to 3 year life expectancy.

○ **If a urine dipstick is positive for blood, but a urine analysis is negative for RBCs, what is the probable disease?**

Rhabdomyolysis. Severe muscle damage can result in free myoglobin in the blood. Very high levels can lead to acute renal failure.

○ **What is the most common neoplasm in men under 30?**

Seminomas. This is also the most common type of testicular neoplasm. Peak incidence is between ages 20 and 40 with a smaller peak occurring below age 10. Ninety to 95% are germinal tumors. However, only 60 to 70% are germinal in children. Cryptorchidism is a significant risk factor for this cancer.

O   **What is the best tumor marker for testicular cancer?**

Placental alkaline phosphatase (PLAP). Seventy to 90% of patients with testicular cancer have elevated PLAP. Other tumor markers are a-fetoprotein and ß-hCG.

O   **Testicular torsion is most common in which age group?**

14-year-olds. Two-thirds of the cases occur in the second decade. The next most common group is newborns.

O   **T/F: Testicular torsion frequently follows a history of strenuous physical activity or occurs during sleep.**

True.

O   **T/F: Forty percent of patients with testicular torsion have a history of similar pain in the past that resolved spontaneously.**

True.

O   **What is the definitive treatment for testicular torsion?**

Bilateral orchiopexy in which the testes are surgically attached to the scrotum.

O   **What is an important difference between testicular teratomas in children and adults?**

In children, teratomas are benign lesions. In adults, they may metastasize.

O   **What is the most common cause of urethritis in males?**

Neisseria gonorrhoeae (gonococcal urethritis) or *Chlamydia trachomatis* (nongonococcal urethritis). Gonorrhea presents with a purulent discharge from the urethra, whereas *Chlamydia* is generally associated with a thinner, white mucous discharge. Treatment should cover both gonorrhea and *Chlamydia* because there is a high incidence of coinfection. Ceftriaxone for gonorrhea and doxycycline or tetracycline for *Chlamydia* are the drugs of choice.

O   **What is the most common cause of urinary tract infections (UTIs)?**

E. coli (80%). *E. coli* is also the most common cause of pyelonephritis and pyelitis because of its ascension from the lower urinary tract. *Staphylococcus saprophyticus* accounts for 5 to 15% of UTIs.

O   **Varicoceles are most common in which side of the scrotum?**

The left. Varicoceles are a collection of veins in the scrotum. These patients have a higher incidence of infertility, presumably because of the increased temperature of the testes surrounded by the warm blood of the varicocele. Incidentally, the left testes is the first to descend and also hangs lower than the right in the majority of men. Hernias are also more common on the left side, too.

O   **What is the mnemonic that refers to the correctable causes of urinary incontinence?**

D   delirium

I   infection
    atrophic urethritis and atrophic vaginitis
P   pharmaceuticals: sedatives, hypnotics, alcohol, diuretics and anticholinergics
P   psychologic disorders: depression, psychosis
E   endocrine disorders: hyperglycemia, hypercalcemia
R   restricted mobility
S   stool impaction

○   **What is the most common malignant renal tumor in children?**

Wilms' tumor is a highly malignant tumor of mixed histology. A suspected hereditary form of Wilms' tumor that is transmitted as an autosomal dominant disorder accounts for about 40 % of all tumors. An abdominal mass is the presenting complaint in these children with peak ages at diagnosis of 1 to 3 years.

○   **What is the most common cancer in young adult males?**

Testicular cancer is one of the leading cancers in incidence in young adult males with an average age of about 32 years. There is a significantly increased incidence of carcinoma developing in cryptorchid testes.

○   **The labs from a patient with hematuria show depressed levels of C3. What etiologies should you suspect?**

Chronic infection, lupus, post-streptococcal glomerulonephritis or membranoproliferative glomerulonephritis.

○   **What is the classic presentation of post-streptococcal glomerulonephritis (PSGN)?**

Sudden development of gross hematuria, hypertension, edema and renal insufficiency following a throat or skin infection with group A beta-hemolytic streptococcus. Patients frequently also have generalized complaints of fever, malaise, lethargy, abdominal pain, etc.

○   **How early in the development of "strep throat" will antibiotic therapy decrease the risk for PSGN?**

Antibiotics have not been found to decrease the risk for PSG.

○   **What is the most common form of lupus nephritis?**

Diffuse proliferative nephritis (WHO class IV). Unfortunately, this is also the most severe form.

○   **The biopsy of the kidney from a 24 year old male with nephrotic syndrome shows increased mesangial cells and, on immunofluorescence, C3 deposits in the mesangium. What is the man's diagnosis and prognosis?**

This man has membranoproliferative glomerulonephritis (a type of chronic glomerulonephritis). Prognosis is poor, with many patients progressing to end stage renal failure.

○   **What is the most common manifestation of Goodpasture's disease?**

Hemoptysis. These patients usually develop pulmonary hemorrhage before any signs of renal failure develop.

○   **What is the diagnostic triad of the nephrotic syndrome?**

Edema, hyperlipidemia, and proteinuria with hypoproteinemia.

❍   **How is renal tubular acidosis (RTA) classified?**

Into one of three types: Type 1-distal RTA, Type II-proximal RTA, or Type IV-mineralocorticoid deficiency.   There is no type III.

❍   **What are the mechanisms for the different types of RTA?**

In Type I, there is a deficiency in the secretion of the hydrogen ion by the distal tubule and collecting duct. In Type II, there is a decrease in the bicarbonate reabsorption in the proximal tubule.

❍   **Which isolated form of RTA will be most likely to lead to renal failure?**

Distal (Type I), though most cases of Type I RTA have an excellent prognosis.

❍   **A patient with nephrogenic diabetes insipidus has a serum sodium level of 117 mEq/l. How do you determine how much NaCl to administer to keep the risk of cerebral edema at a minimum?**

Amount of NaCl to add in mEq/l = 0.6 x wt. (in kg) x (140 - serum sodium).

❍   **What percentage of kidney transplants donated from a relative (usually a parent) are still functional after three years?**

75-80%.

❍   **Patients born with what disease is more likely to have horseshoe kidneys?**

Turner's syndrome.

❍   **What type of RTA usually presents as an isolated condition?**

Type I - distal RTA.

❍   **What are the characteristic acid-base electrolyte abnormalities associated with type I and type II RTA?**

Hypokalemic, hyperchloremic metabolic acidosis.

❍   **What are the characteristic acid-base/electrolyte abnormalities associated with type IV RTA?**

Hyperkalemic, hyperchloremic metabolic acidosis.

❍   **What is the underlying cause of type IV RTA?**

Decreased sodium reabsorption secondary to lack of aldosterone effect.

❍   **What diseases are associated with type IV RTA?**

Diseases of the adrenal gland; most commonly Addison's disease and Congenital Adrenal Hyperplasia.

❍   **What is the antihypertensive of choice in patient with chronic diabetic nephropathy?**

Angiotensin-converting enzyme inhibitors are preferred.

❍   **What treatments are used to ameliorate bleeding in a uremic patient?**

Dialysis may lessen bleeding as may DDAVP, cryoprecipitate or even platelet transfusions. Estrogens may lessen bleeding from angiodysplasia.

O   **What medications may be associated with hemolytic uremic syndrome?**

Mitomycin, estrogens and cyclosporin are known culprits.

O   **What does acute renal failure in a patient with alcoholic cirrhosis and a urine sodium of less than 10 suggest?**

Pre-renal azotemia or hepatorenal syndrome.

O   **Acute renal failure caused by Wegener's granulomatosis may respond best to what treatments?**

This is usually rapidly progressive GN and responds to high dose steroids and cyclophosphamide.

O   **Total and persistent anuria with renal failure should prompt a work up for what?**

These patients are presumed to be obstructed until proven otherwise.

O   **What co-morbid factors are likely to increase the risk of contrast induced ATN?**

Azotemia, diabetic nephropathy, CHF, multiple myeloma and dehydration.

O   **What are the causes of high levels of PTH in CRF?**

Hyperphosphatemia, hypocalcemia due to deficiency of vitamin D and parathyroid receptor resistance.

O   **What is the etiology of CRF associated with cerebral berry aneurysms?**

Adult Polycystic kidney disease is associated with cerebral berry aneurysms.

O   **What are the indications for emergent dialysis in ARF?**

Intractable acidosis, intractable hyperkalemia, intractable volume overload, BUN over 80-100, encephalopathy, pericarditis, uremic bleeding and certain intoxications.

O   **What is the major therapy used to treat allergic interstitial nephritis not responding to discontinuation of the culprit medication?**

Corticosteroids

O   **Sudden ARF, seen after initiation of ACE inhibitors, should prompt a work up for what diseases?**

ACE inhibitors are likely to cause ARF in patients with bilateral renal artery stenosis or renal artery stenosis in a solitary kidney.

O   **What type of ARF is usually seen with rhabdomyolysis?**

Acute tubular necrosis.

O   **Chronic renal failure with hypertension, small shrunken kidneys and gout at an early age should suggest what?**

Lead nephropathy should be considered.

○   **What factors predispose one to acute papillary necrosis?**

Analgesic abuse, sickle cell disease, diabetes mellitus, and alcoholism are usual predisposing factors.

○   **What major renal toxicity is seen with amphotericin B?**

Tubulointerstitial disease with a distal hypokalemic renal tubular acidosis and hypomagnesemia.

○   **Acute renal failure seen after use of cocaine may be due to what?**

Rhabdomyolysis leading to ATN.

○   **What are the major complications seen after placement of percutaneous venous catheters for hemodialysis or CVVH?**

Bleeding, infection with or without bacteremia are the usual complications. Pneumothorax may complicate catheters placed in the subclavian position. Venous stenosis is another potential hazard of these catheters when placed in the subclavian vein.

○   **What type of acute renal failure is seen in a patient with SLE?**

SLE with diffuse proliferative GN is likely to cause renal failure, nephrotic syndrome, hematuria and cylinduria. This may be treated with steroids and pulse IV cyclophosphamide.

○   **Which bacterium is associated with magnesium ammonium phosphate uretero lithiasis?**

Proteus, a bacterium that produces urease. These are infected stones and need to be removed. Antibiotics will help treat the UTI and will generally cease stone formation and urinary acidification. A urease inhibitor like acetohydroxamic acid will also prevent stone growth.

ENVIRONMENTAL

○ **At what altitude does acute mountain sickness typically develop?**

8000 feet. This may seem very low, when the death zone is over 25,000 feet

○ **What organ is most commonly affected in a radiation accident?**

The skin. Burns may take up to 2 weeks to become clinically apparent.

○ **What is the LD50 for a radiation victim?**

Within 60 days: 450 rads. LD90: 700 rads.

○ **What is the clinical significance of fixed, dilated pupils in a near drowning victim?**

Don't give up the ship! Ten to twenty percent of patients presenting with coma and fixed, dilated pupils recover completely. Asymptomatic patients should be observed for a minimum of 4 to 6 hours.

○ **What are the expected blood gas findings of a near drowning victim?**

Poor perfusion and hypoxia resulting in metabolic acidosis.

○ **Are abdominal thrusts, such as the Heimlich maneuver, indicated in a near drowning victim?**

No. Near drowning victims usually aspirate small quantities of water and no drainage procedure is helpful.

○ **A patient presents with two small puncture wounds surrounded by a halo lesion with a circular area of pallor surrounded by a ring of erythema. What is the diagnosis?**

Black widow spider envenomation.

○ **Describe the presentation of black widow spider envenomation versus scorpion envenomation.**

Black widow victims typically stay in one position for a few seconds to a few minutes before moving. They also have a halo lesion. Scorpion victims present with a constant writhing and abnormal eye movements.

○ **What are the indications for administering antivenin in a black widow spider envenomation?**

Severe pain, dangerous hypertension, pregnant women with moderate to severe envenomations, and pregnant women threatening abortion who are mildly symptomatic after an envenomation. Antivenin should be avoided in patients taking ß-adrenergic blocking agents because anaphylaxis will be difficult to treat if it occurs.

○ **What is the recommended treatment for brown recluse spider envenomations?**

Benign neglect. Dapsone, 25 to 100 mg orally for 1 to 2 weeks, has previously been recommended to prevent ulceration if started early, but recent studies have called this into question. It is especially useful if the face or the digits are involved. Dapsone is contraindicated in pregnant patients and in patients with G-

6-PD deficiency. Steroids, vasodilators, and antibiotics are generally not helpful. Avoid NSAIDs because this medication may induce bleeding. Early wide excision is ineffective, unnecessary, expensive, and it may result in increased disability or worsen scarring.

○   **Can a scratch from a rattlesnake result in a serious envenomation?**

Yes. However, up to 25% of rattlesnake bites do not result in envenomation.

○   **At what point should fasciotomy be considered for a rattlesnake bite victim?**

Only after increased compartment pressure that is unresponsive to limb elevation has been documented. Provide antivenin, 5 to 10 vials, and mannitol, 1 to 2 g/kg IV.

○   **Which patients, bitten by a rattlesnake, will develop serum sickness following antivenom administration? What is the treatment?**

Most patients who receive more than 5 vials will develop serum sickness. Symptoms may range from mildly viral-like to severe urticarial rash and arthralgias. Treatment includes antihistamines, corticosteroids, and analgesics.

○   **A patient presents with a bite wound that was inflicted while he was in a mental ward. What bacterium is likely?**

Eikenella corrodens is common in hospitalized and institutionalized patients. Most community acquired human bite infections are due to *Staphylococcus aureus* or *Streptococcus*.

○   **What is the frequency of eye injuries in lightning strike victims?**

Fifty percent develop structural eye lesions. Cataracts are the most common and develop within days to years. Unreactive dilated pupils may not equal death because transient autonomic instability may occur.

○   **What is the most common otologic injury in lightning strike victims?**

Tympanic membrane rupture (50%). Hemotympanum, basilar skull fracture, and acoustic and vestibular deficits may also occur.

○   **What is the most common arrhythmia found in patients with hypothermia?**

Atrial fibrillation. Other ECG findings include PAT, prolongation of the PR, QRS, or QT waves, decreased P wave amplitude, T wave changes, PVC's, or humped ST wave segment adjacent to the QRS complex (Osborn wave).

○   **What is the first line medical treatment of ventricular fibrillation for hypothermic patients?**

Bretylium, not lidocaine.

○   **A 14 year old baseball player is pulled off the field complaining of light-headedness, headache, nausea, and vomiting. Upon examination, the patient has a HR of 110, RR 22, BP of 90/60, and is afebrile. Profuse sweating is noted. What is the diagnosis?**

Heat exhaustion. Treat with IV fluid.

○   **A 27 year old marathon runner presents confused and combative. Her temperature is 105°F. Why must renal function be monitored?**

This patient has heatstroke. Rhabdomyolysis may occur 2 to 3 days after injury. Recall that in heatstroke, volume depletion and dehydration may not always occur.

❍ **What is the treatment for heatstroke?**

Cool sponging, ice packs to groin and axilla, fanning, and iced gastric lavage. Antipyretics are not useful.

❍ **A 12 year old boy presents with fatigue, fever, headache, pruritic rash, and joint aches. Examination reveals multiple sites of lymphadenopathy. The patient cannot recall any past medical problems. Just as you are about to leave the room, scratching your head, Mom says "Oh, he was stung by a bee 2 weeks ago. What is your diagnosis?**

Serum-sickness-like delayed reaction.

❍ **How should a honeybee's stinger be removed?**

Scrape it out. Squeezing with a tweezers or finger may increase envenomation.

❍ **A 4 year old presents with an itching lesion on the legs and waist. Upon examination, you find hemorrhagic puncta surrounded by urticarial and erythematous patches following a zig-zag pattern. Your treatment?**

Starch baths at bedtime are used to treat pruritus of flea bites.

❍ **A color-blind, 36 year old Texan presents with a history of snake bite. He says the snake was as big as a telephone pole, had fangs like a lion, and was striped like a zebra. On examination, you find ptosis, slurred speech, dysphagia, myalgia, and dilated pupils. What snake bit this man?**

Most likely a coral snake.

❍ **An Osborn (J) wave seen on ECG is associated with what disorder?**

Hypothermia.

❍ **Hypothermia is defined as a core temperature below:**

35°C.

❍ **Heat loss can occur via radiation, convection, conduction, and evaporation. Which of these accounts for the greatest loss?**

Radiation. However, if the patient is not perspiring, convection accounts for the greatest loss, and if immersed, conduction does.

❍ **A 4 year old bites into an extension cord and receives a burn on the lips. What specific concern do you have?**

Delayed rupture of the labial artery may occur 3 to 5 days after injury.

❍ **How is a sodium metal wound debrided?**

Cover with mineral oil and excise retained metal fragments.

❍ **Is lightning AC or DC?**

DC. It may cause asystole and respiratory arrest.

○ **What type of arrhythmia is expected with AC shock?**

Ventricular fibrillation.

○ **How long should an asymptomatic lightning strike victim be monitored?**

Several hours as CHF may be delayed.

○ **What neurologic injury may be expected in a lightning injury?**

Lower and upper extremity paralysis due to vascular spasm.

○ **What lab workup should be considered for a lightning victim?**

CBC, BUN/Cr, UA (check myoglobin), CPK-MM, MB, ECG, and CT if change in sensorium.

○ **What are the signs and symptoms of CO poisoning?**

Headache, nausea, vomiting, flu-like symptoms, syncope, tachypnea, tachycardia, coma, circulatory vascualar collapse, and respiratory failure. Presentation depends on degree of CO poisoning.

○ **What is the most common cause of death in CO poisoning?**

Cardiac arrhythmias.

○ **How is topical phenol exposure treated?**

Isopropyl alcohol, glycerol, or polyethlene glycol mixture are used in the emergency department for carbolic acid exposure. Water and olive oil can be useful in the field.

○ **In which two plant ingestions is ipecac contraindicated?**

Jequirity bean (alkaline) and hemlocks (may induce seizures).

HEMATOLOGY AND ONCOLOGY

○ **What four types of blood loss indicate a bleeding disorder?**

1) Spontaneous bleeding from many sites.
2) Bleeding from non-traumatic sites.
3) Delayed bleeding several hours after trauma.
4) Bleeding into deep tissues or joints.

○ **What common drugs have been implicated to acquired bleeding disorders?**

Ethanol, ASA, NSAIDs, warfarin, and antibiotics.

○ **Mucocutaneous bleeding, including petechiae, ecchymoses, epistaxis, GI, GU, and menorrhagia, indicate what coagulation abnormalities?**

Qualitative or quantitative platelet disorders.

○ **Delayed bleeding and bleeding into joints or potential spaces, such as the retroperitoneum, suggest what type of bleeding disorder?**

Coagulation factor deficiency.

○ **What is primary hemostasis?**

The platelet interaction with the vascular subendothelium that results in the formation of a platelet plug at the site of injury.

○ **What four components are required for primary hemostasis?**

1) Normal vascular subendothelium (collagen).
2) Functional platelets.
3) Normal von Willebrand factor (connects the platelet to the endothelium via glycoprotein Ib).
4) Normal Fibrinogen (connects platelets to each other via glycoprotein IIB-IIIA).

○ **What is the end-product of secondary hemostasis (coagulation cascade)?**

Cross-linked fibrin.

○ **What is the principle physiologic activator of the fibrinolytic system?**

Tissue plasminogen activator (tPA). Endothelial cells release tPA, which converts plasminogen, adsorbed in the fibrin clot, to plasmin. Plasmin degrades fibrinogen and fibrin monomer into fibrin degradation products (FDPs—once called fibrin split products) and cross-linked fibrin into D-dimers.

○ **Below what platelet count is spontaneous hemorrhage likely to occur?**

< 10,000/mm3.

❍   **It is generally agreed that most patients with active bleeding and platelet counts < 50,000/mm3 should receive platelet transfusion. How much will the platelet count be raised for each unit of platelets infused?**

10,000/mm3.

❍   **What patients with thrombocytopenia are unlikely to respond to platelet infusions?**

Those with antiplatelet antibodies (ITP or hypersplenism).

❍   **How can an overdose of warfarin be treated? What are the advantages and disadvantages of each treatment?**

Fresh frozen plasma (FFP) or Vitamin K. However, if there are no signs of bleeding, temporary discontinuation may be all that is necessary. Treatment depends on the severity of symptoms, not the degree of prolongation of the prothrombin time (PT).

FFP advantages: Rapid repletion of coagulation factors and control of hemorrhage
FFP disadvantages: Volume overload, possible viral transmission

Vitamin K advantages: Ease of administration
Vitamin K disadvantages: Possible anaphylaxis when given IV; delayed onset of 12 to 24 hours; effects may last up to 2 weeks, making anticoagulation of the patient difficult or impossible.

❍   **What is the only coagulation factor not synthesized by hepatocytes?**

Factor VIII.

❍   **Which four hemostatic alterations are seen in patients with liver disease?**

1) Decreased protein synthesis leading to coagulation factor deficiency
2) Thrombocytopenia
3) Increased fibrinolysis
4) Vitamin K deficiency

❍   **What five treatments are available to bleeding patients with liver disease?**

1) Transfusion with Packed RBC's (maintains hemodynamic stability)
2) Vitamin K
3) Fresh frozen plasma
4) Platelet transfusion
5) DDAVP (Desmopressin)

❍   **What hemostasis test is most often prolonged in uremic patients?**

Bleeding time.

❍   **What treatment options are available to patients with renal failure and coagulopathy?**

1) Dialysis
2) Optimize hematocrit (by recombinant human erythropoietin or transfusion with PRBCs)
3) Desmopressin
4) Conjugated estrogens

Cryoprecipitate and platelet transfusions if hemorrhage is life threatening.

○   **What are the clinical complications of DIC?**

Bleeding, thrombosis, and purpura fulminans.

○   **Which three laboratory studies are most helpful in diagnosing DIC?**

1) Prothrombin time (prolonged)
2) Platelet count (usually low)
3) Fibrinogen level (low)

○   **What are the most common hemostatic abnormalities in patients infected with HIV?**

Thrombocytopenia and acquired circulating anticoagulants (causes prolongation of the PTT).

○   **What is the pentad of Thrombotic thrombocytopenic purpura (TTP)?**

1) Fever
2) Thrombocytopenia
3) Neurologic symptoms
4) Renal insufficiency
5) Microangiopathic hemolytic anemia (MAHA)

○   **What is the leading cause of death in hemophiliacs?**

AIDS.

○   **What is the most common inherited bleeding disorder?**

Von Willebrand disease.

○   **Seventy to 80% of patients with von Willebrand disease have type I. What is the currently approved mode of therapy for bleeding in these patients? What is the dose?**

DDAVP, 0.3 μg/kg IV or subcutaneously every 12 hours for 3 to 4 doses.

○   **What is the most common hemoglobin variant?**

Hemoglobin S (valine substituted for glutamic acid in the sixth position on the ß-chain).

○   **Which clinical crises are seen in patients with sickle cell disease?**

1) Vasoocclusive (thrombotic)
2) Hematologic (sequestration and aplastic)
3) Infectious

○   **Which is the most common type of sickle cell crisis?**

Vasoocclusive (average: 4 attacks/year).

○   **What percentage of patients with sickle cell disease have gallstones?**

75% (only 10% are symptomatic).

○   **What is the only painless type of vasoocclusive crisis?**

CNS crisis (most commonly cerebral infarction in children and cerebral hemorrhage in adults).

○   **What are the four mainstays of therapy for a patient in sickle cell crisis?**

1) Hydration
2) Analgesia
3) Oxygen (only beneficial if patient is hypoxic)
4) Cardiac monitoring (if patient has history of cardiac disease or is having chest pain)

○   **What is the most commonly encountered sickle hemoglobin variant?**

Sickle cell trait.

○   **What is the most common human enzyme defect?**

Glucose-6-phosphate dehydrogenase (G-6-PD) deficiency.

○   **What drugs should be avoided in patients with G-6-PD deficiency?**

1) Drugs that induce oxidation
2) Sulfa
3) Antimalarials
4) Pyridium
5) Nitrofurantoin

○   **What is the most useful test to ascertain hemolysis and a normal marrow response?**

The reticulocyte count.

○   **What is the most common morphologic abnormality of red cells in hemolytic states?**

Spherocytes.

○   **What is the most common clinical presentation of TTP (thrombotic thrombocytopenic purpura)?**

Neurologic symptoms including headache, confusion, cranial nerve palsies, coma, and seizures.

○   **What syndrome is suggested in child who is 6 months to 4 years old with an antecedent URI, fever, acute renal failure, microangiopathic hemolytic anemia (MAHA), and thrombocytopenia?**

Hemolytic uremic syndrome.

○   **What malignancy is most frequently associated with MAHA?**

Gastric adenocarcinoma.

○   **What is the most common worldwide cause of hemolytic anemia?**

Malaria.

○   **What components of whole blood are used for transfusion?**

1) RBCs
2) Platelets

3) Plasma
4) Cryoprecipitate

○   **How much will the infusion of 1 unit of PRBCs raise the hemoglobin and hematocrit in a 70 kg patient?**

Hemoglobin: 1 g/dL. Hematocrit: 3%.

○   **What are the three conditions under which the transfusion of PRBCs should be considered?**

1) Acute hemorrhage (blood loss > 1500 mL)
2) Surgical blood loss > 2 L
3) Chronic anemia (Hgb < 7 to 8 g/dL, symptomatic, or with underlying cardiopulmonary disease)

○   **What five factors indicate the need to type and cross-match blood in the emergency department?**

1) Evidence of shock from any cause
2) Known blood loss > 1,000 mL
3) Gross GI bleeding
4) Hgb < 10; Hct < 30
5) Potential of surgery with further significant blood loss

○   **What are the five contents of cryoprecipitate?**

1) Factor VIII C
2) Von Willebrand factor
3) Fibrinogen
4) Factor XIII
5) Fibronectin

○   **What is the first step in treating all immediate transfusion reactions?**

Stop the transfusion.

○   **What infection carries the highest risk for transmission by blood transfusion?**

Hepatitis C (1/3300 units).

○   **What is the current recommended emergency replacement therapy for massive hemorrhage?**

Type-specific, uncrossmatched blood. Type O negative, whereas immediately life-saving in certain situations, carries the risk of life-threatening transfusion reactions.

○   **In current practice, what blood components are routinely infused along with PRBCs in a patient receiving a massive transfusion?**

None. The practice of routinely using platelet transfusion and fresh frozen plasma is costly, dangerous, and unwarranted.

○   **What is the only crystalloid fluid compatible with PRBCs?**

Normal saline.

○   **What condition should be suspected in a patient with multiple myeloma who presents with paraparesis, paraplegia, and urinary incontinence?**

Acute spinal cord compression. This condition occurs primarily with multiple myeloma and lymphoma, it is also encountered with carcinomas of the lung, breast, and prostate.

O   **What are the two most common neoplasms that cause pericardial effusion and tamponade?**

Carcinoma of the lung and breast.

O   **A 48 year old male smoker presents with a headache, swelling of the face and arms, and a feeling of fullness in his face and neck. He is noted to have JVD upon physical examination and papilledema upon funduscopic examination. What is the most likely diagnosis?**

Superior vena cava syndrome.

O   **What is the most common cause of hyperviscosity syndrome?**

Waldenstrom macroglobulinemia.

O   **What should be considered in a patient who presents in a coma and with anemia and rouleaux formation in the peripheral blood smear?**

Hyperviscosity syndrome.

O   **Vitamin K dependent factors of the clotting cascade include:**

X, IX, VII and II. Remember 1972.

O   **A classic hemophiliac suffers a major head injury. What treatment should be given?**

Give factor VIII, 50 U/kg.

O   **What is von Willebrand's disease?**

An autosomal dominant disorder of platelet function. It causes bleeding from mucous membranes, menorrhagia, and increased bleeding from wounds. Patients with von Willebrand's disease have less (or dysfunctional) von Willebrand's factor.

Von Willebrand's factor is a plasma protein secreted by endothelial cells and serves 2 functions: (1) It is required for platelets to adhere to collagen at the site of vascular injury which is the initial step in forming a hemostatic plug. (2) It forms complexes in plasma with factor VIII which are required to maintain normal factor VIII levels.

O   **What factors are deficient in classic hemophilia, Christmas disease, and von Willebrand's disease, respectively?**

Classic hemophilia: Factor VIII
Christmas disease: Factor IX
Von Willebrand's disease: Factor VIIIc and von Willebrand's cofactor

O   **What pathway involves factors VIII and IX?**

Intrinsic pathway.

O   **What effect does deficiency of factors VIII and IX have on PT and on PTT?**

Deficiency leads to an increase in PTT.

○   **What pathway does the PT measure? What factor is unique to this pathway?**

Extrinsic pathway. Factor VII.

○   **What blood product is given when the coagulation abnormality is unknown?**

Fresh frozen plasma.

○   **What agent can be used to treat mild hemophilia A and von Willebrand's disease type 1?**

D-Amino-8, D-arginine vasopressin (DDAVP) induces a rapid rise in factor VIII levels.

○   **Where is a parotid gland tumor most likely to develop?**

The superficial lobe, which is located just below the ear lobe. Forty percent of parotid gland tumors are malignant. All tumors, benign or malignant, should be removed.

○   **What is the most common type of malignant parotid gland tumor?**

Mucoepidermoid carcinoma. Other types of malignant tumors are acinic cell carcinoma, adenocarcinoma, malignant mixed tumor, adenoid cystic carcinoma, and epidermoid carcinoma.

○   **What age and ethnic group is at greatest risk for esophageal cancer?**

Elderly African-Americans. Their risk is four times higher than in elderly Caucasian-Americans. Other ethnic groups at higher risk include Chinese, Iranians, and South Africans.

○   **Which are the most common cancer cell types of the esophagus?**

Squamous carcinoma, occurring most frequently in African Americans, while adenocarcinoma is most common type in Caucasian Americans.

○   **Where does esophageal cancer most commonly metastasizes to?**

Lungs, liver, and bones.

○   **Which types of cancer metastasize to bone?**

Prostate, thyroid, breast, lung, and kidney. (Remember: "P.T. Barnum Loves Kids").

○   **A hard mass in the upper outer quadrant of the right breast of a 45 year old woman is detected. What are the next steps?**

Mammogram followed by an excision biopsy. A negative needle aspiration alone cannot rule out malignancy. False negative rates for fine needle biopsy are 3-30%.

○   **What is the most common histologic type of breast cancer?**

Infiltrating ductal carcinoma (70-80%). Subtypes are colloid, medullary, papillary, and tubular.

○   **A 30 year old female comes to you worried that she has breast cancer in both breasts. She is concerned because of a yellowish, green discharge from her nipples, soreness in the upper outer quadrants of her breasts, what she calls a "lumpy" feeling upon self examination, and mild swelling that seems to come and go. Further questioning reveals that her pain begins 1 week before she**

menstruates, then disappears when her menses is over. Understandably concerned, your patient wants to know when she can start chemotherapy. What do you tell her?

Hold off on the chemo! She most likely has fibrocystic breast changes. Put her mind at rest, and let her know that fibrocystic changes are not a pre-malignant syndrome.

○   **What is the most common lung cancer in non-smokers?**

Adenocarcinoma. Smoking is a great risk factor for all lung cancers, with the exception of adenocarcinoma.

○   **A 44 year old gentleman presents with a deep, dull pain in the center of his abdomen that radiates to his back and will not go away. He states he has not "felt like himself" for a few weeks and that he has been kind of depressed. He also notes that he has lost a lot of weight; about 30 pounds in 3 weeks. On physical examination, you palpate an enlarged liver and an abdominal mass in the epigastrium. What is your diagnosis?**

Most likely pancreatic cancer. The ability to palpate a mass suggests that the disease has progressed too far to be surgically resectable. Carcinoma of the pancreas can only be resected in 20% of patients. Depression often occurs before the onset of other symptoms.

○   **Where is the most common anatomic and histologic location of pancreatic cancer?**

Head of the pancreas (80%). Pancreatic cancer is generally adenocarcinoma and located in the ducts.

○   **What gender and age group most commonly presents with pancreatic cancer?**

Middle aged men.

○   **What is the 5 year survival rate for pancreatic carcinoma?**

2 to 5%. Symptoms generally do not show up until the tumor has metastasized or spread to local structures.

○   **What is the most common endocrine tumor of the pancreas?**

An insulinoma. However, only 10% are malignant. Gastrinomas are the second most common and have a malignancy rate of 50%. Vipomas and glucagonomas are also endocrine tumors of the pancreas.

○   **Glucagonomas arise from which type of cells?**

Alpha cells. The majority are malignant. Increased plasma glucagon is diagnostic.

○   **Pheochromocytomas produce what compounds?**

Catecholamines. This group of chemicals result in increased blood pressure, perspiration, heart palpitations, anxiety, and weight loss.

○   **Where are the majority of pheochromocytomas located?**

Ninety percent are found in the adrenal medulla. The remainder are located in other tissues originating from neural crest cells.

○   **What is the pheochromocytoma rule of 10's?**

10% are malignant; 10% are multiple or bilateral; 10% are extra-adrenal; 10% occur in children; 10% recur after surgical removal and 10% are familial.

○   **Where does hepatic cancer most commonly metastasize to?**

The lungs (bronchiogenic carcinoma).

○   **Clinically, how is right sided colon cancer differentiated from left sided?**

Right sided lesions present with occult bleeding, weakness, anemia, dyspepsia, palpable abdominal mass, and dull abdominal pain. Left sided lesions present with visible blood, obstructive symptoms, and noticeable changes in bowel habits. Pencil thin stools are also common.

○   **Is a villous, tubulovillous, or tubular adenoma more likely to become malignant?**
40% of villous adenomas will become malignant, compared to 22% of tubulovillous adenomas and 5% of tubular adenomas.

○   **Which are more likely to turn malignant, pedunculated or sessile lesions?**

Sessile.

○   **Where are the majority of colorectal cancers found?**

In the rectum (30%), ascending colon (25%), sigmoid colon (20%), descending colon (15%), and transverse colon (10%).

○   **Where are soft tissue sarcomas most often found?**

In the lower extremities. They are fairly rare. The most common sarcomas are liposarcomas, leiomyosarcomas, fibrosarcomas, rhabdomyosarcomas, and malignant fibrous histiocytomas.

○   **What percentage of those with familial polyposis will go on to develop colorectal carcinoma?**

100%. Due to the imminent development of cancer, such patient should be advised to have a total colectomy and ileostomy.

○   **A 64 year old male presents with jaundice, upper GI bleeding, anemia, a palpable non-tender gallbladder, a palpable liver, and rapid weight loss. What is your diagnosis?**

This is the clinical picture of a tumor of the ampulla of Vater.

○   **Which cell markers can be used to follow the progression of germinal tumors of the testes?**

Serum α-fetoprotein or human chorionic gonadotropin. HCG may be elevated in both seminomas and non-seminomas, but α-fetoprotein will never be elevated in seminomas.

○   **Serum acid phosphatase is a common cell marker used to follow prostate cancer. What other diseases can cause the serum acid phosphatase level to rise?**

Benign prostatic hypertrophy, bone tumors, multiple myeloma, and urinary retention.

○   **What lab result indicates bony metastasis?**

Increased alkaline phosphatase.

○   **What percentage of palpable prostate nodules are malignant?**

50%. Surgical cure of patients who present with asymptomatic nodules and no metastasis is attempted with radical prostatectomy or radiation therapy.

○   **Why are red cell transfusions rarely required to treat iron deficiency anemia?**

Nucleated red blood cells and reticulocytes appear in the blood stream within 72 hours after starting oral iron replacement.

○   **What are the three major proteins that inhibit clotting?**

Antithrombin III, Protein C, and Protein S.

○   **What does deficiency of antithrombin III, protein C or protein S increases the risk of?**

Venous thrombosis.

○   **Why should warfarin, as an <u>initial</u> treatment for venous thrombosis secondary to protein C deficiency, be avoided?**

It may, by inhibiting the synthesis of protein C, lead to paradoxical hypercoagulability. Always treat with heparin before warfarin.

○   **What is the most important aspect of treating DIC?**

Attempting to correct the underlying disorder (usually septic shock).

○   **What is the characteristic bone marrow finding in idiopathic thrombocytopenic purpura (ITP)?**

Increased or normal megakaryocytes.

○   **What are the potential treatment modalities for ITP?**

Gammaglobulins, steroids, radioactive phosphorus, fresh frozen plasma and plasmapheresis.

○   **How do gamma globulin and steroids work in the treatment of ITP?**

They block the uptake of antibody-coated platelets by splenic macrophages.

○   **Under what circumstances is a bone marrow aspirate crucial in the diagnosis and treatment of ITP?**

If treatment with steroids is planned, a bone marrow aspirate must be performed to rule out leukemia. Steroid treatment can delay the diagnosis of an occult leukemia.

○   **What are the signs and symptoms of splenic sequestration crisis?**

Pallor, weakness, lethargy, disorientation, shock, decreased level of consciousness, enlarged spleen.

○   **What is the treatment of splenic sequestration crisis?**

Rapid infusion of saline and transfusion of red cells or whole blood.

○   **In anemia, which way is the oxygen dissociation curve shifted?**

The right (affinity of hemoglobin for oxygen is decreased).

○ **What is the progression of biochemical and hematological events in iron deficiency anemia?**

Decreased serum ferritin, then decreased serum iron and total iron binding capacity, followed by a fall in MCV and MCH, and a rise in RDW. Thrombocytosis may occur.

○ **What are the most common sites for bleeding in patients with hemophilia?**

Joints, muscles, and subcutaneous tissue.

○ **There is simultaneous activation of coagulation and fibrinolysis in what pathologic condition?**

Disseminated intravascular coagulation.

○ **What are some common ischemic complications of DIC?**

Renal failure, seizures, coma, pulmonary infarction, and hemorrhagic necrosis of the skin.

○ **What are the common lab findings in DIC?**

Decreased platelets, increased PT and PTT, decreased fibrinogen and increased FSP (Fibrin split products).

○ **What is the most common familial and congenital abnormality of the red blood cell membrane?**

Hereditary spherocytosis.

○ **What are the major complications of hereditary spherocytosis?**

Hyperbilirubinemia in the newborn period, hemolytic anemia, gallstones, and susceptibility to aplastic and hypoplastic crises secondary to viral infections.

○ **Hemosiderosis from chronic transfusion therapy for thalassemia can be successfully treated with:**

Subcutaneous deferoxamine via pump.

○ **A cure for thalassemia major is possible with what treatment?**

Bone marrow transplant.

○ **What is the incompatibility risk of typed blood, screened blood and fully crossmatched blood?**

The risk of incompatibility of ABO/Rh-compatible blood is 0.1% if the patient has never been transfused. The risk increases to 1.0% if the patient has had a previous transfusion. Adding a negative antibody screen decreases the risk to 0.06%. Fully crossmatched blood should carry a risk less than 0.05%.

○ **What is the most common blood group? What percentage of blood is Rh positive?**

The most common blood group is type O; 45% of whites, 49% of African-Americans, 79% of Native Americans and 40% of Orientals are blood type O. Approximately 85% of the population are Rh positive and 15% Rh negative.

○ **At what hematocrit level is the oxygen treatment capacity maximum?**

It occurs at a hematocrit of 30%.

○   **What does Prothrombin Time (PT) measure? How is it performed?**

PT measures the extrinsic and common pathways of the coagulation system.   The time to clot formation is measured after the addition of thromboplastin. If the concentration of factors V, VII, IX, and X are significant lower than usual, the PT may be prolonged.

○   **What does Activated Partial Thromboplastin Time (PTT) measure? How is it performed?**

PTT measures the intrinsic and common pathways of the coagulation cascade.   After the blood sample is exposed to celite for activation and a reagent is added, the clot formation is measured. When factors II, V, VIII, IX, X, XI, XII, or fibrinogen are deficient, the PTT may be prolonged.

○   **What are the indications for the administration of FFP?**

*   Replacement of isolated factor deficiencies.
*   Reversal of coumadin effect.
*   Treatment of pathological hemorrhage in patients who have received massive transfusion.
*   Use in antithrombin III deficiency.
*   Treatment of immunodeficiencies.

○   **What are the indications for cryoprecipitate administration?**

Treatment of congenital or acquired fibrinogen, and factor VIII deficiencies. Cryoprecipitate can also be administered prophylactically for nonbleeding perioperative or peripartum patients with congenital fibrinogen deficiencies or for Von Willebrand's disease that is unresponsive to desmopressin (DDAVP).

○   **Is it necessary to administer ABO-specific platelets?**

The administration of ABO-specific platelets is not required because platelet concentrates contain few red blood cells. However, the administration of pooled platelet components of various ABO types can transfuse plasma containing anti-A and/or anti-B, resulting in alloimmunization and a weakly positive direct antiglobulin test.

○   **What are the indications for platelet transfusion?**

Platelets should be administered to correct thrombocytopenia or platelet dysfunction (thrombocytopathy). Perioperative factors to consider for the transfusion of platelets for counts between 50-100 x 109/L are the type of surgery, anticipated and actual blood loss, extent of microvascular bleeding, presence of medications (e.g. aspirin) and disorders (e.g. uremia) known to affect platelet function and coagulation. The prophylactic administration of platelets is not recommended in patients with chronic thrombocytopenia caused by increased platelet destruction (e.g., idiopathic thrombocytopenic purpura).

○   **What is the potassium load with transfusion?**

It depends on the age of the blood. The potassium load in 1 week old whole blood is 4.5-4.8 mEq/unit. With the transfusion of 20 units of 1 week old whole blood, the potassium load is 60 mEq (presuming no urinary output). If these 20 units are 21 days old, the potassium load is 110 mEq.

○   **What is the incidence of transmission of HIV types I and II with transfusion?**

The most recent estimates are 1 in 450,000 to 1 in 600,000. Prior to the implementation of testing for HIV-I p24 antigen in 1996, approximately 18 to 27 infected donor units, not detected by testing, were made available for transfusion annually. Antigen testing reduces that number by 25%.

O **What is the incidence of hemolytic transfusion reactions (HTR)?**

1 in 33,000 units. The HTR is potentially life threatening and often regarded the most serious complication of transfusions. Fifty one percent of 256 transfusion associated deaths reported to the US Food and Drug Administration between 1976 and 1985 resulted from acute hemolysis following the transfusion of ABO-incompatible blood or plasma.

O **What are the types of HTR's and what is the pathophysiology of each one?**

HTR's are divided in two types of reactions: 1) intravascular hemolysis and 2) extravascular hemolysis. Intravascular hemolysis occurs when the antibody coated RBC is destroyed by the activation of the complement system. Extravascular hemolysis destroys antibody coated RBC's via phagocytosis by macrophages in the reticuloendothelial system. In most HTR's, some RBC's are probably destroyed by both mechanisms.

O **What is the treatment for HTR's?**

The transfusion should be stopped immediately. Hypotension should be treated with fluids, inotropes or other blood as appropriate. Renal output should be maintained with crystalloids, diuretics or dopamine, as necessary. Component therapy should be used if DIC develops.

O **What causes febrile reactions to blood and what are the incidences?**

The febrile reaction is the most common mild transfusion reaction and occurs in 0.5% to 4% of transfusions. It is caused by alloantibodies (leukoagglutinins) to white blood cell, platelet or other donor plasma antigens. Fever is presumably caused by pyrogens liberated from lysed cells. It occurs more commonly in previously transfused patients.

O **What is the MOPP regimen of drugs used to treat?**

Hodgkin's lymphoma. MOPP stands for Mechlorethamine, Oncovin, Prednisone, and Procarbazine.

O **After a course of chemotherapy, your patient has had a course of fever, neutropenia and granulocytopenia for over a week, despite antibiotic usage. What should you do now?**

Add Amphotericin B for a presumed fungal infection while continuing your search for the source of the infection.

O **What is the mechanism of action of methotrexate?**

It inhibits the enzyme dihydrofolate reductase.

O **A patient on chemotherapy for his Burkitt's lymphoma is found to be hyperkalemic, hypocalcemic, hyperphosphatemic, and hyperuracemic. What is the presumptive diagnosis?**

Tumor lysis syndrome.

O **What percent of children with acute lymphoblastic leukemia (ALL) are cured by conventional chemotherapy?**

70%.

○   **What is graft versus host disease (GVHD)?**

Engraftment of immunocompetent donor cells into an immunocompromised host, resulting in cell-mediated cytotoxic destruction of host cells if an immunologic incompatibility exists.

○   **When does acute GVHD present and what are the typical manifestations?**

Acute GVHD typically occurs around day 19 (median), just as the patient begins to engraft, and is characterized by erythroderma, cholestatic hepatitis, and enteritis.

○   **What is the clinical definition of chronic GVHD (cGVHD)?**

As early as 60-70 days status-post engraftment, the patient exhibits signs of a systemic autoimmune process, manifesting as Sjogren's syndrome, systemic lupus erythrematosus, scleroderma, primary biliary cirrhosis, and commonly experiences recurrent infection with encapsulated bacteria, fungus, or viruses.

○   **How long is immunosuppressive treatment required for BMT recipients?**

Usually 6 -12 months or until a state of tolerance is attained.

○   **Treatment with methotrexate may result in what complications and how is it treated?**

Methotrexate may worsen renal impairment, resulting in fluid retention and may aggravate existing mucositis. In these situations, rescue of the dihydrofolate reductase system with leucovorin is indicated.

○   **What drugs may exacerbate the nephrotoxicity of cyclosporine?**

Aminogylcosides, amphotericin B, acyclovir, digoxin, furosemide, indomethacin, and trimethoprim.

○   **What are the long term effects of corticosteroid treatment?**

Growth failure, Cushingoid appearance, hypertension, cataracts, GI bleeding, pancreatitis, psychosis, hyperglycemia, osteoporosis, aseptic necrosis of the femoral head, and suppression of the pituitary-adrenal axis.

○   **What are the most common types of infections seen post transplant engraftment (day 0-30)?**

Oral thrush, bacterial sepsis, catheter infections, fungal infections, pneumonia, and sinusitis.

○   **What are the most common types of infections seen in post transplant postengraftment (day 30-100)?**

CMV and EBV infection, viral hepatitis, toxoplasmosis, diffuse interstitial pneumonia, and cystitis.

○   **What are the most common types of infections seen posttransplant postengraftment (day 100-365)?**

Varicella, herpes, CMV, toxoplasmosis, *Pneumocystis carinii* pneumonia, viral hepatitis, and common bacterial infections.

○   **What are the most common cancers of the small bowel?**

Adenocarcinoma, followed by carcinoid, lymphoma, and leiomyosarcoma. The small bowel is not a common site for malignancy and accounts for only 2% of all GI malignancies.

○   **Where are the majority of benign tumors of the small bowel located?**

60% are in the ileum, 25% in the jejunum, and 15% in the duodenum.

○   **What carcinoid tumors have the highest rate of metastasis?**

Ileal carcinoids. Malignancy is highly dependent on the size of the tumor: only 2% of tumors under 1 cm in diameter are malignant, while 80 to 90% of tumors > 2 cm are malignant.

○   **What is the most common childhood malignancy?**

Acute lymphoblastic leukemia. Leukemia accounts for one-third of all cancers diagnosed in the pediatric population. ALL accounts for 75% of all acute leukemias and AML acounts for 25%.

○   **What do ALL and AML stand for?**

Acute Lymphoblastic Leukemia and Acute Myelogenous Leukemia.

○   **When is ALL most common?**

ALL peaks between ages 3 and 5, and again around age 30.

○   **What are some signs and symptoms of leukemia?**

Fatigue, petechia, bleeding, purpura, lymphadenopathy, hepatosplenomegaly, bone and joint pain, low grade fever, and pallor.

○   **Petechia and bruising occur with platelet counts below what number? Internal hemorrhage occurs with count below what number?**

< 20,000/mm^3 and < 10,000/mm^3 respectively.

○   **What are some metabolic complications of leukemia?**

Hypercalcemia, hyperuricemia and syndrome of inappropriate antidiuretic hormone.

○   **How is hyperleukocytosis treated?**

IV hydration, alkalinization, allopurinol and antileukemic therapy.

○   **What is the malignant cell in Hodgkin's disease?**

The Reed-Sternberg cell.

○   **What are the peak age groups for Hodgkin's disease?**

13 to 35 and 50 to 75.

○   **What are the signs and symptoms of Hodgkin's disease?**

Painless supraclavicular or cervical lymphadenopathy, hepatomegaly, splenomegaly, unexplained fever, and night sweats.

○   **What are indications for lymph node biopsy?**

Nodes that continue to enlarge after 2 – 3 weeks, that do not return to normal size after 5 – 6 weeks or nodes associated with mediastinal enlargement on chest x-ray.

○   **How are childhood cases of non-Hodgkin lymphomas different from adult cases?**

They grow rapidly, are rarely nodular, and are as likely to be T-cell lymphomas as B-cell lymphomas.

○   **What is the most common presentation of B-cell lymphomas?**

Abdominal masses.

○   **What is the most common presentation of T-cell lymphomas?**

Anterior mediastinal masses.

DERMATOLOGY

○ **A 76 year old, slender female with no history of diabetes or other endocrine problem is found to have acanthosis nigricans upon routine examination. What is a probable diagnosis?**

Underlying malignancy. Acanthosis nigricans is often a marker for malignancy, especially of the GI tract. It is the velvety brown hyperpigmentation and thickening of the flexures common in the axilla and the groin. It is also associated with obesity, diabetes, and endocrine disorders.

○ **What is the most common skin malignancy?**

Basal cell carcinoma. Eighty to 90% of these lesions are found on the head and neck. Basal cell carcinoma appears as a pearly telangectasia with a central ulceration. These may spread locally, but they rarely metastasize.

○ **What percentage of patients have recurrences of basal cell carcinoma within 5 years?**

36%. Metastasis to distant sites, however, is rare.

○ **What are Beau lines?**

Transverse grooves in the nailbed that are caused by the disruption of the nailbed matrix secondary to systemic illness. 1 Illnesses can actually be dated by these lines as nails grow 1 mm per month.

○ *Candida albicans* **infections of the skin are most commonly located where?**

The intertriginous areas, i.e., in the folds of the skin, axilla, groin, under the breasts, etc. *Candida albicans* appears as a beefy, red rash with satellite lesions.

○ **What is a carbuncle?**

A deep abscess that interconnects and extends into the subcutaneous tissue. Carbuncles commonly occur in patients with diabetes, folliculitis, steroid use, obesity, heavy perspiration, and in areas of friction.

○ **Patients with untreated orbital or central facial abscesses are at risk for developing what serious complication?**

Cavernous sinus thrombosis.

○ **A father is worried that his 5 year old will contract chicken pox because she was playing with a neighborhood friend that has chicken pox. The neighbor child had crusty lesions all over his body. If this was the only day she played with the neighbor, will she develop chicken pox too?**

No. Chicken pox is only contagious from 48 hours before the rash breaks out and until the vesicles have crusted over.

○ **What are the most common causes of allergic contact dermatitis?**

Poison ivy, poison sumac, poison oak, ragweed, topical medications, nickel, chromium, rubber, glue, cosmetics, and hair dyes.

○   **A mother brings her 14 year old boy to you a week after you prescribed ampicillin for his pharyngitis. Mom says he developed a rash over his torso, arms, legs, and even the palms of his hands. Upon examination, the patient has a erythematous, maculopapular rash. What might the child have other than pharyngitis?**

Infectious mononucleosis. In almost 95% of patients with Epstein Barr viruses that are treated with ampicillin, a rash will develop. The rash and subsequent desquamation will last about a week.

○   **Ecthyma most commonly presents on what body parts?**

The lower legs. Ecthyma is similar to impetigo but can also be associated with a fever and lymphadenopathy. The most common infecting agent is *Staphylococcus aureus*. This infection is most prevalent in moist warm climates.

○   **What is the most common bullous disease?**

Erythema multiforme. The typical erythema multiforme lesion is the iris lesion (a gray center with a red rim). These lesions are symmetrical and most frequently found on the distal extremities spreading proximally. Patients may also develop plaques, papules, and bullous lesions. The disease is most common in children and young adults.

○   **What is the most common cause of erythema multiforme?**

Repetitive minor herpes simplex infections (90%). Drug reactions are the second most common cause of erythema multiforme. The rash generally erupts 7 to 10 days after a bout of herpes.

○   **Where is the most common location of erythema nodosum?**

The shins. They can also be found on the extensor surfaces of the forearms. Erythema nodosum are erythematous subcutaneous nodules that result from inflammation of subcutaneous fat and small vessels.

○   **A patient presents with a raised, red, small, and painful plaque on the face. Upon examination, a distinct, sharp, advancing edge is noted. What is the cause?**

Erysipelas which is caused by group A streptococci. When the face is involved, the patient should be admitted.

○   **What type of reaction is erythema multiforme (EM)?**

Hypersensitivity. Bullae are subepidermal, the dermis is edematous, and a lymphatic infiltrate may be present around the capillaries and venules. In children, infections are the most important cause; in adults, drugs and malignancies are common causes. EM is often noted during epidemics of adenovirus, atypical pneumonia, and histoplasmosis.

○   **What are the causes of exfoliative dermatitis?**

Chemicals, drugs, and cutaneous or systemic diseases. Usually scaly erythematous dermatitis involves most or all of the surface skin. It can be recognized by erythroderma with epidermal flaking or scaling. Acute signs and symptoms include low-grade fever, pruritus, chills, and skin tightness. The chronic condition may produce dystrophic nails, thinning of body hair, and patchy hyperpigmentation or hypopigmentation. Cutaneous vasodilation may result in increased cardiac output and high-output cardiac failure. Splenomegaly suggests leukemia or lymphoma.

○   **What is a furuncle?**

A deep inflammatory nodule that grows out of superficial folliculitis.

○ **What is hidradenitis suppurativa?**

Chronic suppurative abscesses located in the apocrine sweat glands of the groin and/or axilla. *Proteus mirabilis* overgrowth is common.

○ **Your neighbor brings her 4 year old girl to you because she has a terrible rash. The child's face is patched with vesiculopustular lesions covered in a thick, honey-colored crust. Just 2 days ago, these lesions were small red papules. What is your diagnosis?**

Impetigo contagiosa. This is most common in children and usually occurs on exposed areas of skin. Treat the child by removing the crusts, cleansing the bases, and prescribing systemic antibiotics (erythromycin, cephalosporin, or dicloxacillin).

○ **Which organism is probably responsible for the above child's infection?**

50 to 90% of impetigo contagiosa cases are caused by *Staphylococcus aureus*. ß-Hemolytic *Streptococcus* is the second most common infecting agent. This latter organism is the sole affecting agent in 10% of cases. It can also be coinfecting with *Staphylococcus aureus*.

○ **You are hanging out in the locker room after being beaten by your racquet ball opponent. You feel like insulting him, so you call him an insipid homosapien with androgenic alopecia and tinea cruris. What have you just said?**

You just told him he was a stupid, balding human with jock itch.

○ **What is the Koebner phenomenon?**

The development of plaques in areas where trauma has occurred. Just a scratch can trigger the development of a plaque. This condition is most common in patients with psoriasis and lichen planus.

○ **What are the ABCDE's of melanomas?**

Asymmetry
Border irregularity
Color variation
Diameter > 6 millimeters
Elevation above skin

○ **What age group has the highest incidence of melanoma?**

30 to 50 year olds.

○ **A patient has dysplastic nevus syndrome and is concerned because her aunt has just been diagnosed with melanoma. What is the patient's risk of also developing melanoma?**

100%.

○ **What are the most common locations of melanomas in African Americans? In Caucasian Americans?**

African Americans: hands, feet, and nails. Caucasian Americans: back and lower legs.

○ **Differentiate between pigmented and dysplastic nevi.**

Pigmented nevi are benign moles that are uniform in appearance. They are most common in sun exposed areas and warrant biopsy if they grow suddenly, change color, bleed, or begin to hurt.

Dysplastic nevi are not uniform in appearance and are frequently as large as 5 to 12 mm in diameter. 50% of malignant melanomas originate from the melanocytes in moles.

❍   **What are the most common causes of onychomycosis?**

Trichophyton rubrum and *T. mentagrophytes.*

❍   **What is a pilonidal abscess?**

An abscess that occurs just above the gluteal fold as a result of an ingrowing hair that induces a foreign body granuloma reaction. When the sinus is plugged, and cannot drain, it forms an abscess. Treatment is incision and drainage followed by referal to a surgeon for definitive surgical excision.

❍   **Where does a perirectal abscess originate?**

In anal crypts burrowing through the ischiorectal space. They may be perianal, perirectal, supralevator, or ischiorectal. Perianal abscesses that involve the supralevator muscle, ischiorectal space, or rectum require operative drainage.

❍   **What is the most common cause of secondary pyodermia?**

Similar to impetigo and ecthyma, this superinfection of the skin is caused predominantly by Staphylococcus aureus (80 to 85%). Other responsible organisms *are Streptococcus, Proteus, Pseudomonas,* and *E. coli.*

❍   **A 17 year old female has a rash on her elbows and knees. Upon examination you find several clearly demarcated erythematous plaques covered with silvery scales that can be removed with scraping. These lesions are on her extensor surfaces only in the areas previously mentioned. Examination of her nails reveals pitting in the nailbed. What is her diagnosis?**

Psoriasis. This is an intermittent disease that may either spontaneously disappear or be life long. There may be associated arthritis in the distal interphalangeal joints; otherwise, the disease is limited to the skin and nails. Treat with skin hydration therapy and by topical mid-potency steroids. Remember: "Silvery scales and pitting nails."

❍   **A 12 year old female complains of intense itching in the webs between her fingers; it worsens at night. Upon close examination you see a few small, squiggly lines 1 cm x 1 mm where the patient has been scratching. What is the diagnosis?**

Scabies. Scabies are due to the mite Sarcoptes scabiei hominis. A single application of 5% permethrin cream is curative for children over 2 months old. Scabies are spread by close contact; therefore, all household contacts should also be treated.

❍   **A 60 year old patient presents with greasy, red, scaly, plaques in his eyebrows, eyelids, and nose that are spreading to the naso-labial folds. In what population is this disease most likely to occur?**

The above patient has seborrheic dermatitis. This condition can occur in anyone, but it is a common problem in patients with HIV and Parkinson's disease. The infant form of the disease is cradle cap.

❍   **A 72 year old female has a painful red rash with crops of blisters on erythematous bases in a band-like distribution on the right side of her lower back which spread down and out towards her hip. What is your diagnosis?**

Shingles or herpes zoster disease. This is due to the reactivation of a dormant varicella virus in the sensory root ganglia of a patient with a history of chicken pox. The rash is in the distribution of the dermatome, in this case L5. It is most common in the elderly population or in patients who are immunocompromised. Treatment is with acyclovir and oral analgesics.

O   **Where is the most common site of herpes zoster eruption?**

The thorax. Unlike chicken pox, shingles can recur.

O   **A patient with shingles extending to the tip of his nose is at risk for what?**

Corneal ulceration and scarring. Lesions on the tip of the nose indicate that the nasociliary branch of the ophthalmic nerve is affected and the cornea is at risk. This is a medical emergency and needs immediate referral.

O   **Which of the following is the premalignant lesion that can lead to squamous cell carcinoma: seborrheic keratosis or actinic keratoses?**

Actinic keratosis. The two can be differentiated:

Actinic keratosis: An isolated red-brown macule or papule with a rough yellow-brown scale over it. Seborrheic keratosis: A benign, well-circumscribed, brownish papule with a greasy, warty appearance.

O   **What drugs are most often implicated in Toxic epidermal necrolysis (TEN)?**

Sulfas, penicillins, cephalosporins, anticonvulsants, allopurinol, phenylbutazone, sulfonylureas, barbiturates and NSAIDS.

O   **What areas does staphylococcal scalded skin syndrome (SSSS) usually affect?**

The face around nose and mouth, neck, axillae, and groin. The disease commonly occurs after upper respiratory tract infections or purulent conjunctivitis. Nikolsky's sign is present when lateral pressure on the skin results in epidermal separation from the dermis.

O   **What is the treatment for SSSS?**

Oral or IV penicillinase-resistant penicillin, baths of potassium permanganate or dressings soaked in 0.5% silver nitrate, and fluids. Corticosteroids and silver sulfadine are contraindicated. Drug-induced TEN carries up to 50% mortality as a result of fluid loss and secondary infection.

O   **A patient presents with fever, myalgias, malaise, and arthralgias has bullous lesions of the lips, eyes, and nose. The patient indicates that eating is painful. What is your diagnosis?**

Stevens-Johnson syndrome. This syndrome has a mortality of 5 to 10% and may have significant complications, including corneal ulceration, panophthalmitis, corneal opacities, anterior uveitis, blindness, hematuria, renal tubular necrosis, and progressive renal failure. Scarring of the foreskin and stenosis of the vagina can occur. Treatment in a burn unit is supportive. Steroids may provide symptomatic relief; however, they are not of proven value and may be contraindicated.

O   **What is the most common cause of Stevens-Johnson syndrome?**

Drugs; most commonly sulfa drugs. Other causes are responses to infections with *Mycoplasma pneumoniae* and herpes simplex virus. The disease is self-limiting but severely uncomfortable.

O   **A patient who was born with a diffuse capillary hemangioma in the distribution of the ophthalmic division of the trigeminal nerve will have what neurological findings?**

Epilepsy (usually generalized seizures), mental retardation, and/or hemiparesis. This is Sturge-Weber syndrome. The patient is born with a hemangioma of the ophthalmic nerve and ipsilateral angiomas of the pia matter and cortex (most commonly in the parieto-occipital area).

O   **Tinea capitis most commonly occurs in what age group?**

Four to 14 years. Tinea capitis is a fungal infection of the scalp that begins as a papule around one hair shaft and then spreads to other follicles. The infection can cause the hairs to break off, leaving little black dot stumps and patches of alopecia. *Trichophyton tonsurans* is responsible for 90% of the cases. Wood's lamp examination will fluoresce only *Microsporum* infections, which are responsible for the remaining 10%. This is also called "ringworm of the scalp."

O   **What are the three most common causes of acute urticaria?**

1) Medicine
2) Arthropod bites
3) Infection

Urticaria, also known as hives or wheels, is a localized swelling due to a cytokine mediated increase in vascular permeability.

O   **What is the most common cause of physical urticaria?**

Dermatographism. In this case, urticaria develops after firm, rapid stroking of the skin with a blunt surface. Such urticaria generally resolves within the hour.

O   **Where is the most common location of verrucae vulgaris?**

The back of the hands or fingers. Common warts are caused by HPV.

O   **Xanthomas are associated with which metabolic disorder?**

Hyperlipidemia. Xanthomas are yellow plaques surrounded by erythematous rings. They are most common on the extensor surfaces of the extremities; however, eruptive xanthomas are most common on the buttocks.

O   **How can the development of decubitus ulcers be prevented?**

Change the patient's position every 2 hours, keep the skin clean and dry, use protective padding at potential sites of ulceration, i.e., heel pads or ankle pads, and keep patients on egg crate mattresses or the equivalent. For diabetics, encourage daily foot examination.

O   **What rash is classically associated with a "herald patch" ?**

Pityriasis Rosea. Most cases begin with a single large, oval patch (herald patch) then a secondary eruption of small oval scaly patches on the trunk in a "Christmas tree" pattern appear. A mild pharyngitis and malaise may accompany the rash.

O   **What is the treatment for Pityriasis Rosea?**

Reassurance. The rash is self limited.

○ **What is the treatment for atopic dermatitis?**

Oral antihistamines, topical steroids, emollients, and avoidance of irritants.

○ **Elevations of which immunoglobulin is common in atopic dermatitis?**

IgE.

○ **What are the two main organisms responsible for Tinea capitis?**

Microsporum canis and *Trichophyton tonsurans*. Of these two, *T. tonsurans* is the most contagious.

○ **How do you make the diagnosis of Tinea versicolor?**

Examination under a Wood's lamp would show yellow fluorescence. Also, a KOH prep is useful in confirming diagnosis.

○ **What is the recommended therapy for Tinea capitis?**

Oral Griseofulvin (15-20 mg/kg/day) and shampooing twice a week with 2.5% Selenium Sulfide.

○ **What is the causative agent of Tinea versicolor?**

Pityrosporum orbiculare (Malassezia furfur), a fungus.

○ **Patients with what conditions are more likely to develop vitiligo?**

Diabetes mellitus, Addison's disease, thyroid disorders and pernicious anemia.

○ **Which areas of the body are normally most affected by vitiligo?**

Areas that are normally hyperpigmented (i.e. face, areolae) and areas subject to friction (i.e. hands, elbows).

○ **What is another name for erythema multiforme major?**

Stevens-Johnson syndrome.

○ **A patient presents with red and tender lateral nailfold on his ring finger with a small adjacent abscess. What is the diagnosis?**

Paronychia.

○ **What is the drug of choice for head lice?**

Permethrin (Nix).

○ **What is the treatment of choice for scabies?**

5% Permethrin cream.

○ **An 31 year old female presents with a maculopapular rash on her trunk and upper legs. The rash is in lines along the long axis of the ovoid lesions. The patient states that one week ago, she had only one lesion, which was round and "about as wide as a golf ball". What is your diagnosis?**

Pityriasis rosea.

○   **Patients on which antibiotic are most likely to have photoallergic drug reaction?**

Tetracycline and sulfonamides.

○   **An obese 1 year old male with a history of IDDM reports dark patches in the groin and axilla. What is the most likely diagnosis?**

Acanthosis nigricans, which may be caused by insulin resistance.

○   **What is the treatment for scalp lesions of seborrheic dermatitis?**

Antiseborrheic shampoo (i.e. coal tar, selenium sulfide).

GERIATRICS

○ **What percentage of the elderly are ambulatory?**

90%.

○ **What percentage of the elderly live in nursing homes?**

10%.

○ **What may result from the administration of an aminoglycoside or cephalosporin to an elderly patient who is dehydrated?**

Acute renal failure secondary to tubulointerstitial injury. This may also occur if the above mentioned drugs are given to an elderly patient on furosemide or with preexisting renal disease.

○ **What is the most common cause of hearing loss in the elderly?**

Presbycusis. Other causes include neoplasms, noise exposure, ototoxic drugs, and otosclerosis.

○ **Presbycusis is a hearing loss at which end of the audible range?**

The high end (4000 to 8000 Hz).

○ **What is the most common form of incontinence in the elderly?**

Urge incontinence. It is more common in females and is due to detrusor hyperreflexia or decreased sensory capabilities.

○ **Is the incidence of epidural and subdural hematomas higher or lower in elderly patients?**

Epidural hematomas are less common and subdural hematomas are more common.

○ **What geriatric population is at greatest risk for esophageal cancer?**

Elderly African Americans have a risk 4 times that of elderly Caucasian Americans. Other populations at risk include Chinese, Iranians, and South Africans.

○ **Who has a higher rupture rate in appendicitis, the very young or the very old?**

The very old. The rupture rate for geriatric patients is 65 to 90% with an associated mortality of 15%. The pediatric population has a rupture rate of 15 to 50% and an associated mortality rate of 3%.

○ **What is sundown syndrome?**

Hallucinations and delusions that occur at night time because of decreased sensory stimulation.

○ **What is the most common cause of large bowel obstruction in the elderly?**

Fecal impaction. Other causes are stenosing diverticula, neoplasms, and volvulus colon. Adhesions are rarely a cause of obstruction in the large bowel.

O   **The most common causes of dysphagia in the elderly population include:**

Hiatal hernia, reflux esophagitis, webs/rings, and cancer.

O   **An elderly patient with chronic COPD is most likely to contract what kind of pneumonia?**

H. influenzae pneumonia. Ampicillin is the drug of choice. This population is at risk and should be vaccinated.

O   **Giant cell arteritis is a chronic inflammation of the large blood vessels. What arteries are most commonly involved?**

The carotid and the cranial arteries. Blindness may result in 20% of afflicted patients. Treat with high dose corticosteroids.

O   **What are the common neurologic signs and symptoms of giant cell arteritis?**

Amaurosis fugax, deafness, depression, and paralysis. Amaurosis fugax is the most dangerous because it can lead to permanent monocular or binocular blindness.

O   **What is the Trendelenburg test for varicose veins?**

Raise the leg above the heart, then quickly lower it. If the leg veins become distended immediately after this test, there is valvular incompetency.

O   **What is the most common cause of cataract development?**

Old age. Cataracts occur congenitally, from medication or from trauma. Slit lamp examination may show absent red reflex and a gray clouding of the lens.

O   **What is the most common cause of blindness in the elderly?**

Senile macular degeneration. Such patients experience a gradual loss of central vision. The macula appears hemorrhagic or pigmented. This is due to atrophic degeneration of the retinal vessels that results in leaking vessels, fibrosis, and scarring of the retina.

O   **What is the most common nontraumatic cause of dementia?**

Alzheimer's disease. At 65, 10% of the population has Alzheimer's; by 85, 50% does. Multi-infarct dementia is the second most common cause of nontraumatic dementia.

O   **What is the first symptom of Alzheimer's disease?**

Progressive memory loss. This is followed by disorientation, personality changes, language difficulty, and other symptoms of dementia.

O   **What is the prognosis for patients with Alzheimer's disease?**

Alzheimer's is an irreversible disease. Death occurs 5 to 10 years after presumptive diagnosis.

O   **Differentiate between dementia and delirium.**

Dementia: Irreversible, impaired functioning secondary to changes and deficits in memory, spatial concepts, personality, cognition, language, motor and sensory skills, judgment, or behavior. There is no change in consciousness.

Delirium: A reversible, organic mental syndrome reflecting deficits in attention, organized thinking, orientation, speech, memory, and perception. Patients are frequently confused, anxious, excited, and have hallucinations. A change in consciousness may be evident.

O   **How frequently should a patient at high risk for pressure ulcers be repositioned?**

Every 2 hours.

O   **What is the most common complication of a pressure ulcer?**

Sepsis.

O   **What drugs are used to treat stress incontinence?**

α-Adrenergic agonists and estrogen.

O   **What is the most common presenting symptom in Parkinson's disease?**

Tremor. The brain lesion is located in the substantia nigra.

O   **List, by order of initiation, drugs used for the treatment of Parkinson's disease?**

Start with amantadine (Symmetrel) and trihexyphenidyl (Artane); if this fails, use a combination of levodopa and carbidopa. Pergolide and bromocriptine can be used to treat episodes of immobility.

O   **What is the drug of choice for treating depression in the elderly?**

Nortriptyline.

O   **A 65 year old African American has hypertension and gout. What medications should be prescribed?**

Although diuretics are the most effective drugs for the treatment of hypertension in this race, the patient has gout, which will be exacerbated by the use of diuretics. ACE inhibitors or calcium channel blockers are better choices for this patient.

O   **What is the mortality rate for geriatric patients who have sustained a hip fracture?**

25% will die in the first year following the fracture.

O   **What is the most common cause of community acquired pneumonia in the elderly?**

Streptococcus pneumoniae.

O   **How do you clinically differentiate between polymyalgia rheumatica and polymyositis?**

In polymyositis, there is proximal muscle pain, weakness, and tenderness, and elevated muscle enzymes. In contrast, polymyalgia rheumatica presents with an elevated sed rate (also seen in giant cell arteritis, which is associated with polymalgia rheumatica).

O   **What are the two pathologic findings used to confirm the diagnosis of Alzheimer's disease?**

The quantity of neurofibrillary tangles and senile plaques. Other findings include neuronal loss and amyloid degermation.

○　**What is the most common cause of UTI's in uncatheterized elderly patients?**

E. coli.

○　**In the elderly, what is a common side effect of verapamil?**

Constipation.

○　**Parkinson-like side effects are common with which class of drugs?**

Neuroleptics. Parkinson-like side effects can develop with perphenazine, chlorpromazine, reserpine, haloperidol, metoclopramide, and the illicit meperidine analog MPTP.

○　**In the elderly, what is the most common cause of death resulting from community acquired infections? Institutional? Nosocomial?**

In the community and institutions, it is bacterial pneumonia; in hospitals, it is UTI's.

○　**What is the most common cause of drug induced hallucinations in the geriatric population?**

Propranolol.

○　**Why is it unsafe to place a geriatric patient on digoxin and Lasix?**

Hypokalemia and digoxin toxicity may result.

○　**What percentage of patients with primary Alzheimer's disease will present with secondary depression?**

30 to 35%.

○　**What is the most common cause of abdominal pain in the elderly?**

Constipation.

○　**What is the most common risk factor for Alzheimer's disease?**

A family history of dementia.

○　**An elderly female presents with high blood pressure and a history of CHF. What is the antihypertensive drug of choice?**

ACE inhibitors. They will reduce both preload and afterload.

○　**An elderly male presents with high blood pressure and a history of NIDDM. What is the antihypertensive drug of choice?**

ACE inhibitors. They have renal protective properties.

○　**What is the major risk of tricyclic antidepressants in the elderly?**

Orthostatic hypotension, because this can lead to falls.

○ **An elderly African American male presents with high blood pressure and a history of angina. What is the antihypertensive drug of choice?**

Calcium channel blockers.

○ **What are the most common sources of sepsis in the elderly?**

Respiratory > urinary > intra-abdominal.

○ **Describe the common findings of benign essential tremors?**

Tremulousness of speech and nodding of head. This is an action tremor that is usually familial and is often treated with atenolol, propranolol, diazepam, and alcohol.

○ **What lab values increase with age?**

BUN/Cr, sed rate, thyroxine (T4), and calcium (in females).

○ **What lab values decrease with age?**

Leukocyte count and creatinine phosphokinase.

○ **What is the incidence of morbidity and mortality in patients over 60 who present with syncope?**

1 in 5 will suffer significant morbidity or mortality within 6 months.

○ **What percentage of septic elderly patients do not present with a fever?**

25%.

○ **What drugs are most commonly associated with ADRS in the elderly?**

Analgesics, cardiovascular, and psychotropic drugs.

○ **What are the common adverse drug interactions of cimetidine in the elderly?**

Cimetidine inhibits the metabolism of phenytoin, Coumadin, and theophylline.

○ **What are the common adverse drug interactions of Coumadin?**

Metabolism is inhibited by allopurinol, trimethoprim-sulfamethoxazole, metronidazole, and quinolones.

○ **What is the most common cause of <u>acute</u> abdominal pain in the elderly?**

Acute cholecystitis. Approximately 50% of patients over 65 have gallstones.

○ **Describe the clinical features of appendicitis in the elderly?**

Anorexia and vomiting are less common, and migration of the pain to the RLQ is absent in up to 60% of elderly patients. The elderly account for 50% of the deaths as a result of appendicitis. Half of elderly patients with appendicitis have normal white counts upon presentation.

SURGERY
PEARLS

GENERAL SURGERY

○ **How many days should sutures remain in the following areas: face, scalp, trunk, hands and back, extremities?**

Face: 3 to 5; scalp: 5 to 7; trunk: 7 to 10; hands, back and extremities: 10 to 14.

○ **Which type of needle should be used for skin sutures? Which type should be used for deep tissue sutures?**

For skin, use cutting needles (or reverse cutting needles). For deeper tissues, use taper needles. Taper needles are less likely to cut blood vessels and delicate tissue.

○ **What are lines of Langerhans?**

Lines of tension in the skin that incisions should follow when possible for the best cosmetic results. In the forehead, these lines run horizontally, while in the lower face they run vertically.

○ **Which is more painful to the patient, plain lidocaine or lidocaine with epinephrine?**

Lidocaine with epinephrine because it has a very low pH. To avoid this pain buffer the solution with sodium bicarbonate. The injection should be administered very slowly and subdermally.

○ **Can lidocaine with epinephrine be used on the arm?**

Yes. Lidocaine with epinephrine should not be used on fingers, toes, ears, nose or the penis because the limited vascularity in these regions might be compromised.

○ **Why is epinephrine added to local anesthesia?**

To increase the duration of the anesthesia. Epinephrine also causes vasoconstriction and therefore decreases bleeding. However, epinephrine weakens tissue defenses and increases the incidence of wound infection.

○ **What nerve block is used to anesthetize of the sole of the foot?**

Tibial nerve block. Tibial nerve block does not provide anesthesia to the lateral aspect of the heel and foot.

○ **How should hair be removed prior to wound repair?**

Clip the hair around the wound. A razor preparation can increase the infection rate.

○ **What is the rate of wound infection in the average surgical service?**

4 to 7%. The clean wound infection rate is 2% : clean-contaminated wounds : 3 to 4% : contaminated wounds : 10 to 15% : dirty wounds : 25 to 40%. The wound infection rate is dependent upon the degree of contamination, viability of tissue, blood supply to the tissue, dead space, amount of foreign material, patients' age, concomitant infections, nutrition, and immune system status.

○ **How long can a "clean" wound closure be delayed before proliferation of infection causing bacteria develops?**

6 hours, though the high vascularity of the face and scalp can allow for longer delays in these areas.

○   **What mechanisms of injury create wounds that are most susceptible to infection?**

Compression or tension injuries. They are 100 times more susceptible to infection.

○   **What factors increase the likelihood of wound infection?**

Dirty or contaminated wounds, stellate or crushing wounds, wounds longer than 5 cm, wounds older than 6 hours, and infection prone anatomic sites.

○   **Gabrianna Lucelli, the famous mountain bike racer, comes to your office after stepping on a nail that went right through her favorite, oldest pair of riding shoes. What gram-negative organism might infect her puncture wound?**

Pseudomonas aeruginosa.

○   **Which has greater resistance to infection, sutures or staples?**

Staples.

○   **Which two factors determine the ultimate appearance of a scar?**

Static and dynamic tension on surrounding skin.

○   **Can tetanus develop after surgical procedures?**

Yes. Although most cases of tetanus in the US develop after minor trauma, there have also been numerous reports of tetanus following general surgical procedures, especially those involving the GI tract.

○   **Characterize wounds prone to tetanus.**

Age of wound:	> 6 hours
Configuration:	Stellate wound
Depth:	> 1 cm
Mechanism of injury:	Missile, crush, burn, frostbite
Signs of infection:	Present
Devitalized tissue:	Present
Contaminants:	Present
Denervated and/or ischemic tissue:	Present

○   **How long should one wait before delayed primary closure of a wound?**

Four days. Delayed primary closure will decrease the infection rate. It is used for severely contaminated wounds.

○   **How long does an area of abraded skin or a laceration need have to be kept out of the sun?**

For at least 6 months. Abraded skin can develop permanent hypopigmentation when exposed to the sun.

○   **What organisms are most common in wound infections?**

Staphylococci.

O   **A patient who develops a reddish brown exudate within 6 hours of an appendectomy most likely has a wound infected with what?**

Clostridium. Necrotizing fasciitis, dehiscence, and sepsis may result if not treated promptly.

O   **What is the most likely cause of a postoperative fever which occurs: (1) the day of the operation, (2) 1 to 2 days postoperative, (3) 3 to 5 days postoperative, (4) 5 to 7 days postoperative, and (5) 2 weeks postoperative?**

(1) Metabolic abnormalities
(2) Atelectasis
(3) UTI
(4) Wound infection
(5) DVT or PE
(Remember: "What—Wind—Water—Wound—Walk—Wonder drugs.")

O   **What gas is used to create a pneumoperitoneum during a laparoscopy? Why is this gas used? What are the associated risks?**

Carbon dioxide (CO_2). CO_2 is non-combustible and has a high rate of diffusion which results in a low risk of gas embolism. The use of CO_2 can also result in tachycardia, increased central venous pressure, hypertension, decreased cardiac output, and occasionally, transient arrhythmias due to its rapid rate of absorption into the systemic circulation, which increases PCO_2 and decreases pH.

O   **A 32 year old female is under general anesthesia for a cholecystectomy. Part way into the operation her body tenses up, she develops tachycardia and a fever of 101.8°F. What should you do?**

Administer Dantrolene. This patient is suffering from malignant hyperthermia, a muscular response to general anesthetics that causes the release of calcium. Dantrolene will help prevent renal failure and will inhibit the release of calcium.

O   **What is the maintenance IV fluid rate for a child weighing 30 kg?**

100 mL/kg/day for the first 10 kg + 50 mL/kg/day for the next 10 kg + 20 mL/kg/day for the next 10 kg. This child should receive 1700 mL/day.

O   **What is the appropriate bolus for a dehydrated child weighing 15 kg?**

300 mL (20 mL/kg).

O   **Normal saline and Ringer's lactate have how many mEq/L of sodium, respectively?**

154 mEq/L, 130 mEq/L.

O   **What solutes determine serum osmolality?**

Sodium, glucose, and urea.

O   **What are the laboratory criteria for placing a patient on mechanical ventilation?**

$pO_2 < 70$ on 50% O_2
$pO_2 < 55$ on room air.
$pCO_2 > 50$.
pH < 7.25.
However, a patient's clinical status is still primary consideration.

○   **What is the Whipple procedure?**

Pancreaticoduodenectomy. The procedure involves resection of the distal stomach, pylorus, duodenum, proximal pancreas, and the gallbladder, plus a truncal vagotomy. The jejunum is then anastomosed to the stomach, biliary, and pancreatic ducts. This procedure is used for treating pancreatic, duodenal, ampulla of Vater, and common bile duct cancers.

○   **What are the Billroth I and II procedures?**

The Billroth I anastomosis is a gastroduodenostomy, and the Billroth II is a gastrojejunostomy.

○   **What is the Roux-en-Y operation?**

An end-to-side anastomosis between the distal segment of small bowel and the stomach or esophagus. This forms a Y shape. This procedure is used to treat reflux of bile and pancreatic secretions into the stomach.

○   **Matching transplants:**

1) Autograft   a) Donor and recipient are genetically the same.
2) Heterotrophic   b) Donor and recipient are the same person.
3) Isograft   c) Donor and recipient are of the same species.
4) Orthotopic   d) Donor and recipient belong to different species.
5) Allograft   e) Transplantation to a normal anatomical position.
6) Xenograft   f) Transplantation to a different anatomical position.

Answers: (1) b, (2) f, (3) a, (4) e, (5) c, and (6) d.

○   **What fungal infection is most common in transplant patients?**

Candida albicans.

○   **What transplant organ can be preserved the longest?**

The kidney. Kidneys can be preserved in cold storage for up to 48 hours, the pancreas and liver for 8 hours, and the heart for 4 hours. Viability can be extended by using cold storage solutions, such as Collins solution and UW-Belzer solution.

○   **Differentiate between visceral and parietal pain.**

Visceral pain: Diffuse and poorly localized pain caused by the stretching of a hollow viscus. It is frequently associated with autonomic nervous system responses.

Parietal pain: Sharp and localized pain due to irritation or inflammation of a parietal surface and associated with guarding, rebound, and a rigid abdomen.

○   **What is the most common cause of bleeding in postoperative patients?**

Poor local control.

○   **A fire victim is burned over both legs, his entire back, and his right arm. What percentage of his body is burned?**

63%. Follow the "rule of 9's". Face = 9%. Arms = 9% each. Front = 18%. Back = 18%. Legs = 18% each.

○   **A patient who has been burned over the entire top of his body (arms and torso, front and back) develops severe difficulty breathing and appears to be going into respiratory arrest. What should be done?**

An escharotomy. The patient is most likely suffering ventilatory restriction due to the circumferential eschar about his chest resulting in constriction of the chest cavity. Escharotomies need not be performed with anesthesia, not even a local. Third degree burns destroy the nervous tissue and are thus insensitive to pain.

○   **What is the caloric requirement of a 100 kg firefighter who was burned over 20% of his body?**

3300 Kcal. (25 Kcal/kg of body weight + 40 Kcal/1% burned surface.)

○   **What is the 24 hour fluid resuscitation requirement for the above patient?**

4 L in the first 8 hours (500 mL/hour) and 4 L in the next 16 hours (250 mL/hour). The Parkland formula gives the requirement as 4 mL body weight in kg % burned (4 mL 100 kg 20 8L). Give half the volume in the first 8 hours and the other half in the next 16 hours. Management after this should be based on clinical judgment. Urine output should be maintained at 50 mL/hour in adults and 0.5 to 1 mL/kg/hour in children.

○   **What does an increase in pulmonary arterial wedge pressure indicate?**

Fluid overload. Normal pulmonary wedge pressure is 4 to 12 mm Hg. Higher levels can indicate left ventricular failure, constrictive pericarditis, or mitral regurgitation with stenosis.

○   **A trauma patient has blood at the urinary meatus. What test should be ordered?**

Retrograde urethrogram. Ten milliliters of radiocontrast solution should be injected into the urinary meatus.

○   **What are the two most commonly injured genitourinary organs?**

Kidneys and bladder.

○   **A trauma patient presents with a "rocking horse" type of ventilation. What is the diagnosis?**

Probable high spinal cord injury with intercostal muscle paralysis.

○   **What should be checked prior to inserting a chest tube in an intubated patient with respiratory distress and decreased breath sounds on one side?**

Position of the ET tube.

○   **A trauma patient presents with subcutaneous emphysema. What is the diagnosis?**

Pneumothorax or pneumomediastinum; if emphysema is severe, consider a major bronchial injury.

○   **What rib fracture has the worst prognosis?**

The first rib. First and second rib fractures are associated with bronchial tears, vascular injury, and myocardial contusions.

○   **A patient presents to the emergency department after a motor vehicle accident with hematuria and fractures of the tenth and eleventh ribs. What internal organ might be damaged?**

The spleen is the most commonly injured organ in blunt trauma. However, the spleen is only injured in 10% of penetrating trauma incidents. Be especially suspicious of splenic trauma if the tenth or eleventh ribs are fractured and the patient has hematuria.

○ **For a trauma victim, what test is most helpful for evaluating retroperitoneal organs?**

CT.

○ **How should a DPL be performed on a trauma victim with a fractured pelvis?**

A supraumbilical incision should be made to avoid insertion of the DPL catheter into a contained pelvic hematoma.

○ **What is an absolute contraindication to DPL?**

Nothing. Relative contraindications are clear indication for laparotomy, previous abdominal surgery, and a gravid uterus (use open technique).

○ **What findings represent a positive DPL in blunt trauma?**

RBC > 100,000 cells/mm3, WBC > 500 cells/mm3, bile, bacteria, or vegetable material.

○ **A patient presents with fever and shoulder pain 4 days following a splenectomy. What is the most probable postoperative complication?**

Subphrenic abscess. This condition can cause fever as well as irritation to the diaphragm and to the branch of the phrenic nerve that innervates it.

○ **What organisms are most commonly responsible for overwhelming postsplenectomy sepsis?**

Encapsulated organisms: pneumococcal (50%); meningococcal (12%); *E. coli* (11%); *H. influenzae* (8%); staphylococcal (8%); and streptococcal (7%).

○ **What is a sentinel loop?**

A distended loop of bowel detected by x-ray that lies near a localized inflammatory process. The possibility of pancreatitis or appendicitis should be considered.

○ **Which types of nodules are more likely to be malignant on a thyroid scan, hot or cold?**

Cold. This procedure should not be considered confirmatory. Cysts and benign adenomas can also read as cold. Some types of thyroid cancers will read as "warm" and thus be dismissed. Use caution when interpreting results.

○ **What test should be performed to distinguish a benign cystic nodule from a malignant nodule?**

Fine needle aspiration biopsy and cytological evaluation.

○ **Are epidural hematomas and subdural hematomas more or less common among elderly patients?**

Subdural hematomas are more common. Epidural hematomas are less common.

❍   **When does a subdural hematoma become isodense?**

One to three weeks after the bleed. However, it may not be detectable by CT unless contrast is used.

❍   **What percentage of C-spine fractures can be identified on the lateral x-ray?**

90%.

❍   **Name the function and spinal innervation level of the biceps, triceps, flexor digitorum, interossei, quadriceps, extensor hallucis, biceps femoris, soleus and gastrocnemius, and rectal sphincter.**

Muscle	Action	Spinal Level
Biceps	Forearm flexion	C5–C6
Triceps	Forearm extensors	C7
Flexor digitorum	Finger flexion	C8
Interossei	Finger adduction/abduction	T1
Quadriceps	Knee extension	L3–L4
Extensor hallucis	Great toe dorsiflexion	L5
Biceps femoris	Knee flexion	S1
Soleus and gastrocnemius	Foot plantar flexion	S1–S2
Rectal sphincter	Sphincter tone	S2–S4

❍   **What is the sensory innervation to the nipple, umbilicus, and perianal region?**

Nipple: T4
Umbilicus: T10
Perianal: S2–S4

❍   **What is a solitary thyroid nodule most likely to be?**

A nodular goiter (50%). Other possibilities to consider include cancer (20%), adenoma (20%), cyst (5%), or thyroiditis (5%).

❍   **What is the most common type of thyroid carcinoma?**

Papillary carcinoma (60 to 70% of tumors). It's a good thing too! Papillary carcinoma has the best prognosis; the 10 year survival rate is 89%. Other thyroid carcinomas are follicular (10 to 20%, common in older patients), anaplastic (3 to 5%), and medullary (2 to 5%, often occurring with familial multiple endocrine neoplasia).

❍   **Where is a parotid gland tumor most likely to develop?**

The superficial lobe which is located just below the ear lobe. Forty percent of parotid gland tumors are malignant. All tumors, benign or malignant, should be removed.

❍   **What type of contrast medium should be used to evaluate the esophagus if a traumatic injury is suspected?**

Gastrografin.

❍   **Dysphagia occurs when the esophageal intraluminal diameter is reduced to what size?**

<10 mm. This is a common problem in esophageal cancer. Palliation is achieved by widening the esophageal intraluminal diameter through photoablation of the tumor.

❍   **What age and ethnic group is at greatest risk for esophageal cancer?**

Elderly African Americans.   Their risk is four times higher compared to elderly Caucasian Americans.
Other ethnic groups at higher risk include Chinese, Iranians, and South Africans.

❍   **Cancer occurs more frequently in which third of the esophagus?**

The middle third (50%), followed by the distal third (30%) and the proximal third (20%).

❍   **Which are the most common cancer cell types of the esophagus?**

Squamous carcinoma most frequently in African Americans, while adenocarcinoma is most common type
in Caucasian Americans.

❍   **Which types of cancer metastasize to bone?**

Prostate, thyroid, breast, lung, and kidney. (Remember: "P.T. Barnum Loves Kids.")

❍   **What is Hamman's sign?**

Air in the mediastinum following an esophageal perforation. This condition produces a crunching sound
over the heart during systole.

❍   **What is the most common site of rupture in Boerhaave's syndrome?**

The posterior distal esophagus. Boerhaave's syndrome is a rupture of the esophagus that occurs after binge
drinking and vomiting. Patients experience sudden, sharp pain in the lower chest and epigastric area. The
abdomen becomes rigid, then shock may follow.

❍   **What is the most common acute surgical condition of the abdomen?**

Acute appendicitis.

❍   **What is the most common cause of appendicitis?**

Fecaliths. Fecaliths are found in 40% of uncomplicated appendicitis cases, 65% of cases involving
gangrenous appendices that have not ruptured, and 90% of cases involving ruptured appendices. Other
causes of appendicitis include lymphoid tissue hypertrophy, inspissated barium, foreign bodies, and
strictures.

❍   **How does retrocecal appendicitis most commonly present?**

Dysuria and hematuria (due to the proximity of the appendix to the right ureter). Poorly localized
abdominal pain, anorexia, nausea, vomiting, diarrhea, mild fever, and peritonitis are also common signs.

❍   **What percentage of patients with a pre-operative diagnosis of appendicitis actually have
appendicitis?**

85%. Other postoperative diagnoses commonly include acute mesenteric lymphadenitis, PID, epiploic
appendicitis, ruptured graafian follicle, acute gastroenteritis, and twisted ovarian cysts.

❍   **Differentiate between McBurney's point, Rovsing's sign, the obturator sign, and the psoas sign.**

McBurney's point: Point of maximal tenderness in a patient with appendicitis. The location is two-thirds the way between the umbilicus and the iliac crest on the right side of the abdomen.

Rovsing's sign: Palpation of LLQ causes pain in the RLQ.

Obturator sign: Internal rotation of a flexed hip causes pain.

Psoas sign: These signs are all indicative of an inflamed appendix. Extension of the right thigh causes pain.

○   **Which type of antibiotic should be given to a patient with a perforated appendix prior to surgery?**

A broad spectrum antibiotic effective on both aerobic and anaerobic enteric organisms. Intraoperative cultures can guide further antibiotic therapy.   Antibiotics may be continued for 7 days post-op. If the patient has an uncomplicated appendicitis, i.e. no perforation or gangrene, then 1 preoperative dose of a broad spectrum antibiotic such as cefoxitin or cefotetan is sufficient.

○   **Who has a higher rupture rate in appendicitis, the very young or the very old?**

The very old. The rupture rate for geriatric patients is 65 to 90%; the associated mortality is 15%. The pediatric population has a rupture rate of 15 to 50% with an associated mortality rate of 3%.

○   **What kind of wound closure should be used in a patient with a perforated appendix?**

Delayed primary closure with direct drainage of the infection. Wound infection occurs in 20% of patients with perforated appendices.

○   **A 27 year old man who smokes heavily complains of tingling in his fingers. On examination he has cyanotic digits with ulcers forming. What is the diagnosis?**

Thromboangiitis obliterans or Buerger's disease. This is a disease that effects young smokers (males three times more often than females). Inflammatory changes in the small- to medium-sized vessels cause occlusions. Patients must stop smoking!

○   **Where is the most common site of intracranial aneurysms?**

The circle of Willis (most common in the anterior communicating artery). A ruptured aneurysm presents as a headache followed by altered consciousness.

○   **What are the clinical signs of CSF leakage?**

Raccoon eyes, bruises behind the ears (Battle's sign), otorrhea, and rhinorrhea.

○   **What is the most common type of brain tumor in adults?**

Glioblastoma multiforme (40%). Meningiomas account for 15 to 20%, and metastatic tumors account for 5 to 10%.

○   **Which type of brain tumor occurs most frequently in pediatric patients?**

Medulloblastoma.

○   **What are the most common microorganisms found in brain abscesses?**

The enteric gram-negative bacilli, anaerobes, nocardia, staphylococci, streptococci, and toxoplasma.

○ **How many minutes of cerebral anoxia will result in irreversible brain injury?**

Over 4 minutes.

○ **Matching:**

1) **Neuropraxia**   a) **Damage to the axon, no damage to the sheath.**
2) **Axonotmesis**   b) **Temporary loss of function, no damage to axon.**
3) **Neurotmesis**   c) **Damage to axon and sheath.**

Answers: (1) b, (2) a, and (3) c.

○ **A hard mass in the upper outer quadrant of the right breast of a 45 year old woman is detected. What are the next steps?**

Mammogram followed by an excision biopsy. A negative needle aspiration alone cannot rule out malignancy. False negative rates for fine needle biopsy are 3 to 30%.

○ **What is the most common histologic type of breast cancer?**

Infiltrating ductal carcinoma (70 to 80%). Subtypes are: colloid, medullary, papillary, and tubular.

○ **A 30 year old female comes to you worried that she has breast cancer in both breasts. She is concerned because of a yellowish green discharge from her nipples, soreness in the upper outer quadrants of her breasts, what she calls a "lumpy" feeling upon self-examination and mild swelling that seems to come and go. Further questioning reveals that her pain begins 1 week before she menstruates then disappears when her menses is over. Understandably concerned, your patient wants to know when she can start chemotherapy. What do you tell her?**

Hold off on the chemo! She most likely has fibrocystic breast changes. Put her mind at rest, and let her know that fibrocystic changes are not a premalignant syndrome.

○ **Which is the most common type of non-cystic breast tumor?**

Fibroadenomas. These are most common in women under 25. These tumors are painless, small, mobile and round.

○ **What is the most common lung cancer in non-smokers?**

Small cell carcinoma. Smoking is a great risk factor for all lung cancers with the exception of adenocarcinoma.

○ **What is Westermark's sign?**

Decreased vascular markings on chest x-ray, indicative of pulmonary embolism.

○ **What do muffled heart tones, hypotension, and distended neck veins indicate?**

Pericardial tamponade. This is Beck's triad.

○ **What is the most common tumor in a child's first year of life?**

Wilms' tumor. Hepatoma is the second most common tumor in this age range.

○   **What is the average age for pediatric patients to develop Wilms' tumor?**

3 years old. Cure rates are as high as 90% in patients with no metastasis.

○   **One to two percent of patients with Wilms' tumor will develop secondary malignancies. Which types are most common?**

Hepatocellular carcinoma, leukemia, lymphoma, and soft tissue sarcoma.

○   **What are Grey-Turner's and Cullen's signs?**

Cullen's sign: Periumbilical ecchymosis indicative of pancreatic hemorrhage.
Grey Turner's sign: Flank ecchymosis indicative of pancreatic hemorrhage
Both are caused by dissection of blood retroperitoneally.

○   **Serum amylase is frequently elevated in acute pancreatitis. What other conditions can cause a similar rise in amylase?**

Bowel infarction, cholecystitis, mumps, perforated ulcer, and renal failure. Lipase is more specific. A two hour urine amylase is a more accurate test in pancreatitis.

○   **What are the most common causes of acute pancreatitis?**

Alcoholism (40%) and gallstone disease (40%). The remaining cases of acute pancreatitis are due to familial pancreatitis, hypoparathyroidism, hyperlipidemia, iatrogenic pancreatitis, and protein deficiency.

○   **Name some abdominal x-ray findings associated with acute pancreatitis?**

A sentinel loop (either of the jejunum, transverse colon, or duodenum); a colon cutoff sign (an abrupt cessation of gas in the mid or left transverse colon due to inflammation of the adjacent pancreas); or calcification of the pancreas. About two-thirds of patients with acute pancreatitis will have x-ray abnormalities.

○   **What are Ranson's criteria?**

A means of estimating prognosis for patients with pancreatitis.

At initial presentation - developing within 24 hours:
Age > 55
LDH > 700 IU/L
WBC > 16,000/mm3
AST > 250 UI/L
Serum glucose > 200 mg/dL

48 hours later:
Hematocrit falling > 10%
Increase in BUN > 5 mg/dL
Serum Ca+ < 8 mg/dL
Arterial PO2 < 60 mm Hg
Base deficit > 4 meq/L
Fluid sequestration > 6 L

0 to 2 criteria = 2% mortality
3 to 4 criteria = 15% mortality
5 to 6 criteria = 40% mortality
7 to 8 criteria = 100% mortality

(Editor's note: These are the classic mortality percentages. Current treatment has decreased these rates.)

○   **What is the most common cause of pancreatic pseudocysts in children? In adults?**

Children: trauma. Adults: chronic pancreatitis. Pseudocysts are generally filled with pancreatic enzymes and are sterile. They present about 1 week after the patient has a bout with acute pancreatitis displayed as upper abdominal pain with anorexia and weight loss. Forty percent will regress on their own.

○   **What is the treatment for pancreatic pseudocysts?**

Initial therapy is to wait for regression (4 to 6 weeks). If no improvement occurs, or if superinfection occurs, surgical drainage or excision is required.

○   **A 44 year old gentleman presents with a deep, dull pain in the center of his abdomen that radiates to his back and will not go away. He states he has not "felt like himself" for a few weeks and that he has been kind of depressed. He also notes that he has lost a lot of weight, about 30 pounds in 3 weeks. On physical examination you palpate an enlarged liver and an abdominal mass in the epigastrium. What is your diagnosis?**

Most likely pancreatic cancer. The ability to palpate a mass suggests that the disease has progressed too far to be surgically removed. Carcinoma of the pancreas can only be resected in 20% of patients. Depression often occurs before the onset of other symptoms.

○   **Where is the most common anatomic and histologic location of pancreatic cancer?**

Head of the pancreas (80%). Pancreatic cancer is generally adenocarcinoma and located in the ducts.

○   **What gender and age group most commonly presents with pancreatic cancer?**

Middle-aged men.

○   **What is the 5 year survival rate for pancreatic carcinoma?**

2 to 5%. Symptoms generally do not show up until the tumor has metastasized or spread to local structures.

○   **What is the most common endocrine tumor of the pancreas?**

An insulinoma. However, only 10% are malignant. Gastrinomas are the second most common and have a malignancy rate of 50%. Vipomas and glucagonomas are also endocrine tumors of the pancreas.

○   **Glucagonomas arise from which type of cells?**

Alpha cells. The majority are malignant. Increased plasmin glucagon is diagnostic.

○   **Which type of operation is associated with a higher incidence of common bile duct injury, laparoscopic cholecystectomy or conventional cholecystectomy?**

Laparoscopic.

○   **Pheochromocytomas produce what compounds?**

Catecholamines. This group of chemicals result in increased blood pressure, perspiration, heart palpitations, anxiety, and weight loss.

❍   **If vanillylmandelic acid, normetanephrine, and metanephrine are detected in the urine, what is the likely cause?**

Pheochromocytoma.

❍   **Where are the majority of pheochromocytomas located?**

Ninety percent are found in the adrenal medulla. The remainder are located in other tissues originating from neural crest cells.

❍   **What is the pheochromocytoma rule of 10's?**

10% are malignant; 10% are multiple or bilateral; 10% are extra-adrenal; 10% occur in children; 10% recur after surgical removal; 10% are familial.

❍   **What is the most common benign liver tumor?**

Cavernous hemangioma.

❍   **All types of hepatomas are associated with underlying liver disease except one. Which is it?**

Fibrolamellar hepatomas. These are single nodules in non-cirrhotic livers.

❍   **Hepatic cancer most commonly metastasizes to where?**

The lungs (bronchiogenic carcinoma).

❍   **What is the two year survival rate for patients with liver cancer who have had a liver transplant?**

25 to 30%.

❍   **Where will colorectal cancer most commonly metastasize?**

The liver.

❍   **α-Fetoprotein (AFP) will be elevated in which types of tumors?**

Primary hepatic neoplasms and endodermal sinus or yolk sac tumors of the ovaries and testes. AFP is present in 30% of patients with primary liver cancer. It is not associated with metastatic tumors to the liver, but it is used as a cellular marker in the above mentioned tumors.

❍   **What is the most common cause of portal hypertension?**

Intrahepatic obstruction (90%), which is most often due to cirrhosis. Other causes of portal hypertension are increased hepatic flow without obstruction, i.e., fistulas, and extrahepatic outflow obstruction.

❍   **What are the most commonly isolated organisms in pyogenic hepatic abscesses?**

E. coli and other gram-negative bacteria. The source of such bacteria is most likely an infection in the biliary system.

❍   **Which has a higher mortality rate, amebic or pyogenic liver abscesses?**

Pyogenic. The mortality rate for a singular pyogenic abscess is 25%, and for multiple abscesses up to 70%. Amebic abscesses have mortality rates of only 7% if uncomplicated by superinfection. Amebic abscesses are more likely to be singular in nature while pyogenic abscesses can be singular or multiple.

❍   **What clinical sign can assist in the diagnosis of cholecystitis?**

Murphy's sign : pain on inspiration with palpation of the RUQ. As the patient breaths in, the gallbladder is lowered in the abdomen and comes in contact with the peritoneum just below the examiner's hand. This will aggravate an inflamed gallbladder, causing the patient to discontinue breathing deeply.

❍   **What is the difference between cholelithiasis, cholangitis, cholecystitis, and choledocholithiasis?**

<u>Cholelithiasis:</u> Gallstones in the gallbladder

<u>Cholangitis:</u> Inflammation of the common bile duct often secondary to bacterial infection or choledocholithiasis

<u>Cholecystitis:</u> Inflammation of the gallbladder secondary to gallstones

<u>Choledocholithiasis:</u> Gallstones which have migrated from the gallbladder to the common bile duct

❍   **What percentage of people with gallstones will develop symptoms?**

Only 50%.

❍   **Which ethnic group has the largest proportion of people with symptomatic gallstones?**

Native Americans. By the age of 60, 80% of Native Americans with previously asymptomatic gallstones will develop symptoms, as compared to only 30% of Caucasian Americans and 20% of African Americans.

❍   **What percentage of patients with cholangitis are also septic?**

50%. Chills, fever, and shock can occur.

❍   **What percentage of gallstones can be visualized on ultrasound?**

95%. Ultrasound is the diagnostic procedure of choice in patients with suspected cholecystitis.

❍   **How much bile can held within a distended gallbladder?**

50 mL.

❍   **What is Charcot's triad?**

1) Fever
2) Jaundice
3) Abdominal pain

This is the hallmark of acute cholangitis.

❍   **What is Reynolds' pentad?**

Charcot's triad plus shock and mental status changes. This is the hallmark of acute toxic ascending cholangitis.

○   **What are the majority of gallstones composed of?**

Cholesterol (75 to 95%). The rest are made of pigment.

○   **What are the majority of kidney stones made of?**

Calcium oxalate (60%). The remainder of kidney stones are made of uric acid, calcium oxalate/calcium phosphate, struvite, and cystine.

○   **What percentage of patients with cancer of the gallbladder will also have cholelithiasis?**

90%.

○   **What is the diagnostic test of choice for acute cholecystitis?**

HIDA scan (technetium-99–labeled N-substituted iminodiacetic acid scan). The HIDA scan uses a gamma-ray–emitting isotope that is selectively extracted by the liver into bile. The labeled bile can then be used to determine if there is cystic duct obstruction or extrahepatic bile duct obstruction which is based whether the bile fills the gall bladder or enters the intestine. For practical reasons, the diagnosis is frequently make using clinical impressions, CBC, and ultrasound.

○   **How effective is oral dissolution therapy with bile acids for those with symptomatic gallstones?**

Oral therapy with bile acids can dissolve up to 90% of stones. However, therapy works only on stones smaller than 0.5 mm, made of cholesterol, and floating in a functioning gallbladder. Patients are then treated for 6 to 12 months and 50% have recurrence of gallstones within 5 years.

○   **What are the contraindications to lithotripsy?**

Stones > 2.5 cm, more than 3 stones, calcified stones, stones in the bile duct, and poor overall condition of the patient.

○   **Laparoscopic cholecystectomy is the procedure of choice for removal of gallstones. What is the most common major complication associated with this surgery?**

Injury to the bile duct.

○   **After a cholecystectomy, can gallstones reform?**

Yes. They can recur in the bile ducts.

○   **Where is the most common site for fibromuscular dysplasia?**

The right renal artery. Fibromuscular dysplasia is an arterial disease that causes areas of stenosis and dilation; the artery appears as a link of sausage. Women are more commonly affected than men.

○   **Where are most hernias located?**

In the groin (75%). Incisional and ventral hernias account for 10%, and umbilical hernias account for 3%.

○   **Characterize the majority of inguinal hernias in infants and children (direct or indirect).**

Indirect inguinal hernias.

O   **Differentiate between reducible, incarcerated, strangulated, Richter, and complete hernias.**

Reducible: Contents of hernia sac return to the abdomen spontaneously or with slight pressure when the patient is in a recumbent position.

Incarcerated: Contents of the hernia sac are irreducible and cannot be returned to the abdomen.

Strangulated: Sac and its contents turn gangrenous.

Richter: Only part of the hernia sac and its contents becomes strangulated. This hernia may spontaneously reduce and be overlooked.

Complete: An inguinal hernia that passes all the way into the scrotum.

O   **What are the boundaries of Hesselbach's triangle?**

The triangle is medial to the inferior epigastric artery, superior to the inguinal ligament, and lateral to the rectus sheath. Hesselbach's triangle is the site through which direct hernias pass.

O   **A direct hernia is due to a weakness in what tissue?**

The transversalis fascia that makes up the floor of Hesselbach's triangle. Direct hernias do not pass through the inguinal canal and are often called pantaloon hernias.

O   **Indirect inguinal hernias occur secondary to what defect?**

A failure of the processus vaginalis to close. The resulting hernia can then pass through the inguinal ring.

O   **Which type of hernia is most common in females?**

Direct hernia. Direct hernia is the most common hernia in both women and men.

Note: While femoral hernias are more common in females than in males, they are still less common than direct hernias.

O   **Of all hernias in the groin area, which is most likely to strangulate?**

A femoral hernia. Femoral hernias occur in the femoral canal, an unyielding space between the lacunar ligament and the femoral vein.

O   **Which are more common, sliding or paraesophageal hiatal hernias?**

Sliding hiatal hernias account for 95% of hiatal hernias.

O   **Where is the most common site of duodenal ulcers?**

The duodenal bulb (95%). Surgery is indicated only if perforation, gastric outlet obstruction, intractable disease, or uncontrollable hemorrhage occur.

O   **What is the most common site for gastric ulcers?**

The lesser curvature of the stomach. Surgery is considered earlier in gastric ulcers because of the higher recurrence rate after medical treatment and because of the higher malignant potential.

O   **What are the signs and symptoms of intestinal obstruction in the newborn?**

Maternal polyhydramnios, abdominal distention, failure to pass meconium, and vomiting.

❍   **What amount of residual volume suctioned from the stomach of a newborn is diagnostic of obstruction?**

> 40 mL.

❍   **A newborn's vomit will be stained with bile if the obstruction is distal to what anatomical structure?**

The ampulla of Vater.

❍   **What are the common causes of neonatal obstruction?**

Annular pancreas, Hirshsprung's disease, intestinal atresia, malrotation, volvulus, peritoneal bands, meconium plug, small left colon syndrome, and stenosis.

❍   **Where is the most prevalent location for atresia of the bowel?**

The duodenum (40%), jejunum (20%), ileum (20%), and colon (10%).

❍   **What is the "double bubble" sign?**

The appearance of a distended stomach and duodenum on the x-ray of a patient with duodenal obstruction. This is classically seen in duodenal atresia of the newborn.

❍   **What is the most common cause of bowel obstruction in children?**

Hernia.

❍   **What are the most common causes of small bowel obstruction in adults?**

Adhesions (70%), followed by strangulated groin hernia and neoplasm of the bowel. Twenty percent of acute abdominal surgical admissions are due to obstructions.

❍   **Volvulus of the colon most frequently involves which segment?**

The sigmoid (65%), cecum (30%), transverse colon (3%), and splenic flexure (2%). Volvulus is the cause of 5 to 10% of all large bowel obstructions.

❍   **Where is the most common site of intestinal obstruction secondary to gallstones?**

The terminal ileum. 55 - 60% will have associated air in the biliary tree.

❍   **What is the differential diagnosis for a 65 year old man who has abdominal pain and bloody diarrhea a few days after the repair of an abdominal aortic aneurysm?**

Ischemic colitis is most probable. This condition occurs secondary to a decreased blood flow to the inferior mesenteric artery during the operation. Other differentials include pseudomembranous colitis (assuming the patient was receiving antibiotics) and aortoenteric fistulas (generally a later development).

❍   **Is colovesicular fistula between the colon and the urinary tract more common among men or women?**

Men (3:1) more than women because a woman's uterus lies between her colon and bladder.

❍   **What is Osler-Weber-Rendu syndrome?**

Hereditary hemorrhagic telangiectasias found in the small intestine, mucosal membranes and skin with A-V malformations, most notably in the lung.

○   **How much blood must be lost in the GI tract to cause melena?**

50 mL. Healthy patients normally lose 2.5 mL/day.

○   **What are the most common causes of upper GI bleeding?**

PUD (45%), esophageal varices (20%), gastritis (20%), and Mallory-Weiss syndrome (10%).

○   **What percentage of patients with upper GI bleeds will stop bleeding within hours of hospitalization?**

85%. About 25% of these patients will rebleed within the first 2 days of hospitalization. If no rebleeding occurs in five days, the chance of rebleeding is only 2%.

○   **What are the most common causes of rebleeding in patients with upper GI bleeds?**

PUD or esophageal varices.

○   **What percentage of patients with PUD bleed from their ulcers?**

20%.

○   **How soon after an episode of bleeding has occurred can an ulcer patient be fed?**

12 to 24 hours after the bleeding has stopped.

○   **Which type of ulcer is more likely to rebleed?**

Gastric ulcers are three times more likely to rebleed compared to duodenal ulcers.

○   **What is the surgical treatment of choice for a bleeding peptic ulcer?**

Oversewing the ulcer combined with a bilateral truncal vagotomy and pyloroplasty. Other treatments are proximal gastric vagotomy and Billroth II gastrojejunostomy. The decision to perform surgery is based on the rate of bleed, not on the location of the bleed.

○   **What percentage of patients with large intestinal bleeding will stop bleeding before transfusion requirements exceed two units?**

90%.

○   **If blood is recovered from the stomach after an NG tube is inserted, where is the most likely location of the bleed?**

Above the ligament of Treitz.

○   **Where do the majority of Mallory-Weiss tears occur?**

In the stomach (75%), esophagogastric junction (20%), and distal esophagus (5%).

○   **Where is angiodysplasia most frequently found?**

In the cecum and proximal ascending colon. Lesions are generally singular, bleeding is intermittent and seldom massive.

○ **What is the major cause of death in patients with Hirshsprung's disease?**

Enterocolitis.

○ **Is Hirshsprung's disease more common in males or in females?**

Males (5:1).

○ **Are tumors located in the jejunum and ileum more likely malignant or benign?**

Benign. Tumors of the jejunum and ileum comprise only 5% of all GI tumors. The majority are asymptomatic.

○ **What is the most common remnant of the omphalomesenteric duct?**

Meckel's diverticulum.

○ **What is the Meckel's diverticulum rule of 2's?**

2% of the population has it; it is 2 inches long; 2 feet from the ileocecal valve; occurs most commonly in children under 2; and is symptomatic in 2% of patients.

○ **What is the most likely cause of rectal bleeding in a patient with Meckel's diverticulum?**

Ulceration of ileal mucosa adjacent to the diverticulum lined with gastric mucosa.

○ **What is the most likely cause of cellulitis of the umbilicus in a pediatric patient with an acute abdomen?**

A perforated Meckel's diverticulum.

○ **What is the difference in the prognosis between familial polyposis and Gardner's disease?**

Although both are inheritable conditions of colonic polyps, Gardner's disease rarely results in malignancy, while familial polyposis virtually always results in malignancy.

○ **Clinically, how is right-sided colon cancer differentiated from left-sided?**

Right-sided lesions present with occult bleeding, weakness, anemia, dyspepsia, palpable abdominal mass, and dull abdominal pain. Left-sided lesions present with visible blood, obstructive symptoms, and noticeable changes in bowel habits. "Pencil thin" stools are also common.

○ **The advancement to adenocarcinoma of the colon from adenoma is size dependent. What is the risk of developing cancer if a 1.5 cm polyp is found upon colonoscopic examination?**

10%. The risk for developing adenocarcinoma is 1% if the polyp is less than 1 cm, 10% if it is 1 to 2 cm, and 45% if the polyp is greater than 2 cm.

○ **Is a villous, tubulovillous, or tubular adenoma more likely to become malignant?**

40% of villous adenomas will become malignant, compared to 22% of tubulovillous adenomas and 5% of tubular adenomas.

○   **Which are more likely to turn malignant, pedunculated or sessile lesions?**

Sessile.

○   **Where are the majority of colorectal cancers found?**

In the rectum (30%), ascending colon (25%), sigmoid colon (20%), descending colon (15%), and transverse colon (10%).

○   **A 41 year old patient complains of severe but short rectal spasms but has not noticed any bleeding. He is known to be stressed and overtaxed at work. What is your diagnosis?**

Proctalgia fugax. These short rectal spasms last less than 1 minute and occur infrequently. They are associated with people that are anxious, overworked or have a history of irritable bowel syndrome. No cause is known. Treatment is with analgesic suppositories, heating pads, and relaxation techniques.

○   **A patient complains of severe pain when defecating. He is constipated, has blood-streaked stools and a bloody discharge following bowel movements. What is the diagnosis?**

Anal fissure. Ninety percent of anal fissures are located in the posterior midline. If fissures are found elsewhere in the anal canal, then anal intercourse, TB, carcinoma, Crohn's disease, and syphilis should be considered.

○   **Differentiate between mucosal rectal prolapse, complete rectal prolapse, and occult rectal prolapse.**

Mucosal rectal prolapse: Involves only a small portion of the rectum protruding through the anus and have the appearance of radial folds.

Complete rectal prolapse: Involves all the layers of the rectum protruding through the anus. Clinically, this condition appears as concentric folds.

Occult rectal prolapse: Does not involve protrusion through the anus but rather intussusception.

○   **Which are more painful, internal or external hemorrhoids?**

External. The nerves above the pectinate or dentate line are supplied by the autonomic nervous system and have no sensory fibers. The nerves below the pectinate line are supplied by the inferior rectal nerve and have sensory fibers.

○   **Differentiate between first, second, third, and fourth degree hemorrhoids.**

First degree: Appear in the rectal lumen but do not protrude past the anus.
Second degree: Protrude into the anal canal if the patient strains only.
Third degree: Protrude into the anal canal but can be manually reduced.
Fourth degree: Protrude into the canal and cannot be manually reduced.

Treatment for degrees one and two is a high fiber diet, sitz baths, and good hygiene. The treatment of choice for third or fourth degree hemorrhoids is rubber band ligation. Other treatments are photocoagulation, electrocauterization, and cryosurgery.

○   **Diverticular disease is most common in which part of the colon?**

The sigmoid colon, which accounts for 95% of diverticular disease.

○   **What percentage of patients with diverticula are symptomatic?**

20%.

○   **What percentage of 45 year olds will have diverticula?**

33%, 66% will have diverticular by the age of 85.

○   **What are the signs and symptoms of diverticulitis?**

Abdominal pain, generally in the left lower quadrant, a low grade temperature, change in bowel habits, nausea and vomiting. If perforated, patients may have peritoneal signs and appear toxic.

○   **What is the treatment for diverticulitis?**

Bowel rest and antibiotics. Treatment can be out patient unless there are signs of systemic infection, or perfuration.

○   **What are some extraintestinal manifestations of ulcerative colitis?**

Ankylosing spondylitis, sclerosing cholangitis, arthralgias, ocular complications, erythema nodosum, aphthous ulcers in the mouth, thromboembolic disease, pyoderma gangrenosum, nephrolithiasis, and cirrhosis of the liver.

○   **Kulchitsky cells are the precursors to what tumor?**

Carcinoid. A carcinoid tumor can arise anywhere in the GI tract, but its most frequent site of involvement is the appendix.

○   **What is the probable cause of colovesicular fistulas?**

Sigmoid diverticulitis. Other causes are radiation enteritis, colon carcinoma, and bladder carcinoma. Colovesicular fistulas are diagnosed by cystoscopy.

○   **A 47 year old man complains of impotence as well as pain and coldness in both legs after exercise. What would you expect to find on examination?**

This patient probably has Leriche's syndrome, caused by occlusion of the abdominal aorta secondary to atherosclerosis. Physical examination should reveal weak or absent femoral and pedal pulses, a bruit, thrill, pallor with elevation of the limb, dependent rubor, and a high blood pressure. Treatment is either bypass or thromboendarterectomy.

○   **What is the most commonly obstructed artery in the lower extremity?**

The superficial femoral. It is a branch of the common femoral, which is a branch of the external iliac.

○   **A 64 year old male presents with jaundice, upper GI bleeding, anemia, a palpable non-tender gallbladder, a palpable liver, and rapid weight loss. What is your diagnosis?**

This is the clinical picture of a tumor of the ampulla of Vater.

○   **Testicular torsion occurs most commonly in what age group?**

Teens.

❍   **What is the maximum amount of time a testicle can remain torsed without being irreversibly damaged?**

4 to 6 hours.

❍   **What is definitve treatment for testicular torsion?**

Emergency surgical scrotal exploration.

❍   **What percentage of palpable prostate nodules are malignant?**

50%. Surgical cure of patients who present with asymptomatic nodules and no metastasis is attempted with radical prostatectomy or radiation therapy.

❍   **What are mycotic aneurysms?**

Mycotic aneurysms are true aneurysms that have become infected or false aneurysms that have occurred because of an arterial infection. The femoral artery is the most common site for such aneurysms.

❍   **Where is mesenteric ischemia more serious, in the small or the large bowel?**

The small bowel. Embolization in the superior mesenteric artery affects the entire small bowel. Mortality from small bowel ischemia is 60%. Embolization to the large bowel is not as serious due to collateral circulation. Ischemia of the large bowel rarely result in a full thickness injury or perforation.

❍   **What is an ABI, and why is it significant?**

An ankle/brachial index. The ankle systolic pressure (numerator) is compared to the higher of the 2 brachial arterial pressures (denominator). It is used to determine if arterial obstruction is present.

❍   **What technical factors can affect the accuracy of the ABI?**

Probe pressure, rapid deflation of the BP cuff, arterial wall calcifications, and probe placement, which should be longitudinal to the vessel and at a 30 to 60 degree angle to the skin surface.

TRAUMA SURGERY

○ **What percentage of cervical fractures are visualized on lateral, odontoid, and AP films of the neck?**

Lateral: 90%
Odontoid: 10%
AP: Just a few

○ **On a lateral C-spine, what does "fanning" of the spinous processes suggest?**

Posterior ligamentous disruption.

○ **What are the 3 most unstable C-spine injuries?**

1) Transverse atlantal ligament rupture.
2) Dens fracture.
3) Burst fracture with posterior ligament disruption.

○ **Describe a Jefferson fracture.**

A burst ring of C1, usually the result of a vertical compression force. It is best detected by using an odontoid view.

○ **Describe a hangman's fracture.**

A C2 bilateral pedicle fracture. It is usually caused by hyperextension.

○ **What is a clay-shoveler's fracture?**

In order of frequency, C7, C6, or T1 avulsion fractures of the spinous process. They can be caused by either flexion or a direct blow.

○ **Describe the key features of spinal shock.**

Sudden areflexia which is transient and distal, with a duration of hours to weeks. BP is usually 80 to 100 mm Hg with paradoxical bradycardia.

○ **A trauma patient presents with a decreasing level of consciousness and an enlarging right pupil. What is your diagnosis?**

Probable uncal herniation with oculomotor nerve compression.

○ **The corneal reflex tests what nerves?**

The ophthalmic branch (V1) of the trigeminal (fifth) nerve (afferent), and the facial (seventh) nerve (efferent).

○ **Name 5 clinical signs of basilar skull fracture.**

1) Periorbital ecchymosis (raccoon's eyes).

2) Retroauricular ecchymosis (Battle's sign).
3) Otorrhea or rhinorrhea.
4) Hemotympanum or bloody ear discharge.
5) First, second, seventh, and eighth CN deficits.

○   **A trauma patient presents with anisocoria, neurological deterioration, and/or lateralizing motor findings. What should be the immediate treatment?**

Immediate intubation and hyperventilation. Unless the patient is hypovolemic, infuse mannitol 1 g/kg rapidly. Elevate head of bed 30°. Some authors still recommend dexamethasone, 10 mg, and phenytoin, 18 mg/kg at 20 mg/min.

○   **How is posterior column function tested? Why is it significant?**

Position and vibration sensation are carried in the posterior columns and are usually spared in anterior cord syndrome. Light touch sensation may also be spared. Pain and temperature sensation cross near the level of entry and are carried in the more posterior spinothalamic tract.

○   **Define increased intracranial pressure.**

ICP > 15 mm Hg.

○   **Where is the most common site of a basilar skull fracture?**

Petrous portion of the temporal bone.

○   **What cardiovascular injury is commonly associated with a sternal fracture?**

Myocardial contusions (blunt myocardial injury).

○   **Which valve is most commonly injured during blunt trauma?**

Aortic valve.

○   **What is the differential diagnosis of distended neck veins in a trauma patient?**

Tension pneumothorax, pericardial tamponade, air embolism, and cardiac failure. Neck vein distention may not be present until hypovolemia has been treated.

○   **What is the most sensitive indicator of shock in children?**

Tachycardia.

○   **What initial fluid bolus should be administered to children in shock?**

20 mL/kg.

○   **A radial pulse on examination indicates a BP of at least what level?**

80 mm Hg.

○   **A femoral pulse on examination indicates a BP of at least what level?**

70 mm Hg.

O **A carotid pulse indicates a BP of at least what level?**

60 mm Hg.

O **Do post-traumatic seizures occur more frequently in children or adults?**

Children.

O **What is the most common complaint of patients with a traumatic aortic injury?**

Retrosternal or intrascapular pain.

O **Amputation is often required after vascular injuries to what artery?**

Popliteal artery. Injuries to arteries below the adductor hiatus lead to a loss of limb more frequently than injuries elsewhere.

O **How long does it take to prepare fully crossmatched blood?**

30 to 60 minutes.

O **Is the heat of firing significant enough to sterilize a bullet and its wound?**

No, contaminants from the body surface and viscera can be carried along the bullet's path.

O **What artery is usually involved in an epidural hematoma?**

The middle meningeal artery.

O **Where are epidural hematomas located?**

Between the dura and inner table of the skull.

O **Where are subdural hematomas located?**

Beneath the dura, over the brain, and in the arachnoid. They are caused by tears of pial arteries or of bridging veins. Subdural hematomas typically become symptomatic 24 hours to 2 weeks after injury.

O **What risk is associated with not treating a septal hematoma of the nose?**

Aseptic necrosis followed by absorption of the septal cartilage, resulting in septal perforation.

ORTHOPEDICS

○ **How do you clinically differentiate between acute compartment syndrome, neuropraxia, and arterial occlusion?**

The patient will have normal pulses in neuropraxia, decreased pulses in compartment syndrome (though this is a very rare and insensitive finding), and no pulses in arterial occlusion. Stretching the muscles will cause great pain in compartment syndrome but not in neuropraxia.

○ **What is Finkelstein's test?**

A test used to determine whether a patient has de Quervain's disorder (an entrapment syndrome caused by tenosynovitis of the abductor pollicis longus and extensor pollicis brevis). If pain is elicited when the patient grasps his thumb with the fingers of the same hand and deviates his wrist in the ulnar direction then the test is positive.

○ **What is the most common type of peripheral nerve compression?**

Carpal tunnel syndrome. This syndrome is more often diagnosed in female patients than male. Clinically, the patient will have pain and weakness which worsen at night. Moderate relief will come by shaking the hands. Wrist supports or hydrocortisone and Xylocaine injections may provide relief. If conservative measures do not work, surgical decompression can be performed.

○ **What fingers are most often affected by carpal tunnel syndrome?**

The third and fourth digits. The sensory nerves to these digits are closest to the volar carpal ligament, which compresses the structures in the carpal tunnel.

○ **Describe Tinel's and Phalen's tests.**

Both tests for carpal tunnel syndrome.

Tinel's: Tapping the volar aspect of the wrist over the median nerve produces paresthesias that extend along the index and long finger.

Phalen's: Full flexion at the wrist for 1 minute leads to paresthesia along distribution of median nerve.

○ **What long bone is most commonly fractured?**

The tibia.

○ **Where is the most common site of osteomyelitis of the vertebral column?**

The lumbar spine.

○ **How many cervical vertebrae does a giraffe have?**

7 very large vertebrae.

○ **What is the most common cause of pyogenic osteomyelitis of the vertebral column?**

Staphylococcus aureus, secondary to hematogenous spread.

○   **What population is most likely to develop osteoid osteoma?**

Males under 30 years of age. Osteoid osteoma is a benign musculoskeletal tumor. It is characterized by intense localized pain that is relieved by aspirin. Definitive treatment is surgery.

○   **What are the four muscles of the rotator cuff?**

Supraspinatus, infraspinatus, teres minor, and subscapularis.

○   **What is the cause of boutonnière deformity?**

Disruption of the extensor hood at the PIP joint of the finger.

○   **Describe a gamekeeper's thumb.**

Disruption of the ulnar collateral ligament of the MP joint of the thumb. If stress tests show an opening larger than 20°, surgical repair is indicated.

○   **What is the treatment for a felon?**

10 to 12 years, with time off for good behavior. Actually, a felon is a subcutaneous infection in the pulp space of the fingertip, usually due to *Staphylococcus aureus*. Treat by incising the pulp space.

○   **A 43 year old female complains that her left knee hurts when she walks down stairs or when she bends her knee too far. There has been no trauma or new exercise. What is the probable diagnosis?**

Chondromalacia, which is degeneration of the cartilage of the patella. The cause is unknown.

○   **Describe the leg position of a patient with a femoral neck fracture.**

Shortened, abducted, and slightly externally rotated.

○   **Describe the leg position of a patient with an anterior hip dislocation.**

Hip is abducted and externally rotated. This accounts for 10% of hip dislocations. The mechanism of injury is forced abduction.

○   **Describe the leg position of a patient with a posterior hip dislocation.**

Shortened, adducted, and internally rotated. This accounts for 90% of hip dislocations. The mechanism of injury is force applied to a flexed knee directed posteriorly. This dislocation is associated with sciatic nerve injury (10%) and avascular necrosis of the femoral head.

○   **Describe the leg position of a patient with an intertrochanteric hip fracture.**

Shortened, externally rotated, and abducted.

○   **Describe a typical patient with a slipped capital femoral epiphysis.**

An obese boy, 10 to 16 years old, with groin or knee discomfort increasing with activity. He may also have a limp. The slip can occur bilaterally and best observed on a lateral view of the hip.

O   **What is the most significant complication of a proximal tibial metaphyseal fracture?**

Arterial involvement, especially when there is a valgus deformity.

O   **What is the most common ankle injury?**

Sprains, account for 75% of all ankle injuries. Of these, 90% involve the lateral complex. Ninety percent of lateral ligament injuries are anterior talofibular.

O   **What is the most helpful physical test for anterior talofibular ligament injuries?**

Anterior drawer test. More than 3 mm of excursion might be significant (compare sides); more than 1 cm is always significant.

O   **How are sprains classified?**

First degree: Ligament is stretched, x-ray is normal.

Second degree: Ligament is severely stretched with partial tear, marked tenderness, swelling, and pain; x-ray is normal.

Third degree: Ligament is completely ruptured, there is marked tenderness, and the joint is swollen and/or obviously deformed. X-ray may show an abnormal joint.

O   **A 21 year old female complains of pain and a clicking sound located at the posterior lateral malleolus. A fullness beneath the lateral malleolus is found. What is the diagnosis?**

Peroneal tendon subluxation with associated tenosynovitis.

O   **Traumatic arthritis occurs in what percentage of ankle fractures?**

20 to 40%.

O   **Which bone is most often fractured at birth?**

The clavicle.

O   **What is the most common shoulder dislocation?**

Anterior (95%).

O   **A patient cannot actively abduct her shoulder. What injury does this suggest?**

Rotator cuff tear. The cuff is comprised of the supraspinatus, infraspinatus, subscapularis, and the teres minor muscles and tendons.

O   **Why is a displaced supracondylar fracture of the distal humerus in a child considered an emergency?**

This fracture often results in injury to the brachial artery or the median nerve. It can also cause compartment syndrome.

O   **What are the signs and symptoms for compartment syndrome involving the anterior compartment of the leg?**

Pain on active and passive dorsi-flexion and plantar-flexion of the foot, and hypesthesia paresthesia of the first web space of the foot.

○   **What is the most feared complication of a scaphoid fracture?**

Avascular necrosis. The more proximal the fracture, the more commonly avascular necrosis occurs.

○   **What fracture is frequently missed when a patient complains of an ankle injury?**

Fracture at the base of the fifth metatarsal, caused by plantar flexion and inversion. Radiographs of the ankle may not include the fifth metatarsal.

○   **What life-threatening injury is associated with pelvic fractures?**

Severe hemorrhage, usually retroperitoneal. Up to 6 liters of blood can be accommodated in this space.

○   **What pelvic fracture is most likely to involve severe hemorrhage?**

Severe hemorrhage will occur in 75% of vertical sheer fractures.

○   **Which pelvic fracture is most likely to involve bladder rupture?**

Lateral compression fractures (20%).

○   **Which pelvic fracture is most likely to involve urethral injury?**

Anterior-posterior compression fracture (36%).

○   **Which fracture is associated with avascular necrosis of the femoral head?**

Femoral neck fractures. Avascular necrosis occurs with 15% of non-displaced femoral neck fractures and with nearly 90% of displaced femoral neck fractures.

○   **What is a stress fracture?**

A stress or fatigue fracture is caused by small, repetitive forces that usually involve the metatarsal shafts, the distal tibia, and the femoral neck. These fractures may not be seen on initial radiographs.

○   **What is "nursemaid's elbow"?**

Subluxation of the radial head. During forceful retraction, fibers of the annular ligament that encircle the radial neck become trapped between the radial head and the capitellum. On presentation, children hold their arm in slight flexion and pronation.

○   **Why "tap" a knee with acute hemarthrosis?**

Tapping the knee relieves pressure and pain for the patient and will allow you to ascertain whether fat globules are present, indicating a fracture.

○   **What is the most common site of compartment syndrome?**

The anterior compartment of the leg.

○   **What type of patient receives an Achilles' tendon rupture?**

Middle-aged men. It occurs most commonly on the left side.

○   **What are the most common lower extremity bone injuries in children?**

Tibial and fibular shaft fractures, usually secondary to twist forces.

○   **What are the differences between avulsion of the tibial tubercle and Osgood-Schlatter disease?**

Both occur at the tibial tubercle. Avulsion presents with an acute inability to walk. A lateral view of the knee is most diagnostic; treatment is surgical. Osgood-Schlatter disease has a vague history of intermittent pain, is bilateral 25% of the time, and has pain with range of motion but not with rest; treatment is symptomatic and not surgical.

○   **What is a toddler fracture?**

A spiral fracture of the tibia without fibular involvement. This type of fracture in toddlers is a common cause of limping or refusal to walk.

○   **What is the most commonly fractured carpal bone?**

The scaphoid bone (navicular).

○   **A stress fracture of the second or third metatarsal is suspected but not detected on initial x-rays. How many days after the initial examination should a second x-ray be ordered?**

14 to 21 days.

○   **After a fracture, what are the 3 stages of healing?**

1) Union
2) Consolidation
3) Remodeling

○   **How long after a fracture does callus start to form?**

5 to 7 days.

○   **What is the tarsal-metatarsal joint also called?**

Lisfranc's joint.

○   **The second metatarsal is the locking mechanism for the mid part of the foot. A fracture at the base of the second metatarsal should raise suspicion of what?**

A disrupted joint. Treatment may require ORIF.

○   **A pneumatic tourniquet can be inflated on an extremity to more than a patient's systolic blood pressure for how long without damaging underlying vessels or neurons?**

2 hours.

○   **What basic disorder contributes to the pathophysiology of compartment syndrome?**

Increased pressure within closed tissue spaces compromising blood flow to muscle and nerve tissue. There are three prerequisites to the development of compartment syndrome:

1) Limiting space
2) Increased tissue pressure
3) Decreased tissue perfusion

○ **What are the two basic mechanisms for elevated compartment pressure?**

1) External compression—by burn eschar, circumferential casts, dressings, or pneumatic pressure garments.

2) Volume increase within the compartment—hemorrhage into the compartment, IV infiltration, or edema secondary to injury or due to post-ischemic (postischial) swelling.

○ **Which two fractures are most commonly associated with compartment syndrome?**

Tibia (resulting most often in anterior compartment involvement) and supracondylar humerus fractures.

○ **What are the early signs and symptoms of compartment syndrome?**

1) Tenderness and pain out of proportion to the injury
2) Pain with active and passive motion
3) Hypesthesia (paresthesia), abnormal two point discrimination

○ **What are the late signs and symptoms of compartment syndrome?**

1) Tense, indurated, and erythematous compartment
2) Slow capillary refill
3) Pallor and pulselessness

○ **What are the 6 P's of compartment syndrome?**

1) Pain
2) Pallor
3) Pulselessness
4) Paresthesia
5) Poikilothermia
6) Paralysis

○ **What are the four compartments of the leg?**

1) Anterior
2) Lateral
3) Deep posterior
4) Superficial posterior

○ **With complete rupture of medial or collateral ligaments of the knee, how much laxity can be expected upon examination?**

> 1 cm without endpoint as compared to an uninjured knee.

○ **Which ligament in the knee is the most commonly injured?**

Anterior cruciate ligament, usually from a non-contact injury.

○ **Overall, what is the leading cause of disability for patients under age 45?**

Chronic lower back pain. One percent of the population is totally disabled from back pain, and only 1% require surgery. Patients with lower back pain who do not qualify for surgery have an 80% to 90% chance of recovering within 6 weeks of their injury.

○   **What is a valgus deformity? Varus deformity?**

Valgus deformity is angulation of an extremity at a joint with the more distal part angled away from the midline. Varus deformity is angulation of an extremity at a joint with the more distal part angled toward the midline.

○   **Are dislocations and sprains more common in children or adults?**
Dislocations and ligamentous injuries are uncommon in prepubertal children as the ligaments and joints are quite strong as compared to the adjoining growth plates. Excessive force applied to a child's joint is more likely to cause a fracture through the growth plate than a dislocation or sprain.

○   **What is the order of ossification centers in the elbow?**

Remember the acronym CRITOE. Capitellum, Radial Head, Internal (medial) epicondyle, Trochlea, Olecranon, External (lateral) epicondyle. These ossify at 3-5-7-9-11-13 years, in that order.

OPHTHALMOLOGY AND EENT

❍ **What are cotton wool spots?**

White patches on the retina that are observed upon funduscopic examination. These patches are due to ischemia of the superficial nerve layer of the retina. They are most commonly associated with hypertension but also occur in patients with diabetes, anemia, collagen vascular disease, leukemia, endocarditis, and AIDS.

❍ **Do visual changes in chronic open-angle glaucoma patients begin centrally or peripherally?**

Peripherally. Patients with chronic glaucoma experience a gradual and painless loss of vision. Those with acute or subacute angle glaucoma will have either dull or severe pain, blurry vision, lacrimation, and even nausea and vomiting. The pain may be more severe in the dark.

❍ **Which is more common, chronic open-angle glaucoma or acute closed-angle glaucoma?**

Chronic open-angle glaucoma (90%). Four percent of the population over age 40 has glaucoma.

❍ **What is the most common cause of chronic open-angle glaucoma?**

Outflow obstruction through the trabecular meshwork. Other causes are obstruction of Schlemm's canal and excess secretion of aqueous fluid.

❍ **What is the most common finding upon funduscopic examination of a patient with AIDS?**

Cotton wool spots due to disease of the microvasculature. Other findings are hemorrhage, exudate, or retinal necrosis.

❍ **What percentage of the elderly are hard of hearing?**

What? Twenty-nine percent of people over the age of 65 and 36% of people over the age of 75 suffer hearing loss sufficient to interfere with normal conversation.

❍ **What is the most common type of hearing loss in the elderly?**

Presbycusis. This is an idiopathic, insidious, symmetrical decline in hearing that is associated with aging.

❍ **If a rupture of the round or oval window is suspected in a patient with acute hearing loss, what test might you perform?**

Test for ipsilateral nystagmus by applying positive pressure to the tympanic membrane.

❍ **What systemic sexually transmitted disease is associated with sensorineural hearing loss?**

Syphilis. Seven percent of patients with idiopathic hearing loss test positive for treponemal antibodies.

❍ **Acute tinnitus is associated with toxicity of what medication?**

Salicylates. Other causes of tinnitus are vascular abnormalities, mechanical abnormalities, and damaged cochlear hair cells. Unilateral tinnitus is associated with chronic suppurative otitis, Meniere's disease, and trauma.

O   **Hairy leukoplakia is characteristic of which two viruses?**

HIV and Epstein-Barr virus. Hairy leukoplakia is usually found on the lateral aspect of the tongue. Oral thrush may also be associated with HIV.

O   **What is the most common cause of odontogenic pain?**

Carious tooth. When percussed with a tongue blade, the offending tooth will produce a sharp pain felt in the ear, throat, eyes, temple, or other side of the jaw.

O   **What is the best transport medium for an avulsed tooth?**

Hank's solution, a pH balanced cell culture medium, which may even help restore cell viability if the tooth has been avulsed for more than 30 minutes. Milk is an alternative.   The patient may place the tooth underneath his tongue if aspiration can be prevented

O   **A patient presents three days after tooth extraction with severe pain and a foul mouth odor and taste.   What is the appropriate diagnosis and treatment?**

Alveolar osteitis (dry socket) results from loss of the blood clot and local osteomyelitis. Treat by irrigation of the socket and application of a medicated dental packing or iodoform gauze moistened with Campho-Phenique or eugenol.

O   **What is the most common oral manifestation of AIDS?**

Oropharyngeal thrush. Some other AIDS related oropharyngeal diseases are Kaposi's sarcoma, hairy leukoplakia, and non-Hodgkin's lymphoma.

O   **A 47 year old female presents complaining of excruciating pain described as an "electric shock sensation" located in her right cheek that waxes and wanes. Diagnosis and treatment?**

Tic douloureux. The most significant finding is that the pain follows the distribution of the trigeminal nerve. Minor trigger zone stimulation will often reproduce the pain. Treat with carbamazepine (100 mg bid starting dose and increasing to 1200 mg daily if needed). Refer the patient to a neurologist and a dentist to rule out cerebellopontine angle tumors, MS, nasopharyngeal carcinoma, cluster headaches, polymyalgia rheumatica, temporal arteritis, and oral pathology.

O   **A 3 year old child presents with a unilateral purulent rhinorrhea. What is the probable diagnosis?**

Nasal foreign body.

O   **What potential complications of nasal fracture should always be considered on physical examination?**

Septal hematoma and cribriform plate fractures. A septal hematoma appears as a bluish mass on the nasal septum. If not drained, aseptic necrosis of the septal cartilage and septal abnormalities may occur. A cribriform plate fracture should be considered in a patient who has a clear rhinorrhea after trauma.

O   **What 4 physical examination findings would make posterior epistaxis more likely than anterior epistaxis?**

1) Inability to see the site of bleeding. Anterior nosebleeds usually originate at Kiesselbach's plexus, and are easily visualized on the nasal septum.
2) Blood from both sides of the nose. In a posterior nosebleed, the blood can more easily pass to the other side because of the proximity of the choanae.
3) Blood trickling down the oropharynx.
4) Inability to control bleeding by direct pressure.

O   **A patient returns to the emergency department with fever, nausea, vomiting, and hypotension two days after having nasal packing placed for an anterior nosebleed. What potential complication of nasal packing should be considered?**

Toxic shock syndrome.

O   **A child with a sinus infection presents with proptosis; a red, swollen eyelid; and an inferolaterally displaced globe. What is the diagnosis?**

Orbital cellulitis and abscess associated with ethmoid sinusitis.

O   **A patient with frontal sinusitis presents with a large forehead abscess. What is the diagnosis?**

Pott's puffy tumor. This is a complication of frontal sinusitis in which the anterior table of the skull is destroyed, allowing the formation of the abscess.

O   **An ill appearing patient presents with a fever of 103°F, bilateral chemosis, third nerve palsies, and untreated sinusitis. What is the diagnosis?**

Cavernous sinus thrombosis. This life-threatening complication occurs from direct extension through the valveless veins. Complications of sinusitis may be local (osteomyelitis), orbital (cellulitis), or within the central nervous system (meningitis or brain abscess).

O   **Retropharyngeal abscesses are most common in what age group? Why?**

6 months to 3 years of age. Retropharyngeal lymph nodes regress in size after age 3.

O   **Describe the overall appearance of a child with a retropharyngeal abscess.**

These children are often ill appearing, febrile, stridorous, drooling, and in an opisthotonic position. They may complain of difficulty swallowing or may refuse to eat.

O   **What radiographic sign indicates a retropharyngeal abscess?**

A widening of the retropharyngeal space which is normally 3 to 4 mm, or less than half the width of the vertebral bodies. False widening may occur if the x-ray is not taken during inspiration and with the patient's neck extended. Occasionally, an air fluid level may be noted in the retropharyngeal space.

O   **Retropharyngeal abscesses are most commonly caused by which organisms?**

ß-Hemolytic *Streptococcus*.

O   **A 48 year old male presents with a high fever, trismus, dysphagia, and swelling inferior to the mandible in the lateral neck. What is the diagnosis?**

Parapharyngeal abscess.

O   **Where is the most common origin of Ludwig's angina?**

The lower second and third molar. Ludwig's angina is a swelling in the region of the submandibular, sublingual, and submental spaces, which may cause upward and posterior displacement of the tongue. It is most commonly caused by hemolytic streptococci, staphylococci, and mixed anaerobic/aerobic bacteria.

O   **What are the signs and symptoms of a mandibular fracture?**

Malocclusion, pain, opening deviation or abnormal movement, decreased range of motion, bony deformity, swelling, ecchymosis, and lower lip (mental nerve) anesthesia.

O   **A bilateral mental fracture can lead to what acute complication?**

Acute airway obstruction caused by the tongue because of a loss of anterior support.

O   **A patient was yawning in lecture and is now unable to close his mouth. He is having difficulty talking and swallowing. What is the diagnosis?**

Bilateral dislocation of the mandibular condyles. This can occur if the mouth is opened excessively wide. X-rays can rule out bilateral condyle fractures, which may have a similar clinical appearance.

O   **A 42 year old female presents with dull pain in her right ear and jaw, and a burning sensation in the roof of her mouth. The pain is worse in the evening. She also hears a "popping" sound when opening and closing her mouth. Further examination reveals tenderness of the joint capsule. What is the diagnosis and treatment?**

TMJ syndrome. Treat with physiotherapy, analgesia, a soft diet, muscle relaxants, and occlusive therapy. Apply warm, moist compresses 4 to 5 times daily for 15 minutes for 7 to 10 days.

O   **What radiographic view best reveals a zygomatic arch fracture?**

The modified basal view of the skull. Synonyms include jug-handle view, submental occipital view, or submental vertical view.

O   **What are the signs and symptoms of a fracture of the zygomaticomaxillary complex?**

Subcutaneous emphysema, edema, ecchymosis, facial flattening, subconjunctival hemorrhage, ecchymosis around the orbit, unilateral epistaxis, anesthesia of the cheek upper lip and gum from infraorbital nerve injury, step deformity, decreased mandibular movement, and diplopia.

O   **What two findings are most commonly associated with orbital floor fractures?**

Diplopia and globe lowering.

O   **What plain radiograph views are most helpful in evaluating facial fractures?**

Water's view: Useful for evaluating zygomaticomaxillary complex, orbital blowout, and Le Fort fractures

Modified basal view of the skull: Useful for evaluating zygomatic arch fractures

Panorex: Useful for evaluating mandibular fractures

O   **What 3 clinical signs should lead a physician to consider disruption of the medial canthal ligaments with nasal skeletal fracture?**

1) Widened nasal bridge
2) Intercanthic distance greater than approximately 35 mm
3) Almond-shaped palpebral fissures

○ **A 48 year old presents with pain, itching, and discharge from the right ear. The tympanic membrane is intact. What is the diagnosis?**

Otitis externa. Suction ear and prescribe antibiotic/steroid otic solution for one week. An ear wick may improve delivery of the antibiotic. Suspect malignant otitis externa if the patient is diabetic.

○ **A patient presents with ear pain and fluid filled blisters on the tympanic membrane. What is the diagnosis?**

Bullous myringitis, commonly caused by *Mycoplasma* or a virus. Treat with erythromycin.

○ **A 16 year old boxer presents with right ear pain and swelling after receiving a blow to the ear. What is the treatment?**

The ear should be aseptically drained by incision or aspiration and a mastoid conforming dressing should be applied. ENT follow-up is mandatory. If the ear is not treated appropriately, a cauliflower deformity may result.

○ **A patient presents with a swollen, tender, red left auricle. What is the diagnosis?**

Perichondritis. This is most often caused by *Pseudomonas*.

○ **What is the most common cause of hearing loss?**

Cerumen impaction.

○ **Describe the physical finding of unilateral sensory hearing loss.**

The patient will lateralize and have air conduction greater than bone conduction (i.e., normal Rinne test) indicating no conductive loss. The Weber test will lateralize to the normal ear. The most common cause of unilateral sensory hearing loss is viral neuritis.

○ **Which causes should be suspected in a patient with bilateral sensory hearing loss?**

Noise or ototoxins (e.g., certain antibiotics, loop diuretics, or antineoplastics).

○ **What is the most common neuropathy associated with acoustic neuroma?**

The corneal reflex may be lost due to trigeminal nucleus involvement.

○ **Name some causes of tympanic membrane perforation.**

Air or water blast injuries, foreign bodies in the ear (particularly cotton tip swabs), lightning strikes, otitis media, and associated temporal bone fractures.

○ **A young man who was involved in a bar room brawl complains of ear pain, significantly decreased hearing, and vertigo. A tympanic membrane rupture is determined by examination. What is the concern?**

Injury to the ossicles, temporal bone, or labyrinth. An urgent ENT consult is necessary.

○ **A diver on vacation decided to go scuba diving despite a cold. While descending, she had acute ear pain followed by vertiginous symptoms and vomiting. What happened?**

Middle ear squeeze.   Pressure from the middle ear could not be equalized because of abnormal eustachian tube function resulting from the illness. The middle ear volume decreased until the tympanic membrane retracted to the point of rupture. The inrush of cold water caused vestibular stimulation. This is the most common form of barotrauma in amateur scuba divers. Similar problems may occur on planes.

○   **What organism usually causes pediatric acute otitis media?**

Streptococcus pneumoniae, followed by *Haemophilus influenzae* and *Moraxella catarrhalis*.

○   **Why are preschool children more susceptible to acute otitis media?**

Children have shorter, more horizontal eustachian tubes, which may prevent adequate drainage and allow aspiration of nasopharyngeal bacteria into the middle ear, particularly with URIs.

○   **What is a Bezold abscess?**

A complication of acute mastoiditis.   Infection spreads to the soft tissues below the ear and sternocleidomastoid muscle.

○   **What is the most common cause of sialoadenitis?**

Mumps.

○   **A patient presents with trismus, fever, and an erythematous, tender parotid gland. Pus is expressed from Stensen's duct. What conditions predisposes the patient to bacterial parotitis?**

Any situation which decreases salivary flow including irradiation, phenothiazines, antihistamines, parasympathetic inhibitors, dehydration and debilitation. Up to 30% of cases occur postoperatively.

○   **Where do salivary gland stones most frequently develop?**

80% are submandibular. The least likely is the sublingual gland.

○   **What does grunting versus inspiratory stridor indicate?**

Grunting is specific to lower respiratory tract diseases, such as pneumonia, asthma, and bronchiolitis. Stridor localizes respiratory obstruction to the level at or above the larynx.

○   **What is the most common cause of laryngeal trauma?**

Blunt trauma secondary to a motor vehicle accident.

○   **A patient presents with well demarcated swelling of the lips and tongue. She was started on an antihypertensive agent three weeks ago. What is the most likely agent?**

Angiotensin-converting enzyme inhibitor. Although angioneurotic edema may occur anytime during therapy, it is most likely to occur within in first month when using an ACE inhibitor.

○   **A patient presents with an itching, tearing, right eye. Upon examination large cobblestone papillae are found under the upper lid.   What is the probable diagnosis?**

Allergic conjunctivitis.

○   **A patient is seen with herpetic lesions on the tip of the nose. Why is this a problem?**

The tip of the nose and the cornea are both supplied by the nasociliary nerve. Thus, the cornea may also be involved. This is an ophthalmological emergency.

〇　**A patient presents with conjunctiva and lid margin inflammation. Slit-lamp examination reveals a "greasy" appearance of the lid margins with scaling, especially around the base of the lashes. Diagnosis?**

Blepharitis. This is often caused by a staphylococcal infection of the oil glands and skin next to the lash follicles. Treatment consists of scrubbing with baby shampoo and, after consultation with an ophthalmologist, sulfacetamide drops and steroids.

〇　**A patient presents with a painful red eye. Slit-lamp examination reveals a localized, white, flocculent infiltrate in the anterior chamber. What is this?**

Hypopyon which is an accumulation of white inflammatory exudate in the anterior chamber.

〇　**A welder presents with severe eye pain. What is the expected finding upon slit-lamp examination?**

Diffuse punctate keratopathy (welder's flash) which presents as a multiple pinpoint area of fluorescein uptake representing ruptured corneal epithelial cells.

〇　**A patient presents with a pustular vesicle at the lid margin. What is the diagnosis and treatment?**

Hordeolum (stye). An acute inflammation of the meibomian gland, most commonly of the upper lid. Treat with topical antibiotics and warm compresses. Surgical drainage may be necessary.

〇　**A patient presents with a chronic, non-tender, uninflamed nodule of the upper lid. What is the diagnosis?**

Chalazion. Treat with surgical curettage.

〇　**A patient presents with the sensation of a foreign body in the eye. Slitlamp reveals a dendritic (branch-like) pattern. What is the treatment?**

Antiviral agents and cycloplegics. This is most probably a herpes simplex keratitis. Steroids spell disaster! Emergent opthalmology consultation is indicated.

〇　**A patient presents with sudden onset of vision loss in one eye that quickly returns. This should be diagnosed as?**

Amaurosis fugax. Usually caused by central retinal artery emboli from extracranial atherosclerosis.

〇　**A patient presents with painless vision loss in one eye described as a wall slowly developing in the visual field. What finding do you expect upon examination?**

A gray, detached retina. The patient may also complain of flashing lights in the peripheral visual field or spider webs in the visual field. Inferior detachment is treated with the patient sitting up. Superior detachment is treated with the patient lying flat.

〇　**A patient was hit in the eye during a drunken brawl. He presents 8 hours after the incident with proptosis and visual loss. Examination reveals an intact globe and an afferent pupillary defect. What is the problem?**

Retro orbital hematoma with ischemia of the optic nerve or retina. The pressure of the blood in the orbit exceeds the perfusion pressure resulting in a lack of blood flow and loss of function. Treatment is to release the pressure by lateral canthotomy. A similar situation can occur with orbital emphysema.

○   **Which is worse, acid or alkali burns of the cornea?**

Alkali, because of deeper penetration than acid burns. A barrier is formed from precipitated proteins with acid burns. The exception is hydrofluoric acid and heavy metal containing acids which can penetrate the cornea.

○   **When should an eye not be dilated?**

With known narrow angle glaucoma and with an iris-supported intraocular lens.

○   **Why shouldn't topical ophthalmologic anesthetics be prescribed?**

The anesthetics inhibit healing and decrease the patient's ability to protect his eye due to the lack of sensation.

○   **What is the most common organism in contact lens associated corneal ulcers?**

Pseudomonas.

○   **How can Krazy-Glue (cyanoacrylate) be removed if a patient has stuck their eyelids together?**

Copious irrigation immediately, and then mineral oil. Acetone and ethanol are unacceptable in the eyes. Surgical separation must be done with extreme care to prevent laceration of the lids or globe. Often the patient will have a corneal abrasion, which should be treated in the usual manner.

○   **A very anxious 16 year old male presents, stating that his vision is similar to "looking down a gun barrel." How do you clinically differentiate between physiologic and hysterical scotoma?**

Physiologic: Doubling the distance between the patient and tangent screen (visual screen test) results in doubling of the size of the central visual field.

Hysterical: Visual field remains the same.

○   **What test can a physician use to determine if blindness is of a hysterical origin?**

An optokinetic drum can be used. If nystagmus eye movements occur, the patient is seeing the stripes. Prisms may also be used.

○   **What conditions have been associated with central retinal vein occlusion?**

Hyperviscosity syndromes, diabetes, and hypertension. Funduscopic examination shows a chaotically streaked retina with congested dilated veins. There are superficial and deep retinal hemorrhages, cotton wool spots, and macular edema.

○   **A patient presents with atraumatic pain behind the left eye, a left pupil afferent defect, central visual loss, and a left swollen disc. Diagnosis and potential causes?**

Optic neuritis. This may be idiopathic or may be associated with multiple sclerosis, Lyme disease, neurosyphilis, lupus, sarcoid, alcoholism, toxins, or drug abuse.

◯ **After entering a dark bar, a patient developed eye pain, nausea, vomiting and blurred vision; also, he sees halos around lights. Why would this patient be given mannitol, pilocarpine, and acetazolamide?**

This patient has acute narrow angle glaucoma. The goal of treatment is to decrease intraocular pressure.

1) Decrease the production of aqueous humor with carbonic anhydrase inhibitor.
2) Decrease intraocular volume by making the plasma hypertonic to the aqueous humor with glycerol or mannitol.
3) Constrict the pupil with pilocarpine, allowing increased flow of the aqueous humor out through the previously blocked canals of Schlemm.

◯ **A patient presents with multiple vertical linear corneal abrasions. What should be suspected?**

A foreign body under the upper lid. This pattern is sometimes called an "ice rink" sign.

◯ **How can a physician estimate if the anterior chamber of the eye is narrow?**

Tangential light (as with a penlight) is shone perpendicular to the line of vision across the anterior chamber. If the entire iris is in the light then the chamber is most likely a normal depth. If part of the iris is in a shadow, the chamber is narrow. This can occur with narrow angle glaucoma and with perforating corneal injuries.

◯ **What is the difference between a sympathomimetic and a cycloplegic medication when dilating the eye?**

A sympathomimetic simulates the iris's dilator muscle. The cycloplegic inhibits the parasympathetic stimulation which constricts the iris and inhibits the ciliary muscle. Thus, cycloplegics will cause blurred near vision.

◯ **A patient felt something fly into his eye while mowing the lawn. On examination, there is a brown foreign body on the cornea and a tear drop iris pointing towards the foreign body. What is the diagnosis?**

Perforated cornea with extruded iris. A similar foreign body may appear black on the sclera with scleral perforation.

◯ **A patient presents with a physical finding of a chaotically blood-streaked retina with congested and dilated veins. What is the diagnosis?**

Central retinal vein occlusion. Patients often complain of a painless unilateral decrease of vision.

◯ **Retropharyngeal abscess is most common in what age group?**

Children < 4 years old. Symptoms include difficulty breathing, fever, enlarged cervical nodes, difficulty swallowing, and a stiff neck. Examination may reveal a mass or fullness in the posterior pharyngeal area.

◯ **Peritonsillar abscess is most common in what age group?**

Adolescents and young adults. Symptoms may include ear pain, trismus, drooling, and alteration of voice.

PEDIATRIC PEARLS

○ **A child is born pink with blue extremities, limp, a heartrate of 80 with slow irregular respirations and a grimace. What is this infant's APGAR score?**

4.

Apgar scores	0	1	2
Color	Blue, pale	Pink body, blue extremities	All pink
Muscle tone	Limp	Slight flexion	Active
Heart rate	0	<100	>100
Respirations	None	Slow, irregular	Strong, regular
Response to irritation	None	Some grimace	Strong grimace-cry

○ **What is the moro reflex?**

An extension of the upper extremities at both shoulders and elbows in response to dropping an infant's head to a flat position from a 30 degree incline.

○ **At what age does the moro reflex disappear?**

6 months.

○ **Touching the side of an infants mouth or cheek causes the infant to turn its head in that direction is called the _____ reflex.**

The suck (or rooting) reflex.

○ **Which reflex has the earliest onset?**

The grasp reflex. It can be noted at just 20 weeks gestation.

○ **What are milia?**

Small yellow-white papules typically on the face of newborns. They are transient and are caused by retained sebum.

○ **What is the difference between a cephalhematoma and caput succedaneum?**

A *cephalhematoma* is a unilateral swelling on the scalp caused by subperiosteal hemorrhage.
A *Caput succedaneum* is a swelling on the scalp that extends beyond the suture lines and is caused by the pressure of labor and delivery.

○ **What do decreased femoral pulses on the newborn exam indicate?**

Coarctation of the aorta

○ **What is the normal liver edge in a newborn?**

1 – 2 cm below the right costal margin.

○ **What is the importance of the red reflex in the newborn exam?**

A red reflex means that the infant does not have lens opacities or a retinoblastoma.

○ **What is the Ortolani maneuver?**

Flexing the newborn's hips 90 degrees and abducting the legs until the knees reach the exam table. A click or thump indicates dislocation or developmental dysplasia. Assymetry of the legs, irregular thigh and gluteal folds are also indications of developmental dysplasia.

○ **Why perform a back exam in a newborn?**

To look for signs of neural tube defects such as hairy tufts, hemangiomas and lipomas.

○ **What vitamin must all rewborns receive within an hour of birth?**

Vitamin K1 oxide to prevent vitamin K-dependent hemorrhagic disease and other coagulation disorders.

○ **What vaccination should be given at birth?**

Hepatitis B

○ **Child development: At what age are infants able to perform the following motor skills?**

1) Sit up
2) Walk
3) Crawl
4) Walk up stairs
5) Smile
6) Hold their head up
7) Roll over

Answers: (1) 5 to 7 months, (2) 11 to 16 months, (3) 9 to 10 months, (4) 14 to 22 months, (5) 2 months, (6) 2 to 4 months, and (7) 2 to 6 months.

○ **At what age are infants capable of the following language skills?**

1) "Mama/Dada" sounds
2) One word
3) Naming body parts
4) Combine words
5) Understandable speech

Answers: (1) 6 to 10 months, (2) 9 to 15 months, (3) 19 to 25 months, (4) 17 to 25 months, and (5) 2 years to 4 years.

○ **At what age is a child able to uncover a toy hidden by a scarf?**

9 to 10 months. This is called object permanence, the understanding that "out of sight" is not "out of existence."

❍   **Joe Mississippi (the greatest arm-chair quarterback of all time) comes to you with his 3 year old son distressed, that he can't catch a ball to save his life. You reassure Joe that children are not expected to perform that motor skill until they are how old?**

5 to 6 years.

❍   **How many times a day should a healthy infant eat in the first three months of life?**

6 to 8, on average. The schedule should be dictated by the infant, i.e., when he or she is hungry. By 8 months, meals are consumed only 3 to 4 times a day.

❍   **At what age can a mother switch her child from breast milk or formula to whole cow's milk?**

9 to 12 months. Skim milk should not be given until the child is 2 years old. Non-pasteurized milk should never be given.

❍   **What, if any, nutritional value does cow's milk have over breast milk?**

Cow's milk has a higher protein content than breast milk. Both have the same caloric content (20 kcal/oz). Breast milk has a higher carbohydrate concentration, a greater amount of polyunsaturated fat, and is easier for the infant to digest. And for the obvious immunological advantage, "breast is best."

❍   **A mother who is breast feeding a 2 month old complains of breast pain, swelling, fever, and a red coloration just above her left nipple. She wants to know if she can continue to breast feed her infant. What do you tell her?**

She most likely has bacterial mastitis which is most common in the first 2 months of breast feeding. This is most frequently caused by *Staphylococcus aureus*. The mother should be given antibiotics and may continue breast feeding if she chooses.

❍   **At what age should solid foods be introduced?**

4 to 6 months.   One food should be introduced at a time with 1 to 2 week intervals between the introduction of a new food. In this way, potential allergies can be defined.

❍   **How much weight should an infant gain per day in the first 2 months of life?**

15 to 30 g/day. Newborns commonly lose 10% of their body weight during the first week of life because of a loss of extracellular water and a decrease in caloric intake. Healthy infants double their birth weight in 5 months and triple their weight in a year.

❍   **When do infants begin teething?**

By 6 months. They may become irritable, display a decreased appetite and show excessive drooling. Acetaminophen can be used to control the pain.

O   **What is the American Acadamy of Pediatrics recommended vaccination schedule for the year 2002?**

Vaccine	Birth	1mo.	2mo.	4mo.	6mo.	12mo.	15mo.	18mo.	24mo.	4-6yr.	11-12 yr.
Hepatitis B[1]	-first-	-(only if mom HbsAg (-)-									
		--------second--------									
					-----------third--------------------					
Diphtheria, Tetanus, Pertussis[2]			DtaP	DtaP	DTaP		-----DTaP--------			DTaP	Td
H. influenzae Type b[3]			Hib	Hib	Hib	------Hib----------					
Inactivated Polio[4]			IPV	IPV	---------------------------IPV-------------					IPV	
Pneumococcal Conjugate			PCV	PCV	PCV	----------PCV------------					
Measles, Mumps, Rubella[5]						----MMR #1-----				MMR #2	
Varicella[6]						----------Var-----------					

O   **Which infant immunization will most likely cause a reaction when infants receive standard immunizations?**

The pertussis component of the DTP. Minor reactions (local induration and pain, mild fever) occur in 75% of children who receive the vaccine. This is the most common reaction although reactions can be as severe as shock, encephalopathy, and convulsions.

O   **When should toilet training be started?**

At about 18 months.

O   **Differentiate between the Sabine and Salk vaccinations.**

Both prevent polio. The Sabine (OPV) is a live, attenuated, trivalent poliovirus. The Salk (IPV) is an inactivated, trivalent vaccine.

O   **What are the signs and symptoms of Reye's syndrome:**

The patient is usually between ages 6 to 11 with a prior viral illness and possible use of ASA followed by intractable vomiting. Patient may be irritable, combative, or lethargic, and may have RUQ tenderness. Seizures may occur. Check for papilledema. Lab findings include hypoglycemia and an elevated ammonia level (> 20 times normal). Bilirubin level is normal.

❍   **Describe the stages of Reye's syndrome.**

Stage I: Vomiting, lethargy, and liver dysfunction
Stage II: Disorientation, combativeness, delirium, hyperventilation, increased deep tendon reflexes, liver
            dysfunction, hyperexcitable, tachypnea, fever, tachycardia, sweating, and pupillary dilatation
Stage III: Coma, decorticate rigidity, increased respiratory rate, and 50% mortality rate
Stage IV: Coma, decerebrate posturing, no ocular reflexes, loss of corneal reflexes, and liver damage
Stage V: Loss of DTRs, seizures, flaccidity, respiratory arrest, and 95% mortality rate

❍   **What is the treatment for Reye's syndrome?**

Stages I and II: Supportive.
Stages III to V: ICP must be managed with elevation of the head of the bed, paralysis, intubation,
furosemide, mannitol, dexamethasone, and pentobarbital coma.

❍   **What are the Wessel criteria for the diagnosis of infantile colic?**

33333! Crying or irritability lasting longer than 3 hours a day, 3 days a week, or 3 weeks total, all in an
infant under 3 months old. Colic usually subsides after age 3 months.

❍   **What percentage of infants develop colic?**

25%. The etiology is unknown.

❍   **When does physiological jaundice occur in newborns?**

2 to 4 days after birth. Bilirubin levels may rise to 5 to 6 mg/dL.

❍   **Name some causes of jaundice that occurs in the first day of life.**

Sepsis, congenital infections, ABO/Rh incompatibility.

❍   **When does jaundice caused by breast feeding occur?**

By the seventh day of life. Bilirubin levels can reach 25 mg/dL.

❍   **At what level of total serum bilirubin will scleral and facial jaundice be visible in the newborn?**

6 to 8 mg/dL. Jaundice of the shoulders and trunk occurs at levels of 8 to 10 mg/dL, and jaundice of the
lower extremities is visible at levels of roughly 10 to 12 mg/dL.

❍   **Can direct hyperbilirubinemia in a neonate be considered physiologic ?**

No. It should be thoroughly investigated.

❍   **What are some extrahepatic causes of direct hyperbilirubinemia with obstructive jaundice in
the infant?**

Biliary atresia, common duct stenosis or stone, obstructive tumor, bile or mucous plug, or choledochal cyst.

❍   **What are some intrahepatic causes of direct hyperbilirubinemia with obstructive jaundice in
the infant?**

Cytomegalovirus, toxoplasmosis, rubella, coxsackie virus, syphilis, hepatitis B, Epstein-Barr virus, UTI, Cystic fibrosis, Gaucher disease, glycogen storage disease, hereditary fructose intolerance, alpha 1-antitrypsin deficiency, neonatal hepatitis, Zellweger syndrome, trisomy (17,18, or 21), and hepatic hemangiomatosis.

O   **What are the most common causes of persistant direct hyperbilirubinemia in the neonate?**

Neonateal hepatitis and biliary atresia.

O   **What is the treatment for biliary atresia?**

Surgery. A portoenterostomy between the liver and the porta hepatis and the bowel.

O   **Which type of jaundice causes the highest levels of bilirubin elevation?**

A-O incompatibility.

O   **What is kernicterus?**

A complex of neurological symptoms caused by very high levels of unconjugated bilirubin. This occurs when free bilirubin crosses the blood-brain barrier.

O   **What are some causes of hydrops fetalis?**

Chronic anemia secondary to Rh incompatabilityor homozygous alpha thalassemia
Intrauterine infection
Cardiac disease
Hypoproteinemia
Chromosomal disorders

O   **What are some signs and symptoms of hydrops fetalis?**

Ascites, CHF, anasarca, ascites, pleural effusions, hepatosplenomegaly, and pallor

O   **What is the normal heartrate, respiratory rate and systolic bloodpressure of newborns, 1 month olds, 6 month olds, 1 year olds, 2 – 4 year olds, 5 – 8 year olds, 8 – 12 year olds and >12 year olds?**

	Heart rate	Respiratory rate	Systolic bloodpressure
Newborn	120 – 180	40 – 60	52 – 92
1 month	110 – 180	30 –50	60 – 104
6 mos. –1year	120 – 140	25 – 35	65 – 125
2 – 4 years	100 – 110	20 – 30	80 – 95
5 – 8 years	90 – 100	4 – 20	90 – 100
8 – 12 years	60 – 110	12 – 20	100 – 110
>12 years	60 – 105	12 – 16	100 – 120

O   **What are some signs and symptoms of dehydration?**

Sunken eyes, dry mucous membranes, sunken fontenelle, decreased tears, poor skin turgor, decreased urine output, lethargy, irritability, tachycardia, and hypotension.

O   **What is a child's daily maintenace requirements for water, sodium, potassium and chloride?**

Water   1500ml/m2
Sodium   2 – 3 mEq/kg

Potassium   2 – 3 mEq/kg
Chloride   2 – 3 mEq/kg

○ **External chest compressions should be initiated for a newborn with assisted ventilation who has a heart rate less than _____ beats per minute.**

50 bpm.

○ **How do you perform chest compressions on an infant?**

Two fingers should be placed in the lower third of the sternum or 1 finger width below the intermammary line. The chest should be compressed to a depth of 1/3 – 1/2 the chest (approx. 1/2 – 1 inch). Current guidelines suggest encircling the chest with your hands and using the thumbs to perform compressions. The rate of compression is 100 bpm.

○ **How do you perform chest compressions in a child?**

The heel of the hand is placed 2 finger widthes above the lower edge of the xiphoid and the chest is compressed $1 – 1\frac{1}{2}$ inches. In children under 8 the rate of compression is 100 bpm. Ventilation should be performed every 5th compression.

○ **When does colic most commonly occur?**

In the evenings. Colic is irritability, excessive unconsolable crying bouts, and fussiness in infants aged 1 – 4 months.

○ **What is the treatment for colic?**

As the cause is not known a specific treatment is not indicated. Reassurance to parents that the infant will out grow this stage is appropriate. Rocking, vibrations (going for a car ride), changing formula etc. may be helpful. It is important to always exclude other more serious problems that can cause inconsolable crying before making the diagnosis of colic.

○ **Define SIDS.**

Sudden Infant Death Syndrome is an unexpected death of a previously well infant whose death cannot be explained. SIDS pertains only to infants under 1.

○ **Sudden Infant Death Syndrome (SIDS) is the most common cause of death for infants in the first year of life. It occurs at a rate of 2/1000, or 10,000/year. What are 8 risk factors associated with SIDS?**

1) Prematurity with low birth weight.
2) Previous episode of apnea or apparent life-threatening event.
3) Mother is a substance abuser.
4) Family history of SIDS.
5) Male gender.
6) Low socioeconomic status.
7) Prone sleeping position.
8) Smoking during pregnancy.

○ **SIDS has a bimodal distribution. At what ages do the peaks occur?**

1.5 and 4 months.

○ **In what season is the incidence of SIDS higher?**

In the winter.

○   **Define failure to thrive (FTT).**

Infants who are below the third percentile in height or weight or whose weight is less than 80% of the ideal weight for their age. Almost all patients with FTT are under 5 years old, while the majority of children are 6 to 12 months old. Other disorders commonly confused with FTT include anorexia nervosa, bronchiectasis, cystic fibrosis, congenital heart disease, chronic renal disease, Down syndrome, hypothyroidism, inflammatory bowel disease, juvenile rheumatoid arthritis, HIV, Hirschsprung's disease, tuberculosis, malignancy, and Turner's syndrome.

○   **What is the most common cause of FTT?**

Poor intake is responsible for 70% of FTT cases. One-third of these cases stem from poorly educated parents, ranging from inaccurate knowledge of what to feed a child to overdiluting formula in order to "make it stretch further." While in the hospital, patients are fed 150 to 200 kcal/kg/day (1.5 times their expected intake), which will correct environmental problems associated with poor feeding.

○   **What is the prognosis for patients with FTT?**

Only one-third of patients with environmental FTT have a normal life. The remainder grow up small for their size, and the majority also have developmental, psychological, and educational deficiencies.

○   **What percentage of abused children that are brought to the emergency department will be killed by future abuse?**

About 5%.

○   **Broken bones are found in 10 to 20% of abused children. What radiological clues suggest child abuse?**

1) Spiral fractures, especially prior to the onset of walking.
2) Scapula or sternal fractures.
3) Chip fractures or bucket handle fractures.
4) Epiphyseal-metaphyseal posterior rib fractures in infants.
5) Several fractures in various stages of healing.

○   **What other clinical findings would lead you to suspect child abuse?**

"Accident prone" children, cigarette burns, retinal hemorrhages, subdural hematomas, head contusions in children who are preambulatory, back bruises in children who can't climb, burns on the buttocks or in a stocking glove distribution, and lesions in the shape of familiar objects, e.g., belts and hands.

○   **What is the most common type of hypertension in children?**

Idiopathic or essential hypertension. One percent of pediatric patients and 3% of adolescent patients are hypertensive.

○   **What is the most common cause of secondary hypertension in children?**

Renal disease (polycystic kidney disease, infection, tumors, or congenital vascular abnormalities). Other causes are vascular, endocrine, neurological, or pharmacological in nature.

○   **How should you treat a newborn with cyanotic spells and great difficulty breathing, especially during feeding?**

Surgery. This infant has choanal atresia. The septum between the nose and the pharynx is prohibiting the infant from breathing through his nose and must be surgically removed. Infants are obligate nasal breathers, as we all are, during feeding. Cyanosis is often relieved during crying bouts.

○ **What percentage of African Americans are heterozygous for the sickle cell gene?**

10%. Sickle cell is also common in Greek, Turkish, Arabian, and Indian populations.

○ **What commonly precipitates an aplastic crisis in a sickle cell child?**

Viral infections, most commonly an infection with human parvovirus B19.

○ **What does parvovirus B19 cause?**

Erythema infectiosum (fifth disease).

○ **Between what ages will infants with sickle cell anemia show clinical manifestations of their disease?**

4 to 6 months. Prior to this, the infants are protected by Hb F left over from fetal life. By 4 to 6 months they will develop (1) anemia, (2) jaundice, (3) splenomegaly, and (4) hand-foot syndrome, in which the dorsal surfaces of the hands and feet swell and produce pain because of infarction of the bone marrow of the metacarpal, metatarsal, and phalanges.

○ **What organism is most commonly implicated in childhood sickle cell infections?**

Streptococcus pneumonia (60%). Daily doses of prophylactic penicillin are recommended for those least resistant to encapsulated bacteria.

○ **Which organs are most commonly damaged in sickle cell patients?**

Spleen, lung, liver, kidney, skeleton, and skin.

○ **What is acute chest syndrome?**

Chest pain, hypoxemia and/or infiltrates on chest x-ray in a patient with sickle cell disease.

○ **What is the cause of ACS?**

Pneumonia or pulmonary infarct secondary to vasoocclusion. If pneumonia is the cause *Pneumococcus* is the most common organism.

○ **How is ACS treated?**

With early blood transfusion or exchange transfusion, hydration, oxygen, analgesics and antibiotics.

○ **An hour old, premature infant presents with tachypnea, grunting, chest wall retractions, nasal flaring, and cyanosis. What is a possible diagnosis?**

Hyaline membrane disease, also known as respiratory distress syndrome of the newborn. These patients have atelectasis, intrapulmonary shunting, hypoxemia, and cyanosis.

○ **What is the pathophysiology behind hyaline membrane disease?**

The lungs are poorly compliant because of a lack of sufficient surfactant. These infants are generally preterm and have not developed chemically mature lungs.

O   **What does a chest x-ray of an infant with hyaline membrane disease look like?**

Atelectic with diffuse, fine, granular densities.

O   **What is bronchopulmonary dysplasia?**

Residual chronic lung disease of infancy that persists secondary to neonatal lung disease. It can follow any illness that requires mechanical ventilation.

O   **The incidence of brochopulmonary dysplasia is dependent on what?**

Birth weight. The incidence is over 50% in neonates weighing less than 750 g and 40% for neonates weighing 750 – 1000g.

O   **Describe the clinical features of BPD.**

Respiratory distress, tachypnea, reactive airways, hypoxia, hypercarbia, poor feeding, irritability, lethargy, increased oxygen requirement and occasionally pulmonary edema and cor pulmonale.

O   **Patients with BPD may have chronic hypercarbia. Will administering O_2 diminish their respiratory drive?**

No.

O   **What are some causes of wheezing in an infant?**

Asthma, bronchiolitis, foreign body, bronchopulmonary dysplasia, pneumonia, cystic fibrosis, anaphylaxis, vascular rings, aspiration, mediastinal masses and CHF.

O   **What are the most common triggers for asthma?**

Viral infections

O   **How do you diagnose asthma in a small child?**

Clinically. They will have recurrent episodes of wheezing or persistent cough and generally a family history of asthma, atopy or allergies. Pulmonary function tests are useless until a child is about age 6 since children younger are not able to perform the tests.

O   **What are the indications for a chest x-ray in a known asthmatic?**

Suspicion of consolidation, effusion, pneumothorax or impending respiratory failure. Findings on x-ray are nonspecific such as hyperinflation, peribronchial cuffing and atelectasis.

O   **Pediatric patients presenting with severe asthma may be treated with a high dose of nebulized albuterol. How much albuterol is considered "high-dose," and how frequently may such doses be given?**

0.15 mg/kg (0.03 mL/kg of 0.5%), up to 5 mg. Administer every 20 minutes, up to six times.

O   **What percentage of children with asthma are likely to have symptoms persisting into adulthood?**

50%.

○   **What is the most common cause of bronchiolitis?**

RSV. Other major causes are parainfluenza, influenza, mumps, echovirus, rhinovirus, mycoplasma, and adenoviruses.

○   **What is bronchiolitis?**

An acute inflammation of the lower respiratory tract that results in obstrution of the small airways. Patients present with a prodrome of runny nose, low grade fever and decreased appetite leading to increased respirations, retractions and wheezing.

○   **What is the common age range for bronchiolitis?**

2 to 6 months, when maternal antibody to RSV is waning.

○   **What is the most common cause of stridor in neonates?**

Congenital abnormalities, especially laryngotracheomalacia.

○   **Can the type of stridor localize the level of the obstruction?**

Yes. Inspiratory stridor points to a site of obstruction above the vocal folds; expiratory stridor points to obstruction below the vocal folds .

○   **Define apnea.**

Apnea is a period ofno respirations which lasts >20 seconds.

○   **An 8 month old is brought to your office. The mother says that she suddenly started having trouble breathing. She is afebrile and has no other symptoms. What do you do?**

Rule out foreign body with AP and lateral views of the upper airway. Though this could be the presentation of many respiratory problems sudden onset of symptoms should peak your suspicion for a foreign body. 65% of deaths due to foreign body aspiration are in infants under 1.

○   **If the above patient came to you with known aspiration of a foreign body and severe respiratory distress indicating a complete obstruction what would you do first?**

Turn the child over and give 4 sharp thrusts to the back followed by chest thrusts. If unsuccessful removal of FB via direct laryngoscopy should be performed. If that is unsuccessful, then bronchoscopy should be performed.

○   **What is the most common cause of pneumonia in school aged children?**

Mycoplasma pneumonia. Other causes include *Streptococcus pneumoniae*, parainfluenza virus, and influenza virus. These patients present with a persistent, dry, hacking cough. The chest may sound surprisingly clear, but chest x-ray will revel bilateral infiltrates. Treatment is with erythromycin or tetracycline, depending on the age.

○   **A 3 day old infant has a high fever and is coughing, grunting, and really working for air. Chest x-ray shows a reticulogranular pattern. The birth history is unremarkable. Your probable diagnosis?**

Group A streptococcal pneumonia. The infant most likely contracted this while passing through an infected birth canal. Mortality can be as high as 40%, so early treatment with penicillin G is important. Other causes of pneumonia in newborns are *Listeria monocytogenes*, enteric gram-negative bacilli, *Chlamydia*, rubella, CMV, and herpes.

O   **Contrast pneumonia due to Mycoplasma with pneumonia due to streptococcal pneumonia.**

	S. pneumoniae	M. pneumoniae
Prodrome	Little	Mild fever, malaise, cough, HA
Onset	Rapid	Gradual
URI sx	Tachypnea, cough, occasional pleuritic pain	Little
Associated findings	High fever	Exanthem, arthritis, GI complaints, neurologic complications
Pleural effusion	Occasional	Rare
Lab	Leukocytosis	WBC normal or sl. elevation
Tx	Penicillin	Erythromycin

O   **What is the most common pneumonia in children under 5 years old?**

Respiratory syncytial viral pneumonia (RSV). These children present with a nonproductive cough, rhonchi, rales, wheezing, and possible fever and chills. Bilateral infiltrates, atelectasis, and air trapping are present on chest x-ray. Other common viral pneumonias in this population are parainfluenza virus, adenovirus, and influenza B virus.

O   **What is the most common cause of bacterial pneumonia in pediatric patients?**

Streptococcal. A child will present with productive cough, pleurisy, dyspnea, fever, and chills.

O   **Staphylococcal pneumonia frequently results in pleural effusion or empyema. Which lung is most frequently involved?**

The right lung is involved in 65% of the cases. 80% of these pneumonias are unilateral. 25% of the patients will go on to develop pyopneumothorax.

O   **T/F: GABHS is a frequent cause of pharyngitis in patients under 3 years of age.**

False.

O   **What is the most common cause of pharyngitis?**

Viruses, most commonly, Adenovirus, parainfluenza virus, rhinovirus, herpes symplex virus, RSV, EBV, influenza virus and coxsackie virus.

O   **What is the most common bacterial cause of pharyngitis?**

Above the age of 3 the most common bacterial cause is Group A beta-hemolytic streptococci. Though viruses are still the most common cause of pharyngitis overall.

O   **We know that the streptococcal antigen sampling tests for pharyngitis have a high false-negative rate (sensitivity variable, generally > 50%). What is the false-negative rate for a single throat culture?**

10%.

○   **How long should a school-aged child receive antibiotic treatment for GABHS before returning to school?**

1 day. The child with a true streptococcal infection is not infectious within a few hours of penicillin therapy. The child may not feel well enough to return after one day but is not a risk to others.

○   **Rheumatic fever is preventable if antibiotic therapy is initiated prior to how many days after the start of GABHS pharyngitis?**

9 days.

○   **Is antibiotic therapy warranted for the prevention of post streptococcal glomerulonephritis associated with GABHS?**

No! Poststreptococcal glomerulonephritis is not preventable with antibiotic therapy.

○   **A 5 year old boy is brought to your office by his father who tells you that he has had a 3 day history of fever, chills, and pain when swallowing. Upon examination, he has cervical lymphadenopathy, no cough, and erythematous tonsils with bilateral white exudates. What percentage of patients with this presentation will show group A ß-hemolytic *Streptococcus* upon throat culture?**

Twenty-five percent of patients with the above symptoms and tonsillar exudates have a positive culture. Thirty percent of patients with streptococcus do not have tonsillar exudates. Fifteen to 20% of children have group A ß-hemolytic *Streptococcus* as normal flora in their mouths.

○   **What is the most common cause of tonsillitis?**

Viral (75%). Only 25% of the cases are due to ß-hemolytic Streptococcus.

○   **What are the indications for tonsillectomy?**

Peritonsillar abscess, airway obstruction, seven episodes of documented streptococcal tonsillitis within 1 year, or five documented cases of streptococcal tonsillitis per year for 2 consecutive years.

○   **What is the usual age range for presentation of retropharyngeal abscess?**

6 months to 3 years.

○   **What does a "hot potato voice" suggest in the setting of a sore throat?**

A peritonsilar abscess. Patients generally have ipsilateral otalgia, trismus, dysarthria, fever, drooling and a muffled voice.

○   **What is the clinical presentation of a child with mononucleosis?**

Malaise, fever, headache, fatigue, sorethroat, lymphadenopathy, and splenomegaly.

○   **What age group is most commonly affected by mono?**

Adolescents and young adults. It's the "kissing bug" and these are the people doing the most kissing.

○   **What virus causes mononucleosis?**

The Epstein-Barr virus.

○   **What antibiotic should not be given to patients with mono?**

Ampicillin. Almost all patients taking ampicillin who have mono will develop a generalized maculopapular rash.

○   **What is the treatment for mono?**

NOT Ampicillin! Rest. Patients are also counceled not to participate in contact sports as splenic rupture may ensue. The illness can last weeks to months.

○   **What are the three stages of pertussis?**

1) Catarrhal stage: Rhinorrhea, cough, conjunctivitis (lasts 1 week)
2) Paroxysmal stage: Paroxysms of continuous coughing (lasts up to 6 weeks)
3) Convalescent stage: Coughing decreases (NSS)

○   **What is the treatment for pertussis?**

Patients and household contacts should be treated with erythromycin. Superinfective pneumonias can be serious and should be treated with broader coverage. Immunize household contacts who are less than 7 years old.

○   **Pertussis is most common in what age group?**

Infants less than 6 months old.

○   **What is the classic triad of a child with cystic fibrosis?**

Chronic pulmonary disease, malabsorption and increased electrolytes in the sweat.

○   **What are the most common pathogens infecting the lungs of a child with cystic fibrosis?**

Staphylococcus aureus and *Pseudomonas aeruginosa.*

○   **Cystic fibrosis is an autosomal recessive, inherited, lethal disease. The genetic abnormality in this disease is located on what chromosome?**

Chromosome 7. Defects in the gene that encodes for the cystic fibrosis transmembrane regulator is thought to result in a blocked chloride channel in the epithelial cell membranes, which ultimately results in dehydration of mucus secretions.

○   **What is the diagnostic test of choice in determining if a patient has CF?**

The quantitative pilocarpine iontophoresis sweat test. (The sweat chloride test).

○   **What would you expect the serum chloride, sodium, bicarb and pH of a patient with CF to be?**

Sodium and chloride levels will be low, representing renal compensation for the increased salt losses in the sweat. Bicarb and pH are usually elevated.

○   **What might the chest x-ray of a patient with CF look like?**

Hyperinflated lungs, infiltrates and peribronchial thickening.

❍   **How do most patients with CF die?**

They eventually die of respiratory failure complicated by cor pulmonale.

❍   **What is the most common vasculitis in the pediatric population?**

Henoch-Schonlein Purpura (HSP), which is a temporary allergic disorder of the blood vessels. Patients present with bruises over the lower extremities, abdomen, and buttocks. Bleeding from the GI and GU tract are also common. Associated arthritis occurs in 75% of the cases.

❍   **What is the typical rash of HSP?**

Palpable purpura measuring 1 – 2 mm in diameter, symmetrically distributed generally located on the buttox and thighs. The rash lasts 4 – 6 weeks.

❍   **What other symptoms will a patient with HSP commonly have?**

75% will have arthralgias or arthritis (typically of the feet and hands). Abdominal pain and microcytic hematuria are also common. Rarely, patients will have CNS involvement presenting as seizures and coma.

❍   **How can Henoch-Schonlein purpura be distinguished from idiopathic thrombocytopenic purpura?**

The platelet count is normal in HSP. In HSP, the immune complex reacts with blood vessel walls causing capillary leaking. In ITP, IgG antiplatelet antibodies develop and fix to normal platelets which are then destroyed .

❍   **What is the most common thrombocytopenia in childhood?**

Idiopathic thrombocytopenic purpura. A platelet count and a bone marrow examination will confirm the diagnosis. Acute ITP generally follows an acute infection. 80 to 85% of cases resolve within 2 months. Acute ITP is most common in children aged 2 to 9 years old.

❍   **What other illnesses cause thrombocytopenia in children?**

Leukemia, lymphoma, myeloma, autoimmune collagen vascular disease and drugs (thiazides, quinidine, and sulfa antibiotics).

❍   **What is the treatment for ITP?**

Prednisone, IV gamma globulin and supportive care. If the platelet count is below 50,000 patients should be managed in the hospital. For severe cases refractory to the above management, splenectomy is performed.

❍   **What is the most common cause of aquired acute renal failure in children?**

Hemolytic uremic syndrome (HUS).

❍   **What is the classic triad of HUS?**

Microangiopathic hemolytic anemia, thrombocytopenia and acute renal failure.

O   **What organs other than the kidney can be involved in HUS?**

CNS, lungs, heart, and GI tract can all be involved. When systemic involvement occurs, it is difficult to distinguish HUS from thrombotic thrombocytopenic purpura.

O   **HUS is usually preceeded by an infection, either viral or bacterial. What is the most common bacteria associated with HUS?**

Escherichia coli (0157 :H7)

O   **What is the most common anemia in children?**

Iron deficiency anemia. Most cases are caused by an inadequate intake of iron rather than loss through hemorrhage. It is most commonly seen in infants aged 6 – 12 months who are fed exclusively on breast milk. The infant's rapid growth spurt puts a strain on iron stores. Other causes of Anemia in children are lead poisoning and thalassemia.

O   **What are the signs and symptoms of iron deficiency anemia?**

Asymptomatic, irritability, lethargy, fatigue, pallor, tachycardia or even signs of CHF. Treatment for mild cases is oral iron 6mg/kg/day. For severe cases, transfusions of packed red blood cells are indicated.

O   **Twenty percent of children with meningococcemia die. What is the major cause of death in these patients?**

Shock. Rapid administration of penicillin is the treatment of choice.

O   **What is the most common cause of cellulitis in the pediatric population?**

S. aureus.

O   **What is the most common cause of neonatal conjunctivitis?**

A trick question. Chemical conjunctivitis due to silver nitrate is most common. Silver nitrate drops are given to all neonates to prevent gonorrheal opthalmitis. C. trachomatis is the most common bacterial cause in the first 14 days with a usual incubation period of at least 5 days. C. Trichomatis is resolved with erythromycin, not silver nitrate. Gonococcal conjunctivitis has a shorter incubation and may present as soon as 2 days.

O   **What are the most common causes of otitis media?**

Viral (35%), *Streptococcus pneumoniae* (30 to 35%), *H. influenzae* (20 to 25%), *Moraxella catarrhalis* (10 to 15%), group A streptococci (2%) and *Staphylococcus aureus* (1%). In neonates, gram-negative bacilli account for 20%, but these organisms are rare in older children.

O   **What are some risk factors of otitis media?**

Recent URI, caucasian ethnicity, male gender, craniofacial abnormalities, Down's Syndrome, bottle feeding, daycare, secondhand smoke, and a family history of middle ear disease.

O   **How common is otitis media?**

Very common. By 6 months of age, 35% of children have had one episode of otitis media, and by age 7, 90% of children have had one or more bouts and 40% of children have had 6 or more episodes of acute otitis media. Otitis media most commonly affects children from ages 5 to 24 months.

O   **When does recurrent otitis media most commonly occur?**

In the winter and early spring. A patient must have otitis media three or more times in a period of 6 months or 4 times within 1 year for the disease to be classified as recurrent otitis media.

O   **Name the following condition: fluid collection in the middle ear that is usually painless, no sign of infection, and possible reduction in hearing acuity?**

Serous otitis media, also known as otitis media with effusion (OME). This is an under-used diagnosis.

O   **How useful is the light reflex in evaluation of suspected AOM?**

It is useless. TM mobility is an appropriate diagnostics indicator.

O   **In what age group will you most commomly see croup and epiglottitis?**

Croup: 3 months to 3 years
Epiglottitis: 2 to 7 years (Classically, though with the H.Flu vaccine, it is becoming more common in the adult population.)

O   **What are the most common causes of croup?**

The majority of croup cases are caused by viruses, most commonly parainfluenza virus.

O   **What organism most commonly causes epiglottitis?**

Group A *Streptococcus* has now replaced *H. influenzae* as the leading cause of epiglottitis. This is primarily due to the increased number of infants vaccinated with the Hib vaccine.

O   **What percent of cases of stridor with fever are due to croup?**

90%.

O   **When is croup most common?**

In the winter.

O   **A 3 year old child who had a cold last week and now has developed a brassy cough, mild fever, and seems to have some difficulty breathing. How do you differentiate between croup and epiglottitis in this patient?**

A lateral x-ray of the neck should indicate a swollen epiglottis, though direct visualization with a laryngoscope with appropriate backup intubation equipment is definitive. Avoid agitating the child either through tongue blades, oxygen administration, alteration of position, etc. Intubation equipment should always be handy.

O   **What is the presentation of a patient with epiglottitis?**

Acute onset of high fever, sore throat, dysphagia and respiratory distress, muffled voice, stridor, tripod sitting position, and drool. These children are toxic appearing.

O   **What is the presentation of croup?**

A non specific upper respiratory infection followed gradually by a brassy or barking cough and inspiratory stridor with mild temperatures.

O   **What is the treatment for epiglottitis?**

Oxygen, IV antibiotics (ampicillin and cefotaxime), intubation if necessary.

O   **What is the treatment for croup?**

Cool mist therapy for mild croup. Oxygen, cool mist, racemic epinephrine nebulizer, and corticosteroids for moderate and severe croup. Intubation and hospitalization are warrented for severe cases.

O   **What is the most common primary malignant bone tumor in the pediatric population?**

Osteogenic sarcoma.

O   **In what pediatric population is osteogenic sarcoma most prevelant?**

Male adolescents.

O   **Where do osteomas most frequently occur?**

At the metaphyseal ends of the long bones. Osteomas are most common in the distal femur, followed in order by the proximal tibia, proximal humerus, and proximal femur.

O   **How does the prognosis for Ewing sarcoma differ based upon the location of the tumor?**

Tumors in the distal extremities that have not metastasized have a good prognosis. Tumors of the pelvic bone or proximal femurs have a poor prognosis, as do any tumors with distant metastases.

O   **The star of the local high school basketball team is brought into your office by his dad who says his son has been having pain just below his right knee for the past two weeks. The patient does not recall any trauma and says that the pain gets worse when he plays his games or when he walks down stairs. Upon examination, you notice a mild swelling just over the tibial tuberosity of his right knee. When you press there the patient pulls away and says "Yep, that's the spot." There is no effusion. What is your diagnosis?**

Osgood-Schlatter disease. This is a disease found in active adolescent males. Pain and swelling are caused by a detachment of cartilage over the tibial tuberosity that occurs with overuse of the quadriceps. Treatment is rest, ice and NSAIDS. For severe cases; knee immobilization in extension, physical therapy and no sports or excessive use. The disease is generally self limiting.

O   **A 3 year old girl is brought to your office. She is holding her right arm flexed at the elbow with her forearm pronated. She will not let you near it. What is your diagnosis?**

Subluxation of the radial head, commonly called nursemaid's elbow. This injury commonly occurs when an adult pulls or jerks a child up by the arm.

O   **A mother brings her 200 lb. 14 year old son to you because he has been limping and complaining of knee pain for the past two weeks. What is your diagnosis?**

Slipped capital femoral epiphysis. Hip pain can commonly be referred to the knee, most frequently the medial aspect of the knee. Patients may hold the hip in abduction and external rotation. Internal rotation is severely limited.

O   **What is the most serious complication of SCFE?**

A vasular necrosis of the femoral head.

○   **What is the treatment of SCFE?**

In SCFE the epiphysis slips posteriorly on the femoral neck. Surgical pinning and immobilization are indicated. Some mild cases may be corrected with traction and internal rotation.

○   **What is the classic profile of a patient with a slipped capital femoral epiphysis?**

Slipped capital femoral epiphysis is prevalent in obese males aged 10 to 16 at the peak of their growth spurt. Forty percent of patients presenting with this complaint are obese. African Americans are more commonly affected as compared to Caucasian Americans.

○   **How will a patient with slipped capital femoral epiphysis present?**

Patients usually complain of hip or knee pain and a limp sometimes secondary to trauma. On exam they will have limited medial and rotation, flexion, extension and abduction.

○   **A mother brings her 8 year old boy in to see you because he has been complaining of pains in his legs intermittently for the past two weeks. He recalls no injury and says he only has the pains at night time or if he is playing "really hard." Sometimes the pains even awaken him from sleep. What is a likely diagnosis?**

Growing pains. These pains usually occur in the lower limbs of growing children and are always bilateral. Treatment involves heat and massage.

○   **What is the treatment for nursemaid's elbow?**

Radial head subluxation (a.k.a. nursemaid's elbow) occurs with abrupt axial traction on an extended, pronated forearm. This can occur when caretakers lift a child up by the arm or if a child trips while holding an adults hand. Relocation is done by putting a finger over the radial head while supinating, then flexing, the elbow.

○   **A 3 year old girl returns to your office complaining of a limp and mild pain in her right hip. She was seen by you last week, and you sent her home with the diagnosis of viral syndrome/upper respiratory infection. The patient still has a mild fever (100.5°F). What is your diagnosis?**

Toxic synovitis. This is the most common non-traumatic cause of limp and hip pain in patients between the ages of 3 to 6. This is a transient unilateral (95%) inflammatory arthritis that follows a viral illness within 3 to 6 days. Septic arthritis present with more severe symptoms, such as higher fever, guarding, malaise, and sharp pain.

○   **A father brings his 5 year old son, Willaby, to you because he is limping and complaining of hip pain. Upon examination, you note that his quadriceps appear atrophied on the right side, his right leg is shorter than his left, and he has decreased motion at his hip joint, especially noted on internal rotation and abduction. He is otherwise healthy. What's wrong with Willaby?**

Legg-Calvé-Perthes disease. This disease is an idiopathic, aseptic necrosis of the femoral head. It is most common in boys 4 to 8 years old (male:female = 5:1). It is thought that Legg-Calve-Perthes disease may be the result of an interruption in the blood flow to the femoral epiphysea due to trauma, synovitis, hyperviscosity, or coagulation abnormalities. The exact etiology is unknown.

○   **What is Willaby's prognosis?**

After casting and braces for 1 to 2 years or surgery, 40 to 50% of patients still develop severe degenerative hip disease that requires hip replacement. Younger patients have a better prognosis.

O   **A 12 year old forward on the local soccer team is brought in by her mom complaining of pain in the front of her knee. She denies any trauma or injuries and says that she feels like her knee is made of sand paper because of a grating sensation when she runs or climbs stairs. This grating sensation is reproducible when you ask the patient to do a deep kneebend and is accompanied by some crepitus. Pressing down on the patella induces pain. What is your diagnosis?**

Chondromalacia patellae which is a breakdown of the cartilage. This disease generally manifest in prepubescent children.

O   **Differentiate between a sprain and a strain.**

Sprains: Stretches or incomplete tears of a ligament
Strains: Stretched tendons or muscles

O   **When is the peak incidence of scoliosis?**

Early adolescence. It is most commonly idiopathic in origin. Females are more frequently affected than males.

O   **What is the treatment for scoliosis?**

Less than 15 degree curvature – back exercises and check ups every 6 months
Greater than 20 degrees – bracing, exercise and or surgical stabilization.

O   **Bowed legs, thinning of the skull, thickening of the costochondral junction, and prominences on the wrists and knees is suggestive of what disease?**

Rickets

O   **What will an x-ray of a child's knee who has ricket's look like?**

There will be a widened space between the metaphysis and the epiphysis and the ends of the metaphysis will be cupped and irregular.

O   **Rickets can be due to a lack of or an abnormal metabolism of what vitamin?**

Vitamin D

O   **What are the most common risk factors for inguinal hernias in the pediatric population?**

Male gender and prematurity.

O   **What is extraosseous Ewing sarcoma?**

Ewing sarcoma that arises in soft tissues rather than bone. It is most common in the extremities and paravertebral area.

O   **What are the most common complaints of children with Ewing sarcoma?**

Pain and swelling at the site. Systemic symptoms may also exist.

O   **What is the most common primary malignant bone tumor seen in pediatric patients?**

Osteogenic sarcoma.

○ **Who is most likely to get osteogenic sarcoma?**

Male adolescents.

○ **Where in the body are you most likely to find osteogenic sarcoma?**

50% of cases occur in the knee joint and metastasize to the lungs.

○ **A white pupil or "cat's eye" is indicative of what congenital malignancy?**

Retinoblastoma. This is a tumor arising from neural tissue of the retina. Treatment depends on the extent of the disease and can involve enucleation, radiation and chemotherapy.

○ **Wilms' tumor is most commonly found in what age group?**

1 to 3 year olds. Wilms' tumors (nephroblasomas) are more common in girls (2:1) and generally present as a painless abdominal mass, with fever, decreased appetite, nausea, and vomiting. Forty percent are hereditary. Treatment is surgical resection and chemotherapy.

○ **What is the most common childhood malignancy?**

Acute lymphoblastic leukemia. Leukemia accounts for one-third of all cancers diagnosed in the pediatric population. ALL accounts for 75% of all acute leukemias and AML acounts for 25%.

○ **What do ALL and AML stand for?**

Acute Lymphoblastic Leukemia and Acute Myelogenous Leukemia.

○ **When is ALL most common?**

ALL peaks between ages 3 and 5, and again around age 30.

○ **What are some signs and symptoms of leukemia?**

Fatigue, petechia, bleeding, purpura, lymphadenopathy, hepatosplenomegaly, bone and joint pain, low grade fever, and pallor.

○ **Petechia and bruising occur with platelet counts below what number? Internal hemorrhage occurs with count below what number?**

< 20,000/mm^3 and < 10,000/mm^3 respectively.

○ **What is the malignant cell in Hodgkin's disease?**

The Reed-Sternberg cell.

○ **What are the peak age groups for Hodgkin's disease?**

13 to 35 and 50 to 75.

○ **What are the signs and symptoms of Hodgkin's disease?**

Painless supraclavicular or cervical lymphadenopathy, hepatomegaly, splenomegaly, unexplained fever, and night sweats.

○   **What are indications for lymph node biopsy?**

Nodes that continue to enlarge after 2 – 3 weeks, that do not return to normal size after 5 – 6 weeks or nodes associated with mediastinal enlargement on chest x-ray.

○   **How are childhood cases of non-Hodgkin lymphomas different from adult cases?**

They grow rapidly, are rarely nodular, and are as likely to be T-cell lymphomas as B-cell lymphomas.

○   **What is the most common presentation of B-cell lymphomas?**

Abdominal masses.

○   **What is the most common presentation of T-cell lymphomas?**

Anterior mediastinal masses.

○   **What populations are most likely to have lead poisoning?**

Inner city, lower socioeconomic, African Americans and those living in housing built before 1960.

○   **When patients are symptomatic with lead poisoning what might you see?**

Lethargy, irritability, anorexia, constipation, abdominal pain, vomiting, clumsiness, regression in speech, and decreased hearing. If patients have levels over 70ug/dL, they may have symptoms of lead encephalopathy such as ataxia, seizures and coma.

○   **What percentage of children with lead encephalopathy willl have permanent brain damage?**

70 – 80%.

○   **A child presents in DKA. On average, how dehydrated is this patient likely to be?**

125 mL/kg average fluid volume deficit.

○   **You are managing a child in DKA. After an initial 20 mL/kg bolus with 0.9% NS and careful fluid replacement with 0.45% NS for maintenance and replacement, you are considering switching to D5 0.45% NS. At approximately what glucose level should this change in fluid selection occur?**

250 mg/dL.

○   **What dose of insulin should be used for low-dose, continuous infusion therapy for a child?**

0.1 unit/kg/h of regular insulin.

○   **Insulin is usually mixed in NS at 1 unit/5 mL NS. How much of this fluid should be voided through the tubing to saturate nonspecific binding sites in the plastic?**

50 mL = 10 units.

○   **A child known to have IDDM presents unconscious. What is the correct amount of D50W (in mL/kg) to administer to this patient?**

0.5 mL/kg.

O **Five minutes have passed since administering D50W to the child yet no improvement is noted. Now what should you do?**

Nothing. Clinical response to glucose often takes 10 minutes. Use the time to think of other causes of coma in this patient's differential diagnosis which could be sepsis, meningitis, metabolic abnormalities, poisoning, head injury, or postictal state.

O **Are urinary tract infections more common in boys or girls?**

In the newborn periord they are twice as common in boys but in childhood they are 10 times more common in girls.

O **What is the most common cause of UTI's in children?**

Fecal flora, most commonly *Escherichia coli* which accounts for 80% of UTI's.

O **What is hypospadias?**

A defect in the penis in which the opening of the urethral meatus is on the ventral surface of the penis.

O **Why should boys with hypospadias not be circumsized?**

The treatment for hypospadias, if severe, is surgery. The foreskin of the penis is needed to reconstruct the urethra and should therefore not be taken off in circumcision.

O **Cryptorchidism must be corrected by the age of 2 to decrease the potential for testicular malignancy. True or false?**

False. The risk of malignancy exists regardless of correction or not. The risk of infertility is removed if the testes descend before the age of 2.

O **What is the treatment for cryptorchidism?**

Medical treatment is with hCG. If unsuccessful, an orchiopexy should be performed.

O **A 15 year old boy comes into your office complaining of 12 hours of a swollen, painful, red, testis, with associated nausea, and vomiting. On exam, his affected testis is lying horizontally. The cremasteric reflex is absent and elevating the testis causes more pain. What should you do?**

Call for a urological consult for a presumed torsed testis. While you are waiting you may obtain a UA to rule out infectious causes, try detorsing the testis by turning it outwards towards the thigh (much like opening a book) or sending the patient for a doppler ultrasound. None of this should delay a urology consult as this is a urological emergency.

O **What is Prehn's sign?**

Elevation of the testis leads to improvement in the testicular pain. This is indicative of epididymitis, though not diagnostic.

O **What are the two age peaks for the incidence of testicular torsion?**

Perinatally and during puberty.

O **What is the eponym for congenital aganglionic megacolon?**

Hirschsprung's disease. In this disease, a portion of the distal colon lacks ganglion cells, thus impairing the normal inhibitory innervation in the myenteric plexus. This impedes coordinated relaxation, which can, in turn, cause clinical symptoms of obstruction 85% of the time after the newborn period.

○   **Is Hirschsprung's disease more common in males or females?**

Males by a ratio of 4 :1.

○   **What are the signs and symptoms of toxic megacolon in the first year?**

Decreased number of bowel movements, obstipation, sporatic abdominal distention, decreased appetite, failure to thrive, vomiting and bouts of non bloody diarrhea.

○   **How is toxic megacolon diagnosed?**

Abdominal films showing a dilated colon, barium enema showing dilated colon proximal to the lesion (with a cone shaped transition zone between the two), anal rectal manometry and biopsy of rectal tissue.

○   **Acute enterocolitis with development of "toxic" megacolon is the life-threatening complication of Hirschsprung's disease. Between what ages does this complication most frequently present?**

2 to 3 months. Treatment involves gastric decompression (rectal tube), NPO, IV fluids, and antibiotics.

○   **A one month old frequently vomits directly after and up to several hours after eating. The vomiting is never bloody, bilious, painful or forceful. It appears effortless as small amounts of curdled milk drool out of her mouth. What is a probable diagnosis?**

GERD

○   **What percentage of infants have GERD?**

50%

○   **Do infants with GERD have high, low or normal lower esophageal sphincter pressures?**

Unlike adults with GERD who have low LES pressures, infants generally have normal LES pressures. Their reflux has been explained as transient relaxation of LES at inappropriate times or failure to increase the LES pressure at times of increased gastric pressure. Other factors that cause GERD in infants are delayed gastric emptying, increased intragastric pressure, and impaired esophageal motility.

○   **What non-gastrointestinal symptoms are seen with rotavirus?**

Patients may also have fever and upper respiratory symtoms in addition to vomiting and diarrhea.

○   **What age group does rotavirus most commonly affect?**

Ages 6 months – 2 years. Rotavirus is most common in the fall and winter.

○   **What is a lasting sequella in 50% of infants affected with rotavirus?**

Lactose intolerance. It may last for several weeks after a rotavirus infection.

○   **What signs and symptoms tend to indicate a bacterial pathogen as the cause of diarrhea?**

Fever, acute onset of multiple diarrhea stools/day, and blood in the stool.

○   **What children with gastroenteritis should receive antibiotic treatment?**

Antibiotic therapy for gastroenteritis is limited in utility to children with high or prolonged fevers, those with inflammatory cells present in stool, those with protracted diarrhea, and infants less than 6 months old.

○   **What is the most common cause of obstruction in infants under 1 year of age?**

Intussusception. The classic presentation is vomiting, irritability, currant jelly stool, and a sausage-shaped mass in the RUQ.

○   **Is intestinal intussusception associated with GI bleeding?**

Yes, although the classic history of sudden onset of severe pain that often is relieved as quickly as it arose and is recurrent is more sensitive. The currant jelly stool associated with this disorder is only present in about half of the cases.

○   **What is the classic triad of syptoms associated with intussusception?**

Intermittent abdominal pain, vomiting, and bloody stools.

○   **A sausage shaped mass is found in what percent of patients with intussusception?**

60 – 95%

○   **About how old is the average patient who presents with intussusception?**

60% of cases occur in the first year. Most commonly between the 5th and 9th month.

○   **How is intussusception treated?**

Either with air insufflation or barium enema. If these are unsuccessful then surgical reduction is required.

○   **Is constipation more common in breast fed or formula fed infants?**

Formula fed infants. It is very rare in breast fed infants. Treat by increasing the amount of fluid and/or sugar in the formula, and adding prune juice, fruits, cereal, and vegetables to the baby's diet to increase bulk.

○   **A new mother brings her 3 week old infant boy to your office because he doesn't seem to be growing. He has constipation and intermittent vomiting, "with such force he can almost hit the door," the mother exclaims.   What might you find upon abdominal examination?**

This patient probably has pyloric stenosis. Expect a small, firm, mobile, olive shaped mass in the RUQ or epigastric area. If the stenosed pylorus cannot be palpated, then ultrasound or x-ray will reveal the defect. Treatment is pyloromyotomy.

○   **Pyloric stenosis is most common in what population?**

Male caucasian Americans. The male to female ratio is 5:1, and the defect is 2.5 times as likely in caucasian infants as compared to African American infants.

○   **What is the average age for the onset pyloric stenosis?**

4 weeks. The onset of pyloric stenosis is generally between the second and the fourth week of life. It is rarely diagnosed after 5 months.

❍   **Differentiate between omphalocele and gastroschisis.**

Omphalocele is a herniation of the intestines into the umbilical cord.

Gastroschisis is a herniation of the intestines through the abdominal wall due to a defective closure of the abdominal wall itself.

❍   **Gastroenteritis in the pediatric population occurring in the summer is likely caused by _____, not by _____.**

Enterovirus. Overall, the rotavirus is the most common cause of pediatric gastroenteritis, as it is responsible for more than 50% of the cases of acute diarrhea in this population. Rotavirus gastroenteritis is generally preceded by an upper respiratory infection and is a self-limiting disease that lasts 4 to 10 days. Other causes of gastroenteritis in children are parvoviruses, coxsackie viruses, echoviruses, adenoviruses, and caliciviruses.

❍   **What is the most common bacterial cause of gastroenteritis in the pediatric patient?**

Campylobacter jejuni. This, too, is a self-limiting disease, lasting less than 1 week. These patients appear more sick than those with viral syndromes. Fever, abdominal pain, copious diarrhea, vomiting, and malaise are common complaints. *Campylobacter jejuni* is also the most common bacterial etiology of gastroenteritis in the adult population too.

❍   **A happy, outdoorsy family with the obligatory dog (Spot), went on a summer vacation in the Grand Canyon. The trip was cut short because the whole family (even Spot) suddenly developed watery diarrhea and excessive gas in the abdomen. They have no fevers. What is the most likely parasite ruining this family's fun?**

Giardia lamblia. This organism is commonly contracted from contaminated water or animal contact but can also be spread by person to person contact. Diagnosis is made by microscopic examination of the stool. Treatment is by rehydration and metronidazole. Spot's on his own.

❍   **What is the most common bacterial etiology of pediatric mesenteric lymphadenitis?**

Yersinia enterocolitica

❍   **Where is a neuroblastoma most commonly found?**

This tumor may be found in any part of the nervous system, but it is most common in the adrenal glands. Neuroblastomas occur predominantly in children under 6, and are twice as common in females as males. 90% of neuroblastomas produce hormones, such as epinephrine, which can cause tachycardia and anxiety.

❍   **What is the association between prematurity and hyaline membrane disease?**

There is a positive correlation. At 29 weeks gestation, 60% of newborns will have HMD. By 39 weeks gestation, the incidence has decreased to near 0%. Treatment includes prevention of premature birth, glucocorticoid hormones, for mothers who must deliver prematurely and surfactant replacement.

❍   **What is the most common cause of orbital cellulitis?**

Infection extended from the paranasal sinuses. The causative organisms are usually *H. influenzae*, *Staphylococcus aureus*, group A ß-hemolytic streptococcus and *Streptococcus pneumonia*. This is a serious condition because of the potential for infection to spread causing meningitis, brain abscesses, or cavernous sinus thrombosis.

○   **What is the most common cause of conjunctivitis in the pediatric population?**

Adenovirus.

○   **What is the most common cause of seasonal allergic pediatric rhinitis.**

Ragweed pollen, otherwise known as hay fever. The most common perennial allergens are house dust and house mites, followed by feathers, dander, and mold spores. Removal of the allergen, if possible, is the best treatment. Treat the patient with sodium cromoglycate or intranasal corticosteroids.

○   **What is an allergic shiner?**

Bluish purple rings under the eyes associated with allergies. They result from a decreased or obstructed periorbital venous drainage.

○   **How can you clinically distinguish orbital cellulitis from periorbital cellulitis?**

Only orbital cellulitis will present with proptosis and limited extraocular movements but both will have fever, eyelid swelling, erythema, and leukocytosis.

○   **A 7 year old girl presents with joint pain everywhere, fever, and hard bumps on her elbows and forearm. Three weeks ago she was afflicted with strep throat. Your diagnosis?**

Rheumatic fever. Rheumatic fever is most common in children 5 to 15. It is always preceded by an infection with group A streptococcus. The Jones' criteria are used to make the diagnosis. Patients must meet either two major criteria, or one major and two minor criteria.

Major criteria
Polyarthritis
Carditis
Erythema marginatum
Subcutaneous nodules
Chorea

Minor criteria
Fever
Arthralgia
Prior rheumatic heart disease
Elevated sed rate
Elevated C-reactive protein
Prolonged P-R interval

○   **What does a high pitched systolic , blowing, apical murmur that radiates to the axilla suggest?**

Mitral valve insufficiency. This is the valve most commonly affected by rheumatic heart disease.

○   **What is the treatment for rheumatic fever?**

Bed rest, NSAIDS, penicillin and hospitalization. Patients must have long term folllow up of the ensuing valcular disease as well as check ups for recurrence.

○   **What heart defect is associated with Trisomy 18 syndrome?**

Ventricular septal defect.

O   **What heart defect is associated with Rubella syndrome?**

Patent ductus arteriosus

O   **What percentage of children have heart murmurs?**

50%! Only 10% of children with heart murmurs have pathological heart murmurs.

O   **What is the most common innocent heart murmur?**

Still's murmur, a vibratory murmur heard only in systole. Other innocent heart murmurs are a venous hum, pulmonary flow murmur, and a neonatal pulmonary artery branch murmur.

O   **What are the common characteristics of an innocent heart murmur?**

The patient is otherwise physically healthy with no signs of cyanosis, shortness of breath, or lethargy. The murmur is low frequency, does not radiate, has no associated thrill, is located in the mid-to-lower sternal border (as opposed to higher up), is systolic, and is accentuated by sitting up, exercise, fever, anxiety, or crying.

O   **A normal appearing term neonate presents with tachypnea, cyanosis and CHF.   What is the likely pathology?**

Congenital cardiac pathology. CHF can present symptomatology for VSD, severe aortic coarctation, or transposition of the great vessels. The "hyperoxia" test may help differentiate cardiac etiology. Place the infant on 100% O2; the pO2 will increase < 20 mm Hg with right to left shunting.

O   **What is the most common congenital heart disorder?**

Ventricular septal defects. These defects account for approximately 38% of all congenital heart disorders. Other disorders include atrial septal defects (18%), pulmonary valve stenosis (13%), pulmonary artery stenosis (7%), aortic valve stenosis (4%), patent ductus arteriosis (4%), and mitral valve prolapse (4%).

O   **What is the most common congenital heart disease associated with Down syndrome?**

Septal defects, most commonly endocardial cushion defects. These are inflow ventricular septal defects that have associated abnormalities of the tricuspid and mitral valves.

O   **Name 8 clinical presentations of pediatric heart disease.**

1) Cyanosis
2) CHF
3) Pathologic murmur
4) Cardiogenic shock
5) HTN
6) Tachyarrhythmias
7) Abnormal pulses
8) Syncope

O   **T/F: During childhood, symptoms of aortic stenosis are common.**

False. Even if severe, the left ventricle has the ability to hypertrophy in childhood, compensating for many years.

○ **Describe the three aspects of acute treatment of Tetralogy of Fallot.**

Positioning: Place the patient in a knee-chest position with minimal stimulation such as upright on parents lap

Oxygenation: Deliver high FIO2

Pharmacologic: Morphine 0.1 mg/kg or propranolol 0.1 mg/kg

○ **Name four congenital heart lesions with a right-sided aortic arch.**

1) Truncus arteriosus
2) Transposition of the great vessels
3) Tetralogy of Fallot
4) Tricuspid Atresia

○ **What congenital heart defect is classically associated with a precordial thrill and a high-pitched, harsh pansystolic murmur which is best heard on the left sternal border?**

Ventricular septal defect. Prognosis for VSD is good: 50% of VSDs will close spontaneously within the first year of life.

○ **A newborn with a systolic ejection murmur and widely split S2 probably has which congenital heart malformation?**

Atrial septal defect. This is due to a patent foramen ovale, allowing blood to be shunted back from the left atrium to the right. This results in an increased blood flow through the pulmonary artery and a delay in the closure of the pulmonic valve which causes the split S2.

○ **Coarctation of the aorta is associated with a narrowing of the aortic arch. Where is the narrowing located?**

Just distal to the origin of the left subclavian. This results in hypertensive upper extremities and normotensive lower extremities.

○ **Match the congenital heart defect with the direction of the shunt (i.e., right-to-left or left-to-right).**

1) Ventricular septal defect
2) Patent ductus arteriosus
3) Transposition of the great vessels
4) Tetralogy of Fallot
5) Atrial septal defect
6) Pulmonary stenosis

Answers: (1) L to R, (2) R to L, (3) L to R, (4) R to L, (5) L to R, and (6) R to L

○ **A premature newborn with bounding pulses, a precordial thrill, and a continuous machine-like murmur, heard best just under the left clavicle, most likely has what congenital heart defect?**

Patent ductus arteriosis. This heart defect should be treated with an injection of indomethacin, which produces a closure within a few days. If patency persists, surgery is necessary.

○ **By what age does a child reach half her/his adult height?**

Two years. However, by this time the child will have attained only 20% of his/her adult weight.

○ **How is short stature due to heredity and short stature due to a constitutional delay in growth differentiated?**

Bone age determination. In children with familial short stature, bone ages will be normal. In children with constitutional growth delay, the bone ages will also be delayed, as will sexual maturation.

○   **When is menarche in relation to the female growth spurt?**

Females have menarche just after their peak growth spurt. This is just the opposite of males, who are well on their way through puberty before they hit their peak growth spurt.

○   **What is the first sign of puberty in males?**

Growth of the testes, followed by thinning and pigmentation of the scrotum, growth of the penis, and lastly the development of pubic hair.

○   **A 15 year old adolescent male has developed small breasts. His parents want this situation surgically corrected. What do you recommend?**

Surgery is a consideration if the physical abnormality is causing severe psychological pain or if the breasts have persisted for a long time.   Surgery is not recommended because gynecomastia in adolescents generally lasts only 1 to 2 years. It has been reported that gynecomastia occurs in 36 to 64% of pubertal males.

○   **What drugs can cause gynecomastia?**

Marijuana, hormones, digitalis, spironolactone, cimetidine, ketoconazole, antihypertensives, antidepressants, and amphetamines.

○   **A 5 month old baby appears lethargic yet flinches at every little noise.   Upon physical examination you note, a "cherry red" spot on the macula.   Your prognosis?**

Tay-Sachs disease This is an autosomal recessive disorder affecting the gray matter. Myoclonic and akinetic seizures begin 1 to 3 months after the initial symptoms of decreased alertness and hyperacusis (excessive reaction to noise). Patients usually do not survive past age 4.

○   **What is a Dandy-Walker malformation?**

A congenital malformation in the brain consisting of a dilated cystic fourth ventricle and obstructive hydrocephalus resulting from blockage of the foramen of Magendie and the foramen of Luschka.

○   **You are examining a 5 year old and you notice eight café au lait spots ranging from 6 to 9 mm in diameter, freckles in the axillary region, and a Lisch nodule (pigmented hamartoma of the iris). What disease are you worried about?**

Neurofibromatosis (von Recklinghausen's disease). Neurofibromatosis should be investigated in any child with more than five café au lait spots measuring larger than 5 mm. For adolescents, the spots must measure larger than 15 mm. Neurofibromatosis is an autosomal dominant disease that affects the nervous system, the integument, bone, muscle, and several other organs.

○   **What disease did the Elephant Man have?**

Neurofibromatosis, also known as von Recklinghausen's disease. He developed large, disfiguring, stalk-like tissue tumors. Patients with neurofibromatosis should be screened for visual and hearing diseases.

○   **List three other diseases that affect both the skin and the central nervous system.**

Bourneville disease (Tuberous sclerosis): "Ash leaf" skin lesions, seizures, and mental retardation.

Sturge-Weber syndrome: Port wine stain in trigeminal distribution, glaucoma, and possible seizures.

Ataxia-Telangiectasia (Louis-Bar syndrome): Progressive ataxia, telangiectasis most noticeably on the conjunctiva and ears, lung infections, and malignant lymphomas.

O   **A mother brings her 5 month old infant in to your office because the baby is weak, lethargic, has a fixed gaze, and will not eat; not even his favorite treat, honey on the pacifier. The baby has no fever. What is your diagnosis?**

Infant botulism. Honey is the key word. Botulism spores can lay dormant in honey or formula and are not killed by pasteurization. Once ingested, these spores germinate and produce a toxin that causes the illness. Adult botulism is generally from ingestion of the toxin, not the spores, in foods. Treatment is supportive.

O   **A pediatric patient who has suffered head trauma one week ago now has a seizure. What is the risk that this patient will have another seizure in the future?**

75%. Patients with posttraumatic epilepsy have a high rate of recurrent seizures and should therefore be on chronic anticonvulsant treatment.

O   **A 4 year old boy has red cheeks, a low grade fever, and a maculopapular rash in a lacy reticular pattern that began on his arms and spread to his trunk and legs. The rash has come and gone for the past 2 weeks. What is your diagnosis?**

Erythema infectiosum, also known as fifth disease or "slapped cheek disease." The patient may also have constitutional symptoms, such as pharyngitis, headache, myalgia, coryza, or gastrointestinal problems.

O   **What is the etiology of Fifth disease?**

Parvovirus B19.

O   **What is the treatment for Fifth disease?**

None, it is self – limited. Pregnant women in contact with infected children should be tested as fifth disease in pregnancy has been associated with fetal death and red cell aplasia with fetal hydrops.

O   **A patient is brought in by her father complaining of a high fever for 4 days that was then followed by a macularopapular rash that began on her trunk and spread to her arms and legs. She has no other complaints. What is the prognosis?**

This patient has roseola infantum (exanthem subitum). This is a self limited disease with no treatment and few complications.

O   **An 11 year old is brought in by his mother who says her son has a fever, sore throat and a rash that feels like sandpaper. What is a likely diagnosis?**

Scarlet fever. This illness usually results from a pharyngeal infection with group A streptococcal strains that produce erythrogenic toxin. The rash is an erthematous, finely punctated rash that begins on the trunk and spreads to the extremities. The skin feels like sandpaper. Patients also have Pastia lines and a strawberry tongue. The rash lasts about a week but then the skin desquamates for several more weeks.

O   **What is the treatment for the above patient?**

Penicillin x 10 days.

O   **What are Pastia lines?**

Areas of increased erythema in the folds of the skin.

○   **What other childhood rash may present with a "strawberry tongue"?**

Kawasaki's disease.

○   **What is the most common cause of stomatitis in 1 to 3 year olds?**

Acute herpetic gingivostomatitis caused by the herpes simplex virus.

○   **Six days ago a 5 year old girl had malaise, cough, coryza, photophobia, conjunctivitis, and a mild fever. Four days ago she had small grayish white dots the size of sand grains on her buccal mucosa. Two days ago her fever climbed to 102° F and she developed a morbilliform rash that began on the head and has now spread to the rest of her body. Her history indicates that she has not received her childhood immunizations. What is your diagnosis?**

Measles.

○   **Where are Koplik spots most commonly found?**

Opposite the lower molars on the buccal mucosa. They can be as small as grains of sand and are commonly grayish white with a red areolae and may occasionally bleed. (Remember: "Kops" catch "weasels," which rhymes with measles.)

○   **Describe the rash of measles.**

A maculopapular rash that begins at the hairline and spreads to the rest of the body. Lesions are initially individual but become confluent over time. The rash starts 2 weeks after initial exposure to infection.

○   **What is the treatment for measles?**

Symptomatic.

○   **What are the 3 stages of measles and what are the associated signs and symptoms?**

Incubation stage (10-12 days) which has no signs or symptoms; prodromal (or catarrhal) stage, which is characterized by Koplik spots, low grade fever, coryza and cough; and the final stage consisting of the classic rash and high fever.

○   **When is the child with measles infectious?**

During the prodromal phase until 5 days after the rash has begun.

○   **What are some complications of measles?**

Photosensitivity, pharyngitis, encephalitis, subacute sclerosing panencephalitis and DIC.

○   **What is the most characteristic sign of rubella?**

Adenopathy. Most notably in the retroauricular, postoccipital and posterior cervical chains. The adenopathy usually appears before the rash.

○   **What are some common complications of mumps?**

Orchitis/epididymitis, meningoencephalomyelitis, mild pancreatitis, and unilateral deafness.

○   **What rash is associated with a herald patch?**

Pityriasis rosea. A "herald patch" is exactly that, a single round or oval lesion that "heralds" the impending maculopapular rash called Pityriasis rosea. The second rash to appear is on the trunk. Small crops of mildly itchy, oval scaly patches create a christmas tree pattern. Sometimes the rash may be associated with pharyngitis and malaise.

○   **What is the treatment for pityriasis rosea?**

None. The secondary patches fade in several weeks. Sunlight may hasten the disappearance of the rash.

○   **An 11 year old unimmunized boy was brought to your office by his pregnant mother. He has a 4 day history of fever, cough, and coryza. A pruritic, confluent, and flushing maculopapular rash began on his face 2 days ago and then spread to the rest of his body. Upon examination, you notice he has posterior auricular along with cervical and suboccipital lymphadenopathy. What is your diagnosis?**

Rubella (German measles).

○   **The mother in the above case is 2½ months pregnant. What should you do?**

Council her on the associated risks of congenital defects in her unborn child. If she chooses to carry the baby to term, advise her to stay away from her infected son as there is a prolonged shedding of the virus. In addition, she should receive some passive protection, 0.25 to 0.50 mL/kg serum globulin (ISG) should be given IM within the first week of exposure. NEVER give a pregnant woman rubella vaccine!

○   **Describe the look and timing of the Rubella rash.**

It is a maculopapular to confluent rash that appears and spreads very quickly, sometimes over 24 hours.

○   **Aside from the rash, what are some findings in German measles?**

Rubella can present concomitantly with polyarthritis, splenomegaly, and low grade fever.

○   **When is the child with Rubella infectious?**

One week before, and one week after, the rash.

○   **Of all the wonderful diaper rashes babies get, how is candidal diaper dermatitis distinguished?**

Babies with candidal dermatitis will have satellite lesions away from the groin area. Otherwise, this rash presents as a large, red confluent vesiculopustular plaque with a clearly demarcated border. Treatment is with topical antifungals.

○   **What causes Rocky Mountain spotted fever (RMSF)?**

Rickettsia rickettsii. Characteristic "spots" result from rickettsial invasion of endothelial cells in small blood vessels, including arterioles. Dermacentor andersoni, a wood tick, is the vector.

○   **Why is RMSF in the pediatric section?**

Because two-thirds of RMSF patients are children under age 15.

○   **Describe the rash of RMSF.**

The rash begins as erythematous blanching macules on the wrists, hands, ankles, and feet that spread to the whole body appearing 3 to 5 days after the onset of fever, headache, and chills. As the illness progresses, the rash becomes papular and even purpuric. Conjunctivitis, photophobia, and even signs of meningoencephalitis can occur.

○   **What is the treatment for Rocky mountain spotted fever?**

Chloramphenicol or tetracycline.

○   **Kawasaki's disease is most common in what age group?**

0 to 2 years. 80% of patients with Kawasaki's are less than 4 years old.

○   **What are the diagnostic criteria for Kawasaki's disease?**

Fever for at least 5 days plus 4 of the following:
Polymorphous exanthem on the trunk
Bilateral conjunctivitis
Lesions in the oral cavity
Cervical lymphadenopathy
Peripheral extremity rashes (erthematous initially then desquamating in convalescent phase)

○   **What is the most serious complication of Kawasaki's disease?**

The formation of coronary artery aneurysms, which can rupture or thrombose. Cardiac involvement occurs in 10 to 40% of the children within the first 2 weeks of the disease. Kawasaki's disease is also known as mucocutaneous lymph node syndrome or infantile polyarteritis.

○   **How long does the fever of Kawasaki's disease last?**

2 weeks.

○   **What is the treatment for Kawasaki's disease?**

High doses of aspirin for the acute phase, then low doses once the child is afebrile, and IV gamma globulin.

○   **A 3 month old presents to your office with flaky grayish-white plaques on the buccal mucosa, lips, gingiva and tongue and a decreased appetite. How do you treat this patient?**

Antifungals, anesthetic gel prior to feeding and cool liquids for discomfort. This patient has oral thrush or candidiasis.

○   **When is thrush most common?**

Candidal gingivostomatitis is most common in the first 3 months.

○   **What is the most common skin infection among pediatric emergency patients?**

Nonbullous impetigo caused by group A ß-hemolytic streptococci and *S.aureus*, a bacterial infection of the dermis.

○   **Describe the rash of impetigo.**

Lesions are either vesicopustular or bullous. Vesicopustular lesions begin as small pustules with an erthematous rim. The pustules pop and leave a honey-like exudate which then crusts over. Bullous impetigo begins as red macules that grow to become large fluid filled lesions with erthematous bases. The bullae then rupture and leave a clear coat over the desquamated area.

O **How does impetigo spread?**

Via direct contact.

O **What is the recommended treatment for impetigo?**

Penicillin VK. Mupirocin, a topical therapy, can be used for mild cases.

O **Erysipelas (St. Anthony's fire) is another pediatric exanthem that represents a primary bacterial infection. What organism causes this uncommon cellulitis, usually characterized by pain at the affected site, along with malaise, and fever?**

Erysipelas is also caused by group A ß-hemolytic streptococci. The use of penicillin or erythromycin usually results in rapid improvement. Recurrences are common and can lead to irreversible lymphedema (elephantiasis nostras).

O **A 10 year old is brought to your office because his mother has noticed red, scaly blistering on the top of the child's feet and toes. What is the diagnosis?**

This is probably a case of contact dermatitis that is caused by new shoes. It is most frequent in preadolescents.

O **What rash is associated with rheumatic fever?**

Erythema marginatum. This is a pink, non-pruritic, evanescent rash that covers the trunk and inner surfaces of the arms and legs. It spreads in wavy lines and rings with clear-cut margins. Subcutaneous nodules over bony prominences are also noted.

O **How do you treat head lice?**

Treatment is with permethrin shampoo therapy: Malathion and lindane may also be used but not with infants. A second shampooing should be applied 1 week after the initial treatment.

O **How are lice spread?**

By direct contact. They do not live long on inanimate objects. Outbreaks are more common in the winter.

O **A mother brings her 5 month old in to your office because she noticed small raised papules between the webbing of his fingers. She says he has been scratching there at night time. What is the treatment?**

This child most likely has scabies. Treatment is with a single application of permethrin cream. All close contacts should also be treated as scabies are spread by direct contact. Scabies do not live longer than 24 hours off their host so washing clothes and sheets is not necessary.

O **How is the diagnosis of pinworms made?**

The female pinworm deposits her eggs in the perianal region at night time, hence the intense anal pruritis associated with pinworm infestation. Eggs can be detected by pressing tape to the perianal area. Sometimes the worms themselves can be seen by direct visualization.

O **How do you treat pinworm infestation?**

Oral mebendazole or albendazole.

○ **What are Aschoff bodies?**

Clusters of multinucleated cells found in fragmented collagen fibers of the myocardium. Aschoff bodies are specific to rheumatic fever.

○ **A 3 week old infant presents with greasy scales and yellow crusts in his scalp, under his arms, and in the folds of his neck and groin. These lesions have been present since birth. What is your diagnosis?**

Seborrheic dermatitis. This is an inflammatory disorder of the sebaceous glands that is common in the first month of life and is generally characterized by diffuse scaling in the scalp known as "cradle cap." Treatment for infants is shampooing and topical hydrocortisone cream.

○ **What is the major cause of fever that afflicts infants 0 to 3 months old?**

Virus (95%).

○ **What are the most common causes of meningitis in neonates?**

Group B streptococci and *E. coli*.

○ **What are the most common causes of meningitis in infants and children?**

Streptococcus pneumoniae, *N. meningitidis*, and *H. influenzae*.

○ **What is Brudzinski's sign?**

A sign of meningeal irritation. Passive neck flexion causes involuntary leg flexion.

○ **What is Kernig's sign?**

Neck pain is elicited with passive knee extension in a leg that is flexed 90° at the hip. This is also a sign of meningeal irritation.

○ **What are some signs and symptoms of meningitis?**

Headache, lethargy, stiff neck, irritability, confusion, vomiting, bulging fontanelle, poor feeding, and petechiae.

○ **Describe the CSF features of bacterial vs. viral meningitis.**

	Bacterial	Viral
Opening pressure	Increased	Increased
WBC's	100 – 10,000	10 – 500
Protein	Increased	Mildly increased
Glucose	Decreased	Normal
Gram stain/culture	+ bacteria	No bacteria

○ **What are the contraindications for a lumbar puncture?**

Increased intracranial pressure, shock, cellulitis or abscess over lumbar vertebrae, respiratory failure, or bleeding diathesis.

O   **What is the treatment for meningitis?**

2000 guidelines recommend ampicillin and cefotaxime for neonates to 1 month old, ampicillin + (cefotaxime or ceftriaxone) + dexamethasone for ages 1 – 3 months; and (cefotazime or ceftriaxone) + dexamethasone + vancomycin for ages 3 months to 50 years. In addition, add fluids if shock, anticonvulsants if seizures, and ventilation if respiratory failure.

O   **What is the most common congenital anomaly of the nervous system?**

A myelomeningocele. This occurs when the neural tube fails to close. It is frequently associated with hydrocephalus or Arnold-Chiari malformation.

O   **How might you recognize an infant with fetal alcohol syndrome.**

Small eyes and midface, long smooth philtrum, mild ptosis, flat nasal bridge, short nose, thin upper lip, epicanthal folds, joint contractures and kidney malformations.

O   **What is the typical body habitus of a child with homocystinuria?**

Long thin limbs and fingers, scoliosis, osteoporosis and sternal deformities.

O   **What other features are common to homocystinuria?**

Mild mental retardation, strokes, MI's, and dislocated lenses.

O   **What is PKU?**

An enzyme deficiency that prevents the conversion of phenylalanine to tyrosine. This results in the toxic buildup of phenylacetic acid and phenyllactic acid. Patients with PKU are mentally retarted, hypopigmented, have hypertonicity, tremors and behavior disorders.

O   **Is it possible to prevent retardation in PKU?**

Yes. Newborn screening can detect PKU early enough to be able to start a diet with no phenylalanine.

O   **What is the most common defect in Down syndrome?**

95% of Down syndrome patients have Trisomy 21. The remaining 5 % have either translocation or mosaicism.

O   **What are the characteristic features of a Down syndrome child?**

Epicanthal folds, flat nasal bridge, small nose, mouth, chin and palebral fissures, hypotonia, endocardial cushion and septal defects, GI abnormalities, and low IQ (50).

O   **What birth defects are associated with Trisomy 13?**

Microcephaly with open lesions of the scalp, holoprosencephaly, microphthalmos, colobomata, omphalocele, ambiguous genitalia, severe retardation, congenital heart desease, cleft lip and or cleft palate. 90% of infants with trisomy 13 die before reaching their first birthday.

O   **What birth defects are associated with Trisomy 18?**

Neural tube defects, congenital heart disease, dislocated hips, rocker-bottom feet, overlapping fingers, intrauterine growth retardation, microcephaly, prominent occiput, micrognathia, severe mental retardation, and various CNS malformations. Like trisomy 13, 90% of infants with trisomy 18 die before their first birthday.

O   **When do the symptoms of Duchenne muscular dystrophy begin?**

Between the ages of 2 and 4. Children experience proximal muscle weakness and have delayed walking.

O   **What do most children with Duchenne muscular dystrophy usually die of?**

CHF or pneumonia. Children with this disease do not generally live more than 25 years.

O   **What is Gowes sign?**

A maneuver used to reach a standing position from a laying position in patients with Duchenne muscular dystrophy. First the child pushes off the floor creating an arch (hands and feet on the floor, buttox in the air) the patient then puts his hands on his knees one by one and walks his hands up his thighs until he is able to stand. This is indicative of weak back and pelvic girdle muscles.

O   **Differentiate between hectic, remittent, and intermittent fevers.**

Hectic fevers: Daily temperature elevations that sometimes return to a normal or lower baseline.

Remittent fevers: Daily temperature elevations that return to a lower but not normal baseline.

Intermittent fevers: Daily temperature elevations that return to normal in between fluctuations.

O   **Febrile seizures occur when the patient's temperature does what?**

Rises rapidly. Febrile seizures are more closely related to a rapid rise in temperature rather than in the highest temperature reached. These seizures occur between 6 months and 6 years of age and are thus labeled if they occur within the context of a febrile illness, are less than 15 minutes duration, and are tonic-clonic generalized and simple. They must have no focal neurological defects and be present in a patient with no prior neurological disorders.

O   **What is the risk for recurrent febrile seizures after an episode of a febrile seizure?**

30 to 35%. Control of fevers with acetaminophen and tepid baths is the recommended treatment.

O   **What is the risk of developing epilepsy after a febrile seizure?**

1%.

O   **Phenobarbital is probably the most efficacious drug used to treat febrile seizures. Should all patients with a febrile seizure receive phenobarbital as prophylaxis against future similar seizures?**

Although its use may be warranted in patients who are particularly ill, who have had repeated febrile seizures, or who have underlying neurologic disease, phenobarbital is not recommended as prophylactic treatment.

O   **Neonatal seizures have a broad range of presentations. What are the two most frequent causes of myoclonic seizures?**

Metabolic disorders and hypoxia.

○   **Infantile spasms are usually noted in children 6 months of age. Is it true that these patients have a high rate of developmental disorders?**

Yes. Eighty-five percent of these patients have developmental disorders.

○   **Are infantile spasms a form of seizures?**

Yes. Infantile spasms are attacks in which an infant laying on her back suddenly bends his or her arms, straightens the legs, and arches the neck and back. Such spasms last a few seconds. These spasms may develop into other forms of seizures in adulthood.

○   **Infantile spasms represent a significant disorder and require aggressive evaluation. In addition to anticonvulsants, what hormone plays a role in their management?**

Adrenocorticotropic hormone (ACTH).

○   **How long must a continuous seizure last to be defined as status epilepticus?**

> 20 minutes.

○   **What is the initial drug of choice for a patient in status epilepticus?**

Diazepam, 1 month – 5 years; 0.3 mg/kg IV q 15 – 30 min. maximum 5 mg/dose. > 5 years maximum is 10 mg/dose.

○   **If the diazepam dosage cited above does not break the seizure, what is the next step?**

Phenytoin load, 15 – 20 mg/kg IV

○   **Your patient is still seizing! What is your next step?**

Phenobarbital, 15 mg/kg IV q 15 – 30 min with a maximum of 40 mg/kg

○   **What is a neuroblastoma?**

A malignant tumor arising from the sympathetic neuroblasts in the sympathetic chain and adrenal medulla. Two thirds of the tumors occur in the abdomen and pelvis. The other third occurs in the posterior mediastinum and neck. Symptoms are generally related to impingement on local structures (bowel obstruction, hypertension, radiculopathy etc…)

○   **When do neuroblastomas most commonly occur?**

Before the age of 4.

○   **What are the three most common organisms that cause bacteremia in both immunized and unimmunized children?**

Streptococcus pneumoniae, *N. meningitidis*, and *H. influenzae*.

○   **What are the two most common organisms causing sepsis in the neonate?**

Group B streptococcus and *E. coli*.

○   **What are the three most common organisms causing sepsis after the newborn period?**

H. influenzae, *N. meningitidis* and *Streptococcus pneumoniae*.

❍ **Differentiate sepsis from bacteremia.**

Bacteremia is the symptom of fever with a positive blood culture. Sepsis is bacteremia with focal findings.

❍ **What is the most common condition associated with occult bacteremia in children?**

Otitis media. Other associated conditions are bacterial pneumonia, streptococcal pharyngitis, and most importantly, meningitis.

❍ **What is the appropriate bolus for a pediatric patient in shock?**

20 mL/kg.

❍ **At what rate should the urine output of a pediatric patient be maintained?**

1 to 2 mL/kg/h.

❍ **What drug can be given to pediatric patients with meningitis to decrease sequelae, especially deafness?**

Methylprednisolone (30 mg/kg).

❍ **Which is a more common cause of dysuria among female pediatric patients, UTI or vulvovaginitis?**

Vulvovaginitis.

❍ **What percentage of infants born to HIV infected mothers will have HIV?**

30 to 50%.

❍ **What CMV infection route of transmission is most serious for a newborn?**

Transfusion. Transfusing blood containing the CMV virus can be deadly for newborns who are not protected by maternal antibodies. Other transmission routes are via the birth canal, breast milk, and the home environment. These infections appear benign and generally only result in minor respiratory infections.

❍ **What is the usual presentation of children with a ventricular septal defect?**

The majority of these children are totally asymptomatically, and the defect usually is not diagnosed until they are school age.

❍ **Is wheezing an integral part of asthma?**

No. Thirty-three percent of children with asthma will have only cough variant asthma with no wheezing.

❍ **What are the most common extrinsic allergens that affect asthmatic children?**
Dust and dust mites.

❍ **Which condition must be ruled out when childhood nasal polyps are found?**

Cystic fibrosis.

○   **What is the incidence of meconium ileus in newborn infants with cystic fibrosis?**

Meconium ileus is most commonly seen in infants with cystic fibrosis, but less than 10% of infants with cystic fibrosis have meconium ileus.

○   **What are the McConnochie criteria for the diagnosis of bronchiolitis?**

1) Acute expiratory wheezing
2) Age 6 months or less
3) Signs of viral illness, such as fever or coryza
4) With or without pneumonia or atopy
5) The first such episode

○   **Foreign body aspiration occurs most commonly in which age group?**

One to three year olds.

○   **What is the most common cause of cardiac arrest in children?**

Hypoxia.

○   **What are the most common arrhythmias in pediatric patients?**

Sinus bradycardia and asystole.

○   **Is Graves' disease more common in boys or girls?**

Girls are affected five times as much as boys.

○   **What are the classic signs and symptoms of Graves' Disease?**

Emotional liability, autonomic hyperactivity, exopthalmos, tremor, increased appetite with no weight gain or weight loss, diarrhea, and a goiter in nearly all affected individuals.

○   **What is the definition of precocious puberty?**

The onset of secondary sexual characteristics before age eight in females and nine in males.

○   **How much water should a newborn baby receive in addition to infant formula or breast feeding?**

In normal situations newborns need no additional free water. In fact, excess free water is the major cause for water intoxication in infancy and the development of subsequent hyponatremic seizures.

○   **What are the most common causes of delayed puberty?**

Constitutional growth delay, familial short stature, and chronic illness.

○   **What percentage of teenage girls have eating disorders?**

20%

○   **What is the most common breast tumor in adolescents?**

Fibroadenoma (>90%).

O   **What endocrine abnormalities can lead to galactorrhea in a teenage girl?**

Hypothyroidism and an increase prolactin (i.e. from a pituitary adenoma).

O   **How common are varicoceles?**

Dilation of the veins of the spermatic cords occurs in about 15% of adolescents (usually on the left side).

O   **What is the most common solid tumor in adolescent males?**

Testicular seminoma.

O   **What are the most common viral causes of pneumonia in the otherwise healthy child?**

RSV, influenza, parainfluenza, and adenovirus.

O   **What should you suspect in a child that presents with tender and swollen pectoral nodes?**

Cat-scratch disease.

O   **What is thought to be the mode of inoculation in cat-scratch disease?**

Rubbing the eye after contact with a cat.

O   **What four classes of contact with a patient with meningococcal disease require prophylaxis?**

1.   People who live in the same household
2.   Attendees of the same child care or school in the previous seven days
3.   Those who have been directly exposed to the index case's secretions, such as by kissing or sharing of food
4.   Health care providers whose mucous membranes were unprotected during resuscitation or intubation of the patient.

O   **What is the most effective treatment of allergic rhinitis?**

Topical use of corticosteroid such as beclomethasone nasal spray.

O   **What is the most common congenital anomaly of the penis?**

Hypospadias.

O   **What is the treatment for testicular torsion?**

Prompt surgical exploration. If the testes is explored within six hours of torsion, 90% of gonads will survive after detorsion and fixation.

O   **What are the complications of circumcision?**

Hemorrhage, infection, dehiscence, denudation of the shaft, glandular injury, and urinary retention.

O   **What is the most frequent cause of acute renal failure in childhood?**

Hemolytic-Uremic Syndrome (HUS)

O   **HUS most commonly follows infection with what organism?**

E. coli (0157:H7). The disease is usually a sequelae to about of gastroenteritis caused by this organism

O   **What is the diagnostic triad for HUS?**

Microangiopathic anemia, acute renal failure, and thrombocytopenia (20K- 1 00/kmm3).

O   **A 6 year old male is diagnosed and treated for intussusception. What tumor is associated with this?**

After the age of *5,* it would be unusual to have an intussusception without a lead point. The most likely malignancy would be a non-Hodgkin's lymphoma.

O   **How does cryptorchism effect the risk of testicular malignancy?**

The risk is 30-50 times greater than in a normal testicle. About one-eighth of testicular tumors develop in cryptorchid testes.

O   **What is the most common cause of obstruction in children?**

Hernia.

O   **What is Rendu-Osler-Weber syndrome?**

Hereditary hemorrhagic telangiectasias found in the small intestine.

O   **What findings comprise the shaken baby syndrome?**

Retinal hemorrhage, subdural hematoma, and rib fractures.

O   **What are some causes (according to age) of painful limping?**

1-3   year olds: Infection, occult trauma, or neoplasm
4-10 year olds: Infection, transient synovitis of the hip, Legg-Calve-Perthes disease, rheumatologic disorder, trauma, or neoplasm
11+ year olds: Slipped capital femoral epiphysis, rheumatologic disorder, and trauma.

O   **What is the Ortolani maneuver?**

Gentle abduction with the hip in flexion while lifting up on the greater trochanter which results in reduction of a dislocated hip with an palpable "clunk" as the femoral head slips over the posterior rim of the acetabulum.

O   **What is Legg-Calve-Perthes disease (LCPD)?**

It is an idiopathic avascular necrosis of the capital femoral epiphysis in a child (usually male) aged 2-12 years (mean: 7 years).

O   **What is the treatment for scoliosis?**

Treatment is based on etiology of the scoliosis, degree of deformity, degree of skeletal maturity, and curve progression. Observation is indicated for mild, idiopathic curve (less than 20 degrees) with clinical exam and x-ray every six months. Orthosis is indicated for those in whom the curve is considered acceptable at diagnosis, but whose curve is likely to progress. Surgical correction is usually indicated for curves greater than approximately 40 degrees or those with significant cosmetic deformity.

❍   **You are seeing a child with recurrent episodes of otitis media and cough. What environmental exposure history should you elicit?**

Exposure to cigarette smoke in the household.

❍   **What organism is the most common cause of septic joints in children?**

Staphylococcus aureus.

❍   **What organism is the most common cause of septic joints in adolesents?**

Neisseria gonorrhoeae.

❍   **What is Sampter's Triad?**

Asthma, nasal polyps, and aspirin allergy.

❍   **What is the dose of epinephrine in acute asthma?**

1 mg/kg SC of epinephrine 1:1000, repeated q 20 minutes as needed.

❍   **What is the best single predictor of pneumonia in children?**

Tachypnea

❍   **What is the normal IV maintenance amount for a 25 kg child?**

1600 cc/day or 65 cc/hr. The formula is: 4 ml/kg/hr or 100 ml/kg/day for the first 10 kg; 2 ml/kg/hr or 50 ml/kg/day for the second 10 kg; 1 ml/kg/hr or 20 ml/kg/day for all further kg.

❍   **How does the urine specific gravity help you determine the level of dehydration in a child?**

A urine specific gravity of < 1.020 is found in mild dehydration, 1.030 in moderate, and >1.035 in severe.

❍   **What equipment needs to be ready for resuscitation of a newborn?**

Suction bulb, towels for drying, suction, laryngoscope with a 0-00 Miller blade, umbilical clip, appropriate oxygen mask and small ventilating bag, and a 3.0 uncuffed ET tube. This should suffice for the majority of resuscitations. Rarely are IV access or medications needed, though these should be nearby.

❍   **What is the appropriate endotracheal tube size and laryngoscope size for a 1 year old child? 5 year old?**

ETT 3.5-4.0 with Miller 1, and ETT 5.0 with Miller 2 or Macintosh 2.
The formula is 16 + age in years/4. The size of the ET tube should be roughly the size of the child's pinky.

❍   **What is the definition of apnea in an infant?**

Apnea is either cessation of breathing for more than 20 seconds, or a shorter period associated with cyanosis or bradycardia.

❍   **What is the definition of ALTE?**

An Apparent Life Threatening Event is apnea associated with color change (cyanosis or redness), a loss of muscle tone, and choking or gagging.

○ **Compared to an otherwise healthy infant, how much more likely is a child with a history of ALTE to go on to have SIDS?**

About 3-5 times more likely.

○ **A newly delivered infant has respiratory movement, a closed mouth, but no air audible in the lungs. What is the most likely diagnosis?**

Choanal Atresia

○ **What is the correct workup for a an infant of 16 days with a temperature of 38°C, but appearing well?**

Don't let looks deceive you at this age. A full septic workup, antibiotics and admission are indicated.

○ **In what percentage of patients with ITP was there an antecedent viral illness?**

Roughly 70% of the time. Interval between infection and onset of purpura is usually about 2 weeks.

○ **What is the test of choice for the serological diagnosis of ITP?**

No specific test exists. Platelet count is usually very low (<20k) with megathrombocytes. The WBC and RBC counts are usually normal.

○ **What is the treatment for ITP?**

Infusions of IV gamma globulin (IVIG) at the rate of 1 g/kg/24hr reduces the severity and frequency of thrombocytopenia. Severe cases may benefit from corticosteroids. Unless there is evidence of life threatening hemorrhage, platelet concentrates have minimal effect as they are quickly destroyed.

○ **What is the prognosis for ITP?**

Usually excellent, with >90% of children regaining normal platelet count, though it may take up to a year for them to do so. Most children recover completely within 8 weeks.

○ **What is the therapy for chronic ITP?**

Splenectomy.

○ **What is the order of ossification centers in the elbow?**

Remember the acronym CRITOE. Capitellum, Radial Head, Internal (medial) epicondyle, Trochlea, Olecranon, External (lateral) epicondyle. These ossify at 3-5-7-9-11-13 years, in that order.

PSYCHOSOCIAL PEARLS

○ **What are the components of the multiaxial diagnostic system?**

Axis I: Symptoms and syndromes comprising a mental disorder, including substance abuse/addiction.
Axis II: Personality and developmental disorders underlying the Axis I diagnosis.
Axis III: Physical medical problems/conditions which may or may not contribute to the Axis I diagnosis.
Axis IV: Psychosocial factors.
Axis V: Adaptive ability/disability.

○ **Is violence more likely between family members or non-family members?**

Family members. Twenty to fifty percent of the murders in the US are committed by members of the victims' families. Spouse abuse is as high as 16% in the US.

○ **In what percentage of child sexual abuse cases is the abuser known by the child?**

90%. In 50% of such cases, the mother is also abused.

○ **What is the epidemiology of domestic violence?**

95% of the victims are women. An estimated 4 million women are battered each year. Domestic abuse is the number one cause of injuries to women.   More than half of all women murdered in the US are killed by their intimate partner.

○ **What are the clinical clues for domestic violence?**

Any evidence of injury during pregnancy or late entry into prenatal care. Injuries presenting after significant delay or in various stages of healing; especially to the head, neck, breasts, abdomen, or areas suggesting a defensive posture, such as bruises on the forearms. Vague complaints or unusual injuries, such as bites, scratches, burns, or rope marks.

○ **What is the prevalence of alcoholism in the US?**

Ten to fifteen percent is the lifetime prevalence. Ten percent of men and 3.5% of women are alcoholic.

○ **What age range has the highest prevalence of drinking problems?**

18 to 29 year olds have the greatest prevalence.

○ **Describe the symptoms of alcohol withdrawal and their temporal relations.**

Autonomic hyperactivity: Tachycardia, hypertension, tremors, anxiety, and agitation occurs 6 to 8 hours after patient's last drink.

Hallucinations: Auditory, visual, and tactile occurs 24 hours after patient's last drink.

Global confusion: Occurs 1 to 3 days after patient's last drink.

O   **What is the difference in treatment methods between alcohol withdrawal compared to sedative hypnotic withdrawal?**

Alcohol withdrawal is treated with benzodiazepine, carbamazepine, or paraldehyde. Sedative hypnotic withdrawal is treated with the substitution of a long-acting barbiturate.

O   **What is the most common mental illness in large cities?**

Substance abuse. Substance abuse is prevelant in rural communities as well but the addiction percentages are lower. Incidentally, opiates are predominantly a city drug, while marijuana, alcohol, and amphetamines are found in both the rural and urban settings.

O   **A patient presents with tearing eyes, a runny nose, tachycardia, hair on end, abdominal pains, nausea, vomiting, diarrhea, insomnia, pupillary dilation, and leukocytosis. What is the diagnosis?**

Opiate and/or opioid withdrawal. Treat with methadone or dolophine. Clonidine may blunt some of the side effects.

O   **What is the most effective long-term treatment program for alcoholism?**

Alcoholics Anonymous.

O   **What is the difference between methadone and heroin?**

Methadone causes analgesia, but does not cause euphoria. Habituation occurs with both drugs. The withdrawal symptoms of methadone are less severe, but they last longer.

O   **What are the two most common behavior problems seen by general practitioners?**

Anxiety and depression.

O   **Describe a patient with generalized anxiety disorder.**

Patients afflicted with this disorder appear apprehensive, restless, irritable, and are easily distracted. Patients can also experience muscle tension and fatigue, as well as various autonomic symptoms, such as palpitations, shortness of breath, chest tightness, nausea, or diffuse weakness and numbness.

O   **Name a few substances that might mimic generalized anxiety when ingested.**

Nicotine, caffeine, amphetamines, cocaine, and anticholinergics. Alcohol and sedative withdrawal can also mimic this disorder.

O   **What are eight common <u>medical</u> causes of anxiety or anxiety attacks?**

(1) Alcohol withdrawal, (2) thyrotoxicosis, (3) caffeine, (4) stroke, (5) cardiopulmonary emergencies, (6) hypoglycemia, (7) psychosensory/psychomotor epilepsy, and (8) pheochromocytoma.

O   **Match the aphasia with the anatomy involved.**

1) Broca's aphasia   a) Superior temporal gyrus, posterior third
2) Global aphasia   b) Arcuate fasciculus near the dominant parietal lobe
3) Wernicke's aphasia   c) Middle cerebral artery occlusion
4) Conduction aphasia   d) Left frontal lobe posterior inferior region

Answers: (1) d, (2) c, (3) a, and (4) b.

O   **What accounts for the most referrals to child psychiatrists?**

Attention-deficit/hyperactivity disorder (ADHD). For those of you not paying attention, the answer again is attention-deficit/hyperactivity disorder. ADHD accounts for 30 to 50% of child psychiatric outpatient cases.

O   **The sibling to a female patient with ADHD is at a higher risk for what other disorders?**

Conduct, mood, anxiety, and antisocial disorders, substance abuse, and, of course, ADHD. Relatives of females with ADHD are at a higher risk for these disorders compared to relatives of males.

O   **What chromosomal abnormality do autistic patients commonly have?**

A fragile X syndrome (8%).

O   **What percentage of autistics are mute?**

50%.

O   **Bereavement generally lasts how long?**

6 months. Full melancholic syndrome, hallucinations, and suicidal ideation are not common in bereavement.

O   **Which has an earlier onset, bipolar disorder or unipolar disorder?**

Bipolar. Onset of bipolar disorder is usually in the patient's twenties or thirties; onset of unipolar disorder is usually between ages 35 to 50.

O   **Differentiate between bipolar I, bipolar II, and hypomania.**

Bipolar I: Mania and major depression
Bipolar II: Hypomania and major depression
Hypomania: Mania without severe impairment or psychotic features

O   **Are the majority of affective disorder patients bipolar or unipolar?**

Unipolar (80%).

O   **Which is most commonly the first episode of bipolar disease, mania or depression?**

Mania. Depression is rarely the first symptom. In fact, only 5 to 10% of patients who develop depression first go on to have manic episodes.

O   **First degree relatives of bipolar patients have a greater risk for which mental illnesses?**

Unipolar disorders and alcoholism.

O   **Postural tremor is a major side effect of lithium. How is this side effect controlled?**

Minimize the dose during the work day and give small doses of ß-blockers.

O   **Should people who are physically active have their lithium dosage increased or decreased?**

Increased. Lithium, a salt, is excreted more than sodium in sweat.

○ **T/F: A patient starting lithium will be expected to gain weight.**

True. All psychotropic medications cause weight gain, hence lithium's usefulness in combatting anorexia nervosa.

○ **What is the potential complication associated with treating manic depression and congestive heart failure simultaneously?**

Lithium toxicity. A low salt diet and/or sodium-losing diuretics can cause lithium retention and toxicity.

○ **Lithium toxicity begins at what level?**

14 mg/L. Above this level nausea, diarrhea, vomiting, rigidity, tremor, ataxia, seizures, delirium, coma, and death can occur.

○ **What is the most common clinical symptom of a patient with a borderline personality disorder?**

Chronic boredom. Other symptoms include severe mood swings, volatile relationships, continuous and uncontrollable anger, and impulsiveness.

○ **What findings in a female patient who presents with parotid gland swelling and eroding tooth enamel might you expect?**

Bulimia, which is associated with elevated serum amylase and hypokalemia.

○ **List some common laboratory findings associated with eating disorders.**

Hyponatremia, hypokalemia, hypocalcemia, hypophosphatemia, anemia, hypoglycemia, starvation ketoacidosis, abnormal glucose tolerance, hypothyroidism due to low T3 levels, persistently elevated cortisol due to starvation, low FSH, LH and estrogens, and elevated growth hormone.

○ **What are criteria A through D for the diagnosis of catatonic disorder?**

A: Manifestations of any of the following: echolalia, echopraxia, excessive purposeless motor activity, motor immobility, extreme negativism, resistance to external instruction or movement, or peculiar involuntary movements such as bizarre posturing or grimacing.

B: Evidence from history, examination, and lab findings that the catatonia is a result of a medical condition.

C: Criterion A actions cannot be attributed to another mental condition.

D: Criterion A actions do not occur in a bout of delirium only.

○ **What is the most common cause of catatonia?**

Affective disorder.

○ **The pleasurable effects of cocaine are due to its effect on what?**

DA2 receptors.

O   **What is the treatment for cocaine toxicity?**

Acidify the urine and administer neuroleptics and phentolamine.

O   **In infancy, simple repetitive reactions like nail-biting, thumb-sucking, masturbation, or temper tantrums are manifestations of what psychological reaction?**

Adjustment reactions. These are responses to separation from the caregiver and are often associated with developmental delay.

O   **What is the prevalence of conduct disorder?**

10%. It is more common in boys, and it is hereditary.

O   **Children with conduct disorders will probably develop what adult disorder?**

Antisocial personality disorder. About 40% will have some pathology as adults.

O   **What is conversion disorder?**

An internal psychological conflict that manifests itself through somatic symptoms. Voluntary motor or sensory functions are affected. Examples include weakness, imbalance, dysphagia, and changes in vision, hearing, or sensation. These symptoms are not feigned or intentionally produced. They are also not fully explained by medical conditions.

O   **Delirium is most likely to occur in patients with which types of conditions?**

Those with multiple medical problems, decreased renal function, a high WBC count, and anticholinergic, propranolol, scopolamine, or flurazepam drug use.

O   **Describe dementia.**

Disturbed cognitive function that results in impaired memory, personality, judgment, and/or language. Dementia has an insidious onset, but it may present as acute worsened mental state when patient is facing other physical or environmental stressors.

O   **Describe delirium.**

"Clouding of consciousness" that results in disorientation, decreased alertness, and impaired cognitive function. Acute onset, visual hallucinosis, and fluctuating psychomotor activity are all commonly seen. These symptoms are variable and may change within hours.

O   **Delirium versus dementia: who is more likely to die within a month of onset. Who is more likely to fully recover after onset?**

Patients with delirium are 15 to 30% more likely to die within a month of the onset. They are also more likely to fully recover from their delirium compared to patients with dementia.

O   **What are two major causes of dementia?**

Alzheimer's disease and multi-infarction.

O   **Name some over-the-counter and "street" drugs that may produce delirium or acute psychosis.**

Salicylates, antihistamines, anticholinergics, alcohols, phencyclidine, LSD, mescaline, cocaine, and amphetamines.

○   **What are eight common medical causes of depression?**

(1) Stroke, (2) viral syndromes, (3) corticosteroids, (4) Cushing's disease, (5) antihypertensive medication, (6) SLE, (7) multiple sclerosis, and (8) subcortical dementias such as Huntington's and Parkinson's diseases and HIV encephalopathy.

○   **Name some vegetative symptoms?**

Loss of appetite, lack of concentration, chronic fatigue, agitation, restlessness, inability to sleep, and weight loss.

○   **What is dysthymia?**

Dysthymia is a chronic disorder that last for more than 2 years. The severe symptoms of depression, such as delusions and hallucinations, are absent. Patients with dysthymia have some good days; they react to their environment, and they have no vegetative signs. 10% of patients with dysthymia develop major depression.

○   **What percentage of melancholic episodes are associated with hallucinations and/or delusions?**

20%.

○   **Wild and abundant dreams may result from the withdrawal of what drugs?**

Antidepressants. Other side effects of withdrawal are anxiety, akathisia, bradykinesia, mania, and malaise.

○   **What is a dystonic reaction?**

A very common side effect of neuroleptics seen in the ED. It involves muscle spasms of the tongue, face, neck, and back. Severe laryngospasm and extraocular muscle spasms may also occur. Patients may bite their tongues, leading to an inability to open the mouth, to tongue edema, or to hemorrhage.

○   **How do you treat dystonic reactions?**

Diphenhydramine (Benadryl), 25 to 50 mg IM or IV, or benztropine (Cogentin), 1 to 2 mg IV or PO. Remember that dystonias can recur acutely.

○   **What are the five Kübler-Ross stages of dying?**

1) Denial
2) Anger
3) Bargaining
4) Depression
5) Acceptance

Patients may undergo all, or only a few, of these stages.

○   **Define the following dyspraxias: ideomotor, kinesthetic, and constructional.**

Ideomotor: Patient is unable to perform simple motor tasks despite adequate understanding and sensory and motor strength.

Kinesthetic: Patient is unable to position his extremities on command despite adequate understanding and sensory and motor strength.

Constructional: Patient cannot copy simple shapes despite adequate understanding and sensory and motor strength.

O   **What psychiatric disease is the most hereditary?**

Idiopathic enuresis. If one parent has enuresis, there is a 44% chance that the child will also have the disease. If both parents have it, the likelihood increases to 77%.

O   **By what age do most children stop wetting their beds?**

Age 4. Thirty percent of 4 year olds and 10% of 6 year olds still wet their beds.

O   **What is the medical treatment for idiopathic enuresis?**

Desmopressin nose drops or imipramine. Most cases eventually resolve spontaneously.

O   **What is folie à deux?**

An induced psychotic disorder. A patient who has a close relationship with another patient begins forming the same delusions as that patient.

O   **How should a 12 year old who snorts and shouts obscenities be treated?**

With neuroleptics. Gilles de la Tourette syndrome develops in childhood with facial twitches, uncontrollable arm movements, and tics. The condition worsens with adolescence.

O   **A 24 year old male presents complaining of pleuritic pain, palpitations, dyspnea, dizziness, and tingling in his arms, legs and lips. What is your diagnosis?**

Hyperventilation syndrome. This is frequently associated with anxiety. The tingling is caused by decreased carbonate levels in the blood. This should always be a diagnosis of exclusion.

O   **A 20 year old male is brought to your office by a concerned friend. It appears the patient sleeps excessively, has been inhaling his food like there is no tomorrow, and is getting into fights at bars whenever he goes out. He also has been hypersexual, pursuing every female within a 5-mile radius. What is the diagnosis?**

This is the Kleine-Levin syndrome. It can be treated with stimulants.

O   **Hallucinogens affect what neurotransmitter?**

Serotonin.

O   **Olfactory hallucinations are associated with lesions in what areas of the brain?**

The periuncal or the inferior and medial surfaces of the temporal lobe.

O   **What is a previously healthy patient most likely suffering from when he becomes suddenly and intensely excited, goes into a delirious mania, develops catatonic features, and a high fever.**

Lethal catatonia. Such patients have a 50% death rate without treatment. Treat these patients with ECT.

O   **How is lethal catatonia differentiated from neuroleptic malignant syndrome?**

By the timing of the hyperthermia. In lethal catatonia, severe hyperthermia occurs during the excitement phase before catatonic features develop. In neuroleptic malignant syndrome, hyperthermia develops later in the course of the disease with the onset of stupor.

O   **What is the treatment for a "bad trip" on LSD?**

Constantly remind patients that their perceptions are only distortions due to the drug. This is called "talking down." Chlorpromazine can be used IM for severe or uncontrollable anxiety.

O   **Who is at a greater risk for mood disorders, men or women?**

Women (7:3).

O   **What is an extreme case of factitious disorder?**

Munchausen's syndrome. These patients may actually try to cause harm to themselves (e.g., by injecting feces into their veins) and are very accepting/seeking of invasive procedures. Munchausen by proxy is another example. In this disease, the patient seeks medical care for another, usually a child.

O   **What labs would you expect to be elevated for a patient with Neuroleptic Malignant Syndrome?**

CPK is usually elevated, which correlates with a higher risk of fatality due to myoglobinuria. Serum alkaline phosphatase and serum aminotransferases are elevated. Leukocytosis with a left shift, hyponatremia, and hypokalemia are also present. Treatment for NMS is with dopaminergic agents, muscle relaxants, discontinuation of the neuroleptics, and supportive therapy. The mortality rate is 20%.

O   **What is the difference between low potency and high potency neuroleptics and give examples of drugs in each catagory.**

Low potency neuroleptics have greater sedative, postural hypotensive, and anticholinergic effects. High potency neuroleptics have greater extrapyramidal effects.

Low potency: Chlorpromazine (Thorazine)
Medium potency: Perphenazine (Trilafon)
High potency: Haloperidol, droperidol (Inapsine), thiothixene (Navane), fluphenazine (Prolixin), trifluoperazine (Stelazine)

O   **Why is Haloperidol one of the preferred neuroleptics?**

It can be used IM in emergencies plus it has few side effects. It does, however, have a high frequency of extrapyramidal effects.

O   **What psychiatric disorder is associated with carcinoma of the pancreas?**

Depression.

O   **What is the only neuroleptic with tardive dyskinesia as a side effect?**

Clozapine. Unfortunately, patients taking clozapine can develop agranulocytosis and are at a higher risk for seizures than patients on other neuroleptics. Other side effects include hypotension, anticholinergic symptoms, and oversedation.

O   **You are considering chemical restraint. List your options.**

Benzodiazepines: 1) Lorazepam (Ativan), 1 to 2 mg IV, or 2 to 6 mg orally every 30 minutes
2) Midazolam (Versed), 2 to 4 mg IV every 30 minutes
3) Diazepam (Valium), 5 mg IV or orally every 30 minutes

Sedative hypnotics: 1) Haloperidol (Haldol), 1 to 5 mg IM/IV, titrate to clinical response
2) Droperidol (Inapsine), 1 to 2 mg IV every 30 minutes

Benzodiazepines may be given in combination with the sedative hypnotics above to both hasten and potentiate their effect. Titrate to effect and monitor appropriately.

○ **A patient has ingested a phenothiazine and arrives hypotensive. What intervention(s) may be considered?**

IV crystalloid boluses usually suffice. Severe cases best managed with norepinephrine (Levophed) or metaraminol (Aramine). These pressors stimulate α-adrenergic receptors preferentially. ß-Agonists, such as isoproterenol (Isuprel), are contraindicated due to the risks of ß-receptor-stimulated vasodilation.

○ **What happens when ethanol is combined with an anxiolytic (benzodiazepine)?**

Death can occur due to their combined respiratory depressive effects.

○ **What should be used to treat a hypertensive crisis caused by the combination of MAO inhibitors with a known toxin?**

An α- and ß-adrenergic antagonist, such as labetalol. Also consider nifedipine or nitroglycerin. If unsuccessful, consider IV phentolamine or sodium nitroprusside.

○ **Name some drugs contraindicated in a patient on MAO inhibitors.**

Meperidine (Demerol) and dextromethorphan can cause toxic reactions, such as excitation and hyperpyrexia. The effects of indirect-acting adrenergic drugs are potentiated, including ephedrine, sympathomimetic amines in cold remedies, amphetamines, cocaine, and methylphenidate (Ritalin).

○ **Name the three common MAO inhibitors (chemical and brand name).**

1) Phenelzine (Nardil).
2) Isocarboxazid (Marplan).
3) Tranylcypromine (Parnate).

○ **Obsessive compulsive disorders generally begin before what age?**

25 years old.

○ **What are some common obsessions?**

Dirt and contamination, order and symmetry, religion and philosophy, daily decisions. Unfortunately, compulsion does not relieve the anxiety of the obsession. Serotonin reuptake inhibitors and exposure therapy can be helpful.

○ **A 6 year old boy consistently wets his pants. You tell his mother to reward the child with treats and praise during dry periods. because this will help reinforce the desired behavior. What is this type of conditioning?**

Positive operant conditioning. The basic principles were defined by Pavlov.

○ **What is organic brain syndrome?**

A reversible or irreversible mental condition believed to be caused by either disease or the use of a substance that interrupts normal anatomical, physiological, or biochemical brain functions.

O   **A 20 year old female complains of sudden episodes of palpitations, diaphoresis, lightheadedness, a fear of losing control, a sense of being choked, tremors, and paresthesias. What is the diagnosis?**

Panic disorder. Panic disorders need not be linked to any events, although they are commonly associated with agoraphobia, social phobia, mitral prolapse, and late non-melancholic depression.

O   **What percentage of patients with panic disorder also suffer from major depression?**

50%. Patients who suffer from panic attacks generally have a low self-esteem as well.

O   **Which is the most common type of paraphilia?**

Pedophilia.

O   **Paresis without clonus or anesthesia to midline are examples of what conversion disorder?**

Pseudoneurologic disorder. The findings do not match the medical neuropathophysiology.

O   **PCP most commonly affects what brain system?**

The vestibulocerebellar system. This has a positive analgesic effect. However, the side effects, including dizziness, muscular incoordination, nystagmus, delirium, anxiety, irritability, and catalepsy, weigh heavily against any positive effect.

O   **How is a patient with PCP overdose treated?**

Acidify the urine with cranberry juice or NH4Cl, give a benzodiazepine, and restrain the patient.

O   **Cite an example for each of the following perceptual disturbances: illusion, complete auditory hallucination, functional hallucination, and extracampine hallucination.**

Illusion: A kitten is perceived as a dragon. (The patient misinterprets reality.)

Complete auditory hallucination: The patient claims to hear people talking when no one is around. (Clear voices are reportedly heard. They are perceived as being external to the patient.)

Functional hallucination: The patient hears voices only when cars honk their horns. (Hallucinations occur only after sensory stimulus in the same category as the hallucination.)

Extracampine hallucination: The patient can see people waving from the top of the Eiffel Tower, even though she is in Chicago. (Hallucinations are external to the patient's normal range of senses.)

O   **What is the most common phobia in men?**

Social phobia.

O   **What is the most common specific phobia in children?**

Animal phobia.

O   **At what age will a child understand concrete operations as defined by Piaget?**

6 to 12 years. By this age, a child is able to distinguish that a line of 5 pennies all touching is equal to those same 5 pennies spread out into a longer line.

❍ **Can a person acquire posttraumatic stress disorder (PTSD) if they did not actually witness a disturbing event?**

Yes. According to the DSM-IV, one can experience PTSD if an event, such as a violent personal assault, a serious accident, or the serious injury of a close friend or family member, is learned of indirectly. PTSD can also occur after a person hears of a life-threatening disease affecting a friend or family member.

❍ **A 28 year old female who was raped 6 months ago has been psychologically sound thus far. She now suddenly develops recurrent flashbacks of the rape, nightmares, intense fear, avoidance of all men, a diminished memory of the rape, and an exaggerated startle response. Is this woman experiencing PTSD?**

Yes. This is delayed onset PTSD. The onset of symptoms occurs at least 6 months after the provoking event.

❍ **What are the five criteria for brief reactive psychosis?**

1) Precipitating stressful event.
2) Rapid onset of the psychosis.
3) Affective lability and mood intensity.
4) Symptoms that match the stressful event.
5) Resolution of symptoms once the stressor is removed, generally within 2 weeks.

❍ **What brain lesions sites are most commonly associated with psychosis?**

The temporolimbic system, caudate nucleus, and frontal lobes.

❍ **List some life-threatening causes of acute psychosis.**

WHHHIMP

Wernicke's encephalopathy.
Hypoxia.
Hypoglycemia.
Hypertensive encephalopathy.
Intracerebral hemorrhage.
Meningitis/encephalitis.
Poisoning.

❍ **What signs and symptoms suggest an organic source for psychosis.**

Acute onset, disorientation, visual or tactile hallucinations, age under 10 or over 60, and any evidence suggesting overdose or acute ingestion, such as abnormal vital signs, pupil size and reactivity, or nystagmus.

❍ **When are women at the greatest risk for psychiatric illness?**

The first few weeks post partum. A psychiatric illness most often occurs in patients who are primiparous, have poor social support, or have a history of depression.

❍ **When does post partum psychosis begin?**

Within a week to 10 days following childbirth. A second, smaller peak occurs 5 to 7 months later, correlating with the first menses post partum. The risk of psychosis is lowest during pregnancy.

❍   **What is the difference between schizophrenia and schizophreniform disorder?**

Schizophreniform disorder implies the same signs and symptoms as schizophrenia, yet these symptoms have been present for less than 6 months. The impaired functioning in schizophreniform disorder is not consistent. Schizophreniform disorder is generally a provisional diagnosis with schizophrenia following.

❍   **What are some characteristics of schizophrenia?**

Delusional disorder, hallucinations (usually auditory), disorganized thinking, loosening of associations, disheveled appearance, and the inability to realize thoughts and behavior are abnormal.

❍   **What are the five first rank symptoms of Schneider?**

1) Experiences of influence.
2) Thought broadcasting.
3) Experiences of alienation.
4) Complete auditory hallucinations.
5) Delusional perceptions.

First-rank symptoms occur in 60 to 75% of schizophrenics. They also develop in patients with affective disorder, more commonly during manic stages.

❍   **What are the five criteria for diagnosing schizophrenia?**

1) Psychosis.
2) Emotional blunting.
3) Abscence of affective features or episodes.
4) Clear consciousness.
5) Absence of coarse brain disease, systemic illness, and drug abuse.

❍   **What percentage of patients with schizophrenia become chronically ill?**

60 to 80%. Males are at a greater risk for chronic illness.

❍   **The onset of schizophrenia generally occurs by what age?**

Eighty percent of schizophrenics develop the disease before their early twenties. The disease is very rare after 40.

❍   **What are five causes of schizophrenia?**

1) Viral infection in the CNS.
2) Problem during pregnancy that affects the neuronal development.
3) Head injury.
4) Seizure disorder.
5) Street drugs.

❍   **A patient who is unable to express his anger, has few close friends, is indifferent to praise from others, is absent-minded, and is emotionally cold and aloof probably has which kind of personality disorder?**

Schizoidia.

O **Are first degree relatives of schizophrenics more likely to have schizoidia or schizophrenia?**

Schizoidia (3:1).

O **When is the average onset of separation anxiety?**

Age 9. Children with separation anxiety fear leaving home, going to sleep, being alone, going to school, and losing their parents. 75% develop somatic complaints in order to avoid attending school.

O **Name eight drugs that decrease sexual desire.**

(1) Antidepressants, (2) antihypertensives, (3) anticonvulsants, (4) neuroleptics, (5) digitalis, (6) cimetidine, (7) clofibrate, and (8) high doses or chronic ingestion of alcohol or street drugs.

O **A child reared by a homosexual couple will most likely have what sexual orientation?**

Heterosexual.

O **How does the insomnia of patients with melancholia differ from that of patients with dysthymia?**

Patients with melancholia have a difficulty staying asleep; this is often associated with early morning wakefulness. Patients with dysthymia have trouble falling asleep and have a tendency to oversleep.

O **Which populations have the greatest incidence of insomnia?**

Women and the elderly. Insomnia can involve trouble falling asleep or trouble staying asleep. It is generally initiated by a stressor in the patient's life.

O **In which stage of sleep do we spend the most time?**

Stage 2 accounts for 50% of our sleep. This stage is characterized by sleep spindles and K complexes on EEG. REM accounts for only 25% of our sleep.

O **Is somnambulism more common in children or adults?**

15 to 30% of children sleepwalk, while only 1% of adults do. Sleepwalking begins around age 4 and generally resolves by age 15.

O **Sleepwalking and pavor nocturnus (night terrors) are disturbances of which stage in sleep?**

Stage 4. A stage 4 sleep depressant, such as a long-acting benzodiazapine, is effective in curbing this behavior.

O **Narcolepsy is a disorder of which sleep cycle?**

REM. Attacks of sleep, dreams, and paralysis last anywhere from 10 minutes to 1 hour. Amphetamines and planned naps throughout the day can help.

O **A 30 year old female complains of calf pain, a headache, shooting pain when flexing her right wrist, random epigastric pain, bloating, and irregular menses, all of which cannot be explained after medical examination. What is the diagnosis?**

Somatization disorder, many unexplained medical symptoms involving multiple systems. In order to diagnose a patient with somatization disorder, one must have 4 or more unexplained pain symptoms.

Symptoms generally begin in childhood and are fully developed by age 30. This is more common in women than men.

❍   **Who is more successful at suicide, men or women?**

Males (3:1). However, women attempt suicide 3 times as often as men.

❍   **T/F: Fantasies frequently precede suicidal acts.**

True.

❍   **Major depression and bipolar affective disorder account for what percentage of suicides?**

50%. Another 25% are due to substance abuse, and another 10% are attributed to schizophrenia.

❍   **What percentage of patients with melancholia attempt suicide?**

15%.

❍   **Give examples of the following thought disorders : perseveration, non-sequiturs, derailment, tangential speech, neologism, private word usage, and verbigeration.**

Perseveration: "I've been wondering if the mechanical mechanisms of this machine are mechanically sound. Mechanically speaking, I must understand the mechanisms." (A repetition of certain words or phrases is found in the natural flow of speech.)

Non-sequiturs: Q: "Are you nervous about the upcoming boards?" A: "Why no, the king of France is an excellent king." (The patient's answers are unrelated to the questions asked.)

Derailment: "I first became interested in the study of medicine after mom bought me a toy ambulance. Toys can be very dangerous, especially if they are very small and can be swallowed. I've been having difficulty swallowing lately." (The patient suddenly switches lines of thought, though the second follows the first.)

Tangential speech: A: "Those are nice clothes you're wearing today." B: "Of course I'm wearing clothes today." A: "I mean, I like the outfit you have on." B: "I think everyone should wear clothes, except on Friday, because Friday is casual day at my office." (Conversations are on the right subject matter; however, the responses are inappropriate to the previous questions or comments.)

Neologism: "I'm going to explaphrase (explain by paraphrasing) the meaning of agnonoctaudiophobia (things that go bump in the night)." (Neologisms are meaningless combinations of 2 or more words to invent a new word.)

Private word usage: "I can't believe the loquacious way he is formicating those tripods." (Words and or phrases used in unique ways.)

Verbigeration: "I have been studying, have been studying, have been studying, for hours for hours hours hours." (The patient repeats words, especially at the end of thoughts, thoughts, thoughts, thoughts.)

❍   **What psychiatric problems are associated with violence?**

Acute schizophrenia, paranoid ideation, catatonic excitation, mania, borderline and antisocial personality disorders, delusional depression, posttraumatic stress disorder, and decompensating obsessive/compulsive disorder.

❍   **What are the prodromes of violent behavior?**

Anxiety, defensiveness, volatility, and physical aggression.

○ **Matching:**

1) Hypomania	a) 1 or more hypomanias plus 1 or more major depressive symptoms
2) Melancholia	b) A mild manic episode
3) Bipolar II	c) Deep depression and vegetative characteristics
4) Unipolar mania	d) Manic episodes only
5) Cyclothymia	e) Many mild episodes of hypomania and depression

Answers: (1) b, (2) c, (3) a, (4) d, and (5) e.

○ **A 27 year old male arrives somnolent with vitals of P: 130, R: 26, BP: 170/80, and T: 105°F. You note diffuse muscular rigidity and intermittent focal muscle twitching and/or jerking that lasts for 1 to 2 seconds. As you "work him up", your nurse returns from the waiting area with news from the family that the patient has had a progressive decline of mental status for the last 2 days, after seeing his psychiatrist. The patient has had a history of psychosis for almost a year. What process should be included in your differential diagnosis at this time?**

Neuroleptic malignant syndrome (NMS).

○ **A patient is brought in because she believes butterflies are landing all around her. The butterflies talk to her and tell her to love everyone. She denies suicidal ideation and any desire to harm herself or others. She has no record of harming people in the past. Can this person be institutionalized against her will?**

No. Unless the patient is a danger to herself or others, she cannot be confined to an institution despite questionable mental status.

OBSTETRICS AND GYNECOLOGY PEARLS

○ **Define the normal menstrual cycle?**

The normal menstrual cycle is 28 days with a flow lasting 2-7 days. The variation in cycle length is set at 21-34 days.

○ **In a normal menstrual cycle, when does ovulation typically occur?**

Ovulation in a 28 day cycle occurs on on day 14. The luteal phase of the cycle is normally 14 days long. The estrogenic (proliferative) phase of the cycle can be variable.

○ **Name the hormones, and their source, that are involved in maintaining a normal menstrual cycle?**

From the ovary: Estrogen and progesterone.
From the pituitary: Follicle stimulating hormone (FSH) and luteinizing hormone (LH). From the hypothalamus: Gonadotropin releasing hormone (GnRH)
(Prolactin and Thyroid Stimulating Hormone are also vital in maintaining a normal menstrual cycle).

○ **Describe the effect of estrogen on the endometrium?**

Estrogen causes growth of the endometrium. The endometrial glands lengthen and the glandular epithelium becomes pseudostratified. Mitotic activity is present in both the glands and the stroma.

○ **When does implantation of the fertilized ovum typically occur?**

At approximately postovulatory day 9 (day 23).

○ **What is the life-span of a normal corpus luteum in the absence of pregnancy?**

Approximately 14 days

○ **In a woman of reproductive age, what is the first step in the evaluation of abnormal uterine bleeding following the history and physical examination?**

A pregnancy test

○ **What is the action of oxytocin?**

It stimulates uterine contractions during labor and elicits milk ejection by myoepithelial cells of the mammary ducts.

○ **What is the function of FSH?**

It stimulates maturation of the graafian follicle and its production of estradiol.

○   **What is the function of LH?**

It causes follicular rupture, ovulation, and establishment of the corpus luteum.

○   **The ovarian luteal phase corresponds to what phase of the uterus?**

The secretory phase. The luteal phase begins after ovulation. At this time, the expelled follicle is called the corpus luteum. The corpus luteum secretes estradiol and progesterone which cause secretory ducts to develop in the endometrial lining.

○   **What does a biphasic curve on a basal body temperature (BBT) chart of a 25 year old woman indicate?**

Normal ovulation and the effect of progesterone. A monophasic BBT curve indicates an anovulatory cycle. A temperature that remained elevated following a normal biphasic curve would indicate pregnancy.

○   **What is the most accurate test of ovulation?**

Endometrial biopsy. This will show if there is a secretory phase, thereby indicating ovulation.

○   **What is the cause of mid-cycle spotting or light bleeding?**

The decline in estrogen that occurs immediately prior to the LH surge

○   **Decline in which hormone heralds the onset of menses?**

Normal menses occurs because of progesterone withdrawal

○   **What levels of FSH and LH would you expect in a 63 year old woman who is not on estrogen replacement therapy?**

High levels of both FSH and LH. The ovarian response to FSH and LH is decreased in menopause. Consequently, there is less estrogen and progesterone being produced. Hence, no negative feedback to inhibit the rising FSH and LH.

○   **What is the function of prolactin?**

It initiates and sustains lactation by the breast glands and it may influence synthesis and release of progesterone by the ovary and testosterone by the testis.

○   **What is the main physiological stimulus for prolactin release?**

Suckling of the breast.

○   **What is the most common presenting symptom of a prolactinoma in a woman?**

Secondary amenorrhea

○   **Match the words with their definitions….**

1) Menorrhagia	a) Bleeding between menstrual periods
2) Metrorrhagia	b) Excessive amount of vaginal bleeding or duration of bleeding
3) Menometrorrhagia	c) Excessive amount of blood at irregular frequencies
4) Polymenorrhea	d) Menstrual periods > 35 days apart
5) Oligomenorrhea	e) Menstrual periods < 21 days apart

Answers: (1) b (2) a (3) c (4) e (5) d

○ **What is secondary amenorrhea?**

No menstruation for 6 months or more in a women who previously had regular menses.

○ **What is the most common cause of secondary amenorrhea?**

Pregnancy. The second most common cause is hypothalamic hypogonadism which can be due to weight loss, anorexia nervosa, stress, excessive exercise, or hypothalamic disease.

○ **What are some causes of premature menopause?**

Smoking, radiation, chemotherapy, and anything else that limits the ovarian blood supply.

○ **A 26 year old with secondary amenorrhea and an essentially normal workup is given an IM injection of 100 mg of progesterone and responds with a normal menstrual period. What does this tell you?**

She has a functional endometrium and a normal production of estrogen. Patients producing less than 40 pg/mL of estrogen will not bleed. This test is called the progesterone challenge.

○ **What are the 2 major differential diagnoses in the above patient?**

Premature ovarian failure and hypothalamic dysfunction. Premature ovarian failure can be diagnosed if the serum LH level is greater than 25 mIU/mL; otherwise, the diagnosis is most likely hypothalamic dysfunction.

○ **A patient with secondary amenorrhea fails the progesterone challenge and has a high FSH level. What is the problem?**

Gonadal failure. A low FSH level would be more indicative of hypothalamic dysfunction.

○ **What is the most common cause of dysfunctional uterine bleeding in children?**

Infection. In teenagers, it is most commonly due to anovulation.

○ **What is the most frequent gynecologic disease of children?**

Vulvovaginitis, the cause of which is poor perineal hygiene.

○ **List the differential diagnosis of persistent vaginal bleeding in a preadolescent female.**

Neoplasia.
Precocious puberty.
Ureteral prolapse.
Trauma.
Sexual assault.
Vulvovaginitis.
Exposure to exogenous estrogen.
Shigella infection.
Group A & Beta hemolytic streptococcal infection.
Foreign body in vagina

○ **Without therapy, approximately 50% of females with precocious puberty will not reach what height?**

5 feet

○   **What blood tests would be appropriate in the evaluation of a female child with precocious puberty?**

Serum levels of FSH, LH, prolactin, TSH, estradiol, testosterone, dehydroepiandrosterone sulfate (DHEAS) and HCG

○   **Breast hyperplasia is a normal physiologic phenomenon in the neonatal period and may persist for how many months?**

Up to six months of age

○   **Retrospective historical data derived from adults imply that what percent of women are believed to have been sexually abused as children?**

15-25%. 80% of all cases of sexual abuse of children involve a family member.

○   **What is the most common cause of vaginal bleeding in childhood?**

A foreign body. Patients will have a bloody, foul smelling discharge.

○   **What is the median age for menopause?**

51.

○   **A 37 year old woman, G2 P2 presents with a history of lengthening menses and acquired dysmenorrhea. This problem had been subtly going on for two years and now is a quality of life issue. Examination reveals a top normal size globular shaped uterus. What is the most likely diagnosis?**

Adenomyosis

○   **What is the most common cause of postmenopausal bleeding?**

Atrophic endometrium and/or atrophic vaginitis

○   **In women of reproductive age, what is the most common cause of estrogen excess bleeding?**

Chronic anovulation associated with polycystic ovaries

○   **How does progesterone work at the cellular level to control dysfunctional uterine bleeding when prescribed in pharmacologic doses?**

Progestins are powerful anti-estrogens. They stimulate 17b hydroxysteroid dehydrogenase and sulfotransferase activity. This results in conversion of estradiol to estrone sulfate which is rapidly excreted in the urine. Progestins also inhibit augmentation of estrogen receptors. Additionally progestins suppress estrogen mediated transcription of oncogenes.

○   **A 27 year old woman presents with secondary amenorrhea for 6 months. Appropriate initial evaluation should include?**

Pelvic examination, PAP smear, pregnancy test, prolactin and progestin challenge, plus a TSM level.

○ **What are the common changes associated with estrogen depletion?**

Menstrual cycle changes, cardiovascular disease, osteoporosis, genitourinary atrophy, vasomotor and psychological symptoms

○ **Which hormones decline as a result of menopause?**

Estrogen and androstenedione.

○ **What happens to progesterone production in menopause?**

Progesterone is no longer produced.

○ **What hormone is secreted more by the postmenopausal ovary than the premenopausal ovary?**

Testosterone. Prior to menopause, the ovary contributes 25% of circulating testosterone, and in menopause the ovary contributes 40% of circulating testosterone.

○ **What is the cause of mild hirsutism in menopause?**

Increased free androgen to estrogen ratio as a result of decreased SHBG and estrogen.

○ **What is the leading cause of death for women?**

Heart disease, followed by malignancies, cerebrovascular disease, and motor vehicle accidents.

○ **How many deaths are attributed to cardiovascular disease in women over 50?**

Greater than 50%.

○ **How much does the risk of coronary heart disease increase after menopause?**

It doubles.

○ **What risk factors are associated with bone loss and osteoporosis?**

White and Asian race, thin women, sedentary lifestyle, smoking, coexisting endocrine disease, and age of menopause.

○ **How does estrogen therapy help maintain bone mass?**

Estrogen has a direct effect on osteoblasts, improves intestinal absorption of calcium, and decreases renal excretion of calcium.

○ **Why does vaginitis increase during the postmenopausal years?**

Due to estrogen deficiency, the vaginal pH increases from 3.5-4.5 to 6.0-8.0, predisposing to colonization of bacterial pathogens.

○ **What is the origin of breakthrough bleeding in continuous hormone replacement therapy?**

Progestational dominance resulting in an atrophic endometrium.

○ **What effect does estrogen therapy have on colorectal cancer?**

It significantly decreases the risk of colorectal cancer.

O   **What are contraindications to estrogen therapy?**

Estrogen sensitive cancers, chronically impaired liver function, undiagnosed genital bleeding, acute vascular thrombosis, neurophthalmologic vascular disease, and known or suspected pregnancy.

O   **What effect does estrogen have on Alzheimer's disease?**

Alzheimer's disease is less frequent among HRT users and cognitive function in affected individuals is improved

O   **What predisposes a woman to yeast infections?**

Diabetes, oral contraceptives, and antibiotics.

O   **What is the most common cause of vaginitis?**

Candida albicans.

O   **A patient presents with a 2 day history of vaginal itching and burning. On examination, you note a thin, yellowish green, bubbly discharge and petechiae on the cervix (also known as a "strawberry cervix"). What test do you perform, and what do you expect to find?**

Mix the discharge with saline and view under a microscope. If you see *Trichomonas vaginalis* (mobile and pear-shaped protozoa with flagella), then the patient and her partner should be treated with Metronidazole (Flagyl).

O   **A 20 year old sexually active female presents to your office complaining of a heavy thin discharge with an unpleasant odor. Adding 10% KOH to the discharge produces a fishy odor. What would you expect to see on microscopic examination?**

"Clue cells," which are epithelial cells with bacilli attached to their surfaces. This patient has *Gardnerella* vaginitis. The patient should be treated with Metronidazole (Flagyl).

O   **What is the number one cause of urinary tract infections?**

E. coli. Other causative agents are also gram-negative.

O   **What is the normal pH of the vagina?**

3.8 to 4.4. (A vaginal pH greater than 4.9 indicates a bacterial or protozoal infection.)

O   **What causes condylomata acuminata (venereal warts)?**

Human papilloma virus types 6 and 11.

O   **What subtypes of HPV are associated with cervical cancer?**

HPV types 16, 18, and 31 are risk factors for cervical dysplasia, which can lead to cervical cancer. Multiple sexual partners and early onset of sexual activity are risk factors for cervical cancer, due to HPV infection.

O   **When should you avoid treating a woman with Flagyl?**

If she is in her first trimester, Metronidazole may have teratogenic effects. Clotrimazole (Gyne-Lotrimin) may be used instead. Side effects of Flagyl include nausea, vomiting, and metallic tastes. It acts similarly to disulfiram (Antabuse) and therefore should not be taken with alcohol.

○ **A 30 year old female complains of a painful sore on her vulva that resembled a pimple at first. On examination, you find an ulcer with vague borders and a gray base. Probable diagnosis?**

Gram's stain, culture, and biopsy (used in combination because of the high false-negative rates) should show that *Haemophilus ducreyi* has caused a chancroid. Treatment is erythromycin or ceftriaxone.

○ **Condylomata acuminata frequently occurs in combination with what other STD?**

Trichomonas vaginitis.

○ **What is the most common cause of septic arthritis in young adults?**

Disseminated gonococcal infection.

○ **What is the treatment for gonorrhea?**

Ceftriaxone and doxycycline. The latter is given because half of the patients infected with gonorrhea are simultaneously infected with chlamydia.

○ **What is the predominant organism in a healthy female's vaginal discharge?**

Lactobacilli (95%).

○ **A 34 year old female presents with a maculopapular rash on her palms and soles, states that she had a strange vaginal lesion about a month and a half ago. She complains of headaches and general weakness. On examination, you find she has multiple condyloma lata and lymphadenopathy. What is the diagnosis?**

Secondary syphilis. This develops 6 to 9 weeks after the syphilitic chancre, which will have resolved by this time. If it goes untreated, tertiary syphilis will develop. This can affect all the tissues in the body, including the CNS and the heart. Treatment is with penicillin G.

○ **Is the Stein-Leventhal syndrome a unilateral or bilateral phenomenon?**

Bilateral. Both ovaries are cystic and enlarged with a thickened and fibrosed tunica. Patients are often infertile, obese, and hirsute.

○ **What are the risk factors for pelvic inflammatory disease?**

1) age less than 20
2) multiple sexual partners
3) nulliparity
4) previous history of pelvic inflammatory disease

○ **T/F: A woman with pelvic inflammatory disease (PID) is likely to have an exacerbation of symptoms when she menstruates.**

True. The breakdown of the cervical mucus antibacterial barrier allows bacteria to ascend from the lower tract to the upper tract. Pelvic examination, intercourse, and exercise can all exacerbate symptoms.

○ **What 2 organisms cause most cases of PID?**

Neisseria gonorrhoeae and *Chlamydia trachomatis.*

○   **Which patients with PID should be admitted?**

Admit patients who are pregnant, have a temperature > 38°C (100.4°F), are nauseated or vomiting (which prohibits oral antibiotics), have pyosalpinx or tubo-ovarian abscess peritoneal signs, have an IUD, show no response to oral antibiotics, or for whom diagnosis is uncertain.

○   **What are the criteria for diagnosis of PID?**

All of the following must be present: (1) adnexal tenderness, (2) cervical and uterine tenderness, and (3) abdominal tenderness. In addition, one of the following must be present: (1) temperature > 38°C, (2) endocervix Gram's stain positive for gram-negative intracellular diplococci, (3) leukocytosis > 10,000/mm3, (4) inflammatory mass on ultrasound or pelvic examination, or (5) WBCs and bacteria in the peritoneal fluid.

○   **What percent of patients with pelvic inflammatory disease become infertile?**

10%.

○   **When does an ectopic pregnancy most commonly present?**

6 to 8 weeks into the pregnancy. Patients usually present with amenorrhea and sharp, generally unilateral abdominal or pelvic pain. Rupture of an ampullary ectopic typically occurs at 8 to 12 weeks, allowing adequate time for early diagnosis and treatment prior to rupture in most cases. Isthmic ectopics may rupture earlier at 6 to 8 weeks.

○   **What percentage of pregnancies are ectopic?**

1.5%. Ectopic pregnancies are the leading cause of death in the first trimester.

○   **What is the risk of a repeat ectopic pregnancy?**

10 to 15%.

○   **What is the most common site of implantation in an ectopic pregnancy?**

The ampulla of the fallopian tube (95%). Less common are ectopics in the abdomen, uterine cornua, cervix, and ovary

○   **What are the risk factors for an ectopic pregnancy?**

Prior scarring of the fallopian tubes from infection (i.e., pelvic inflammatory disease or salpingitis), IUDs, a previous ectopic pregnancy, tubal ligation, STD's, changes in circulating levels of hormones, use of fertility medications, and previous abdominal surgery.

○   **How often is an adnexal mass found in women with an ectopic pregnancy?**

Fifty percent of women with an ectopic pregnancy have an adnexal mass on exam.

○   **How do hCG levels differ in women with ectopic pregnancies versus intrauterine pregnancy?**

In 85% of women with ectopic pregnancy, the hCG level is lower than expected.

❍   **Which is <u>most common</u> sign of an ectopic pregnancy by transvaginal ultrasound: adnexal mass or absence of an intrauterine pregnancy?**

The absence of an intrauterine pregnancy at an hCG level >2,000mIU/ml is highly predictive of an ectopic pregnancy. An adnexal mass or gestational sac in the adnexal is less reliable finding and is not always seen in early ectopic pregnancies.

❍   **Does the presence of a thick endometrial stripe on ultrasound indicate an intrauterine pregnancy?**

The endometrium can be thickened due to the hormonal stimulation associated with either an ectopic or intrauterine pregnancy, so this is not a consistent sign of a normal pregnancy

❍   **Does the presence of a gestational sac always rule out an ectopic?**

Up to 15% of women with an ectopic pregnancy can have a "pseudosac" or fluid area (representing blood and mucus) within the cavity. Therefore, it is critical with women at high risk for an ectopic pregnancy to confirm an intrauterine pregnancy with a follow-up ultrasound. This ultrasound will identify the yolk sac ("double ring sign") or fetal pole within the gestational sac.

❍   **What are the indications for laparotomy for treatment of ectopic pregnancy?**

Common indications for laparotomy include an unstable patient, large hemoperitoneum, cornual pregnancy, lack of appropriate surgical tools for laparoscopy. Some authors would also include a large ectopic (>6 cm) and fetal heart tones in the adnexa as indications for laparotomy.

❍   **Who is eligible for methotrexate treatment of an ectopic pregnancy?**

Patients who are hemodynamically stable with unruptured gestations <4 cm in diameter by ultrasound.

❍   **What is the mode of action of methotrexate?**

Methotrexate is a folic acid antagonist.

❍   **What criteria are used for assuring the success of methotrexate?**

With a single does therapy, the hCG levels should fall by 15% between days 4 and 7 after therapy and continue to fall weekly until undetectable.

❍   **Why is the Rh status of a pregnant patient important?**

If the mother is Rh negative, and the fetus is Rh positive, there is a risk of developing Rh isoimmunization and fetal anemia, hydrops, and fetal loss can result. Rh immunoglobulin should be given to all Rh negative patients. The standard dose of Rho GAM is 300 mg.

❍   **Should Rh negative women with ectopic pregnancies be given Rhogam?**

Most authors recommend administration of mini-rhogam (50 micrograms) with any failed pregnancy up to 12 weeks (with full dose Rhogam after 12 weeks)

❍   **How much blood does a standard size pad absorb?**

20 to 30 mL. This is useful to know when trying to estimate blood loss.

❍   **For a gestational sac to be visible on ultrasound, what must the ß-hCG level be?**

At least 6500 mIU/mL for a transabdominal ultrasound, and 2000 mIU/mL for a transvaginal ultrasound.

○   **When can an intrauterine gestational sac be identified by an abdominal ultrasound?**

In the fifth week. A fetal pole can be identified in the sixth week, and an embryonic mass with cardiac motion in the seventh.

○   **What is the most common non-gynecologic condition presenting with lower abdominal pain?**

Appendicitis.

○   **Is appendicitis more common during pregnancy?**

No (1/850). However, the outcome is worse. Prompt diagnosis is important because the incidence of perforation increases from 10% in the first trimester to 40% in the third.

○   **How is the appendix displaced during pregnancy?**

Superiorly and laterally. Diagnosis of appendicitis in pregnant patients may be further complicated by the fact that a normal pregnancy can itself cause an increased WBC. The WBC count usually does not increase beyond the normal value of 12,000 to 15,000. In a pregnant patient, pyuria with no bacteria suggests appendicitis. Pregnant patients may lack GI distress, and fever may be absent or low-grade.

○   **A patient presents with pain in her eyes, canker sores in her mouth, and sores and scars in her genital area. What is the diagnosis?**

Behcet's disease. This is a rare disease involving ocular inflammation, oral apthous ulcers, and destructive genital ulcers (generally on the vulva). No cure is known, but remission may occur with high estrogen levels.

○   **What is Sheehan's syndrome?**

Anterior pituitary necrosis following post partum hemorrhage and hypotension. It results in amenorrhea, decreased breast size, and decreased pubic hair.

○   **What condition usually causes female pseudohermaphroditism?**

Congenital adrenal hyperplasia. The defective adrenals cannot produce normal amounts of cortisol. These patients have normal XX chromosomes, but an excess of endogenous adrenal steroids has virilizing effects.

○   **What causes toxic shock syndrome (TSS)?**

An exotoxin composed of certain strains of *Staphylococcus aureus*. Other organisms that cause toxic shock syndrome are group A streptococci, *Pseudomonas aeruginosa*, and *Streptococcus pneumoniae*. Tampons, IUDs, septic abortions, sponges, soft tissue abscesses, osteomyelitis, nasal packing, and post partum infections can all house these organisms.

○   **What dermatological changes occur with TSS?**

Initially, the patient will have a blanching erythematous rash that lasts for 3 days. 10 days after the start of the infection there will be a full thickness desquamation of the palms and soles.

○   **What criteria are necessary for the diagnosis of TSS?**

All of the following must be present: T > 38.9°C (102°F), rash, systolic BP < 90 with orthostasis, involvement of 3 organ systems (GI, renal, musculoskeletal, mucosal, hepatic, hematologic, or CNS), and negative serologic tests for diseases such as RMSF, hepatitis B, measles, leptospirosis, and VDRL.

○ **How should a patient with TSS be treated?**

Fluids, pressure support, fresh frozen plasma or transfusions, vaginal irrigation with iodine or saline, and antistaphylococcal penicillin or cephalosporin with anti-ß-lactamase activity (nafcillin or oxacillin). Rifampin should be considered to eliminate the carrier state.

○ **What is the most common complication of ovarian cysts?**

Torsion of the ovary. Torsion is more common in small to medium sized cysts and tumors. Emergency surgery is required.

○ **What are the indications for performing a dilation and curettage?**

1) removal of endometrial polyp or hydatid mole
2) termination of pregnancy/incomplete abortion
3) removal of retained placental tissue
4) relief of profuse uterine hemorrhage

○ **What major complication is associated with the performance of a dilation and curettage?**

Perforation of the uterus.

○ **What are the most common indications for hysterectomy?**

According to a 1987 report, the most common indications were leiomyomata (26.8%), prolapse (20.8%), endometriosis (14.7%), cancer (10.7%), and endometrial hyperplasia (6.2%). The remaining 20.7% were done for abnormal bleeding, diseases of the parametrium and pelvic peritoneum, infections and other diseases of the cervix, tubes, and ovaries, obstetrical castastrophe, and other benign neoplasms.

○ **What is the correct terminology regarding hysterectomies (i.e. total, subtotal, vaginal and abdominal?**

The word "hysterectomy" may be modified by the words "total" or "subtotal" to denote whether the cervix is removed or retained, and by "vaginal" or "abdominal" to specify the route of removal. More recently, the nomenclature has been modified to include "laparoscopic hysterectomy" and "laparoscopic-assisted vaginal hysterectomy".

○ **What is the most frequent complication of hysterectomy?**

Infection. The most common organisms are those found in normal vaginal flora. Because the vagina is difficult to cleanse, most experts recommend antibiotic prophylaxis for all patients undergoing vaginal hysterectomy.

○ **What percentage of the female population has endometriosis?**

More than 15%. 7% of these women have it during their reproductive years.

○ **What is the most common site of endometriosis?**

The ovaries (60%).

○ **What is the drug of choice for treating endometriosis?**

Danazol.

O   **What is thought to be the cause of endometriosis?**

Retrograde menstruation.

O   **What are chocolate cysts?**

Endometriomas (cystic forms of endometriosis on the ovary).

O   **What is a Nabothian cyst?**

A mucous inclusion cyst of the cervix (usually asymptomatic and harmless).

O   **How long after the removal of Norplant capsules must patients wait to become pregnant?**

Ovulation usually occurs within 3 months.

O   **What chemical changes may predispose patients taking oral contraceptives to weight gain?**

Increases in low-density lipoproteins, decreases in high-density lipoproteins, and sodium retention.

O   **At what level of smoking does the risk of the pill exceed the risks of having a baby for a 35-year-old?**

35 cigarettes per day. Women who smoke more than 15 cigarettes per day and are over age 35 should not use pills.

O   **How much is menstrual blood flow decreased by OCP use?**

By 60% or more. This results in less iron deficiency anemia.

O   **By how much is the incidence of functional cysts reduced by OCP use?**

80-90%. Oral contraceptives suppress FSH and LH ovarian stimulation.

O   **For women using oral contraceptives for 4 years or less, what is their reduction in risk of ovarian cancer?**

30%. For 12 or more years of use the risk is decreased by 80%.

O   **For women using oral contraceptives for at least 2 years, what is the reduction in risk of endometrial cancer?**

40%. This increases to 60% for 4 or more years of use.

O   **What is the incidence of venous thrombosis in oral contraceptive users?**

10-20/100,000 users.

O   **How effective is breast feeding alone in preventing pregnancy?**

98% for the first 6 months in women who have not resumed their menses.

O   **Are women more likely to gain or lose weight with oral contraceptive use?**

Both are equally likely. Rarely do pills cause a gain of 10-20 pounds or more.

O   **How does DepoProvera work?**

By suppressing FSH and LH levels and eliminating the LH surge. This inhibits ovulation,

O   **What is the effect of progestin on the uterus?**

It results in a shallow atrophic endometrium and a thick cervical mucus. These both result in decreased sperm transport.

O   **What is the delay in return to fertility after DepoProvera?**

6 months to 1 year

O   **What is the risk of ectopic pregnancy in women with an IUD in place?**
5%. Progestasert users have a 6-10 fold increase in ectopic rates compared with copper IUD users

O   **How long after exposure can emergency oral contraceptives be given?**

Up to 72 hours. It is most effective if initiated in 12-24 hours. Emergency contraception provides a 75% reduction in the risk of pregnancy. Patients should have a negative pregnancy test prior to treatment.

O   **What is the rationale for multiphasic oral contraceptives?**

A lower total dose of steroid is administered

O   **What is the association between oral contraceptives and gallbladder disease?**

They accelerate the development of symptoms without increasing the overall incidence of cholelithiasis.

O   **What effect does oral contraceptive use have on the risk of developing cervical cancer?**

Oral contraceptive users as a group are at higher risk for cervical neoplasia. This increased risk may be secondary to sexual habits rather than the pill itself.

O   **A 21 year old female requests counseling because she was taking birth control pills without knowing she was pregnant. Should she abort the pregnancy?**

No. Recent studies have concluded that exposure to progestins and estrogens (as in birth control pills) are not associated with any specific structural abnormalities in the exposed offspring. Earlier studies had revealed an increased incidence of a pattern of malformations called the VACTERR (Vertebral, Anal, Cardiac, Tracheo-Esophageal, Renal, Radial) association, but these were retrospective studies that were later found to be inaccurate.

O   **What are the differences between spontaneous, threatened, incomplete, complete, and missed abortions?**

Spontaneous abortion is loss of the fetus before the 20th week of gestation.

Threatened abortion is uterine cramping or bleeding in the first 20 weeks of gestation without the passage of products of conception or cervical dilatation.

Incomplete abortions are partial abortions in which part of the products of conception are aborted and part remain within the uterus. The cervix is dilated on examination, and dilation and curettage is necessary to remove the remainder of tissue.

Complete abortion is when all the products of conception have been passed, the cervix is closed and the uterus is firm and non tender.

Missed abortion is defined as no uterine growth, no cervical dilation, no passage of fetal tissue, and minimal cramping or bleeding. Diagnosis is made by the absence of fetal heart tones and an empty sac on ultrasound.

○   **What percentage of pregnancies result in spontaneous abortions?**

20 to 25%.

○   **What is the most common cause of spontaneous abortions?**

Chromosomal abnormality.

○   **How do spontaneous abortions most commonly present?**

Abdominal pain followed by vaginal bleeding.

○   **Before what gestational age do most spontaneous abortions occur?**

8 to 9 weeks.

○   **Spontaneous labor will occur within 3 weeks of fetal death in what percentage of patients?**

80%. It may be helpful to induce labor with vaginal suppositories due to the psychological effects of carrying a dead baby.

○   **What is the chance of spontaneous abortion once fetal cardiac activity is established at eight weeks of gestation?**

3-5%.

○   **Suction or vacuum curettage is used to terminate pregnancies at which gestational ages?**

7-13 weeks

○   **What is the most common cause of postabortal pain, bleeding and low grade fever?**

Retained gestational tissue or clot.

○   **Name three independent risk factors for spontaneous abortion.**

Increasing parity, maternal age, and paternal age.

○   **What is the effect of smoking and drinking on the abortion rate?**

Those who smoke more than 14 cigarettes daily have a 1.7 times greater chance of a spontaneous abortion. Those who drink alcohol at least 2 days a week have a twofold greater risk for spontaneous abortion.

○   **What percentage of American couples are infertile?**

15%. 20% of women in the US above 35 are infertile.

○   **What are the numbers for a normal semen analysis?**

> 1 mL in volume (> 20,000,000 sperm) with > 50% motility.

○   **What percentage of infertility is due to the male factor?**

40%. Problems with the cervix, uterus, fallopian tubes, peritoneum, or ovulation account for the remaining 60%.

○   **At what gestational age does hCG peak?**

8-10 weeks

○   **Name four physiologic actions of hCG?**

1. Maintenence of corpus luteum and continued progesterone production
2. Stimulation of fetal testicular testosterone secretion promoting male sexual differentiation
3. Stimulation of the maternal thyroid by binding to TSH receptors
4. Promotes relaxin secretion by the corpus luteum

○   **What secretes ß-hCG? Why?**

Placental trophoblasts secrete ß-hCG to maintain the corpus luteum, which in turn maintains the uterine lining. The corpus luteum is maintained through the sixth to eighth week of pregnancy, by which time the placenta begins to produce its own progesterone to maintain the endometrium.

○   **How soon after implantation can ß-hCG be detected?**

2 to 3 days.

○   **At what rate do ß-hCG levels rise?**

They double every 48 hours.

○   **T/F: During pregnancy, the uterus can grow to be 500 times its pre-pregnant capacity.**

True. In fact, the uterus can grow to be 1000 times its pre-pregnant capacity.

○   **A mother can feel fetal movement by which week of gestation?**

The 16th to 20th week.

○   **A doppler can detect fetal heart tones by which week of gestation?**

The 12th week.

○   **Why should pregnant women rest in the left lateral decubitus position?**

To avert supine hypotension syndrome due to compression of the IVC by the uterus.

○   **Your 28 year old pregnant patient expresses concerns about the ultrasound exam you have prescribed. How do you counsel her?**

Diagnostic ultrasound is safe. Resonance (mechanical vibration of tissue) does not occur and most of the sound energy is converted to heat which is distributed into the tissues. A safe level of tissue ultrasound exposure is equal to or greater than 100 mW/cm2. Most commercial machines product energies of 10-20 mW/cm2 which is very low. At present, there are no known examples of damage to target tissues from conventional usage.

○   **What is Pica?**

This is a craving for eating non-foods such as laundry starch, and clay during pregnancy. If severe, it can result in nutritional deficiencies and anemia. It is also possible that the agent ingested may be toxic to the developing fetus.

○   **What immunizations are contraindicated during pregnancy?**

In general, live virus vaccines are contraindicated during pregnancy. These include measles, mumps, rubella, oral polio, varicella. On the other hand, all toxoids, immunoglobulins and killed virus vaccines are considered safe in pregnancy and should not be withheld, if indicated.

○   **Teenage pregnancies are associated with increased risks of what?**

Maternal complications like gonorrhea, syphilis, toxemia, anemia, malnutrition, low birth weights, and perinatal mortality.

○   **When does the corpus luteum stop producing progesterone in pregnancy?**

7-8 weeks of gestation

○   **At what gestational age does the uterus rise out of the pelvis?**

About 12 weeks

○   **What are the normal physical changes in the cervix during pregnancy?**

Softening and cyanosis

○   **What are the changes in cervical mucus that occur in pregnancy?**

Thick tenacious mucus forms a plug blocking the cervical canal. Increased cervical and vaginal secretions result in thick, white odorless discharge. The pH is between 3.5 and 6.0 resulting from increased production of lactic acid from the action of *Lactobacillus acidophilus*.

○   **What is the average weight gain in pregnancy?**

11 kg (25 lbs). Only 30 % of the maternal weight gain is attributed to the placenta and fetus. Another 30% is attributed to blood, amniotic fluid and extravascular fluid. Another 30 % is attributed to maternal fat.

○   **What is the physiology of the maternal immune system in pregnancy in general terms?**

Pregnancy represents a 50% allograft from the paternal contribution. As a result, there is a general supression of immune function.

○   **What are the normal changes in the auscultative heart examination during pregnancy?**

Exaggerated split S1 with increased loudness of both components, systolic ejection murmurs heard at the left sternal border are present in 90 % of patients, soft and transient diastolic murmurs are heard in 20%, continuous murmurs from breast vasculature are heard in 10%. The significance of murmurs in pregnancy must be carefully evaluated and clinically correlated. Harsh systolic murmurs and all diastolic murmurs should be taken seriously and worked up before being attributed to pregnancy

○   **What is the most common presentation of twins?**

Vertex-vertex. If the first twin is vertex and the second breach, it is still possible to attempt a vaginal delivery because the extra space afforded after the birth of the first baby allows room to manipulate the position of the second.

○   **The average gestational age for singletons is 39 weeks. What is the average gestational age for twins?**

35 weeks. Prematurity is a large risk factor for respiratory distress syndrome. Half of perinatal deaths involving twins are due to respiratory distress syndrome.

○   **Describe the effect pregnancy has on (1) cardiac output, (2) BP, (3) heart rate, (4) coagulation, (5) sed rate, (6) leukocytes, (7) blood volume, (8) tidal volume, (9) bladder, (10) BUN/Cr, and (11) GI.**

1) Cardiac output: Increases (moving the uterus off the IVC increases cardiac output)
2) BP: Falls in second trimester; returns to normal in third
3) Heart rate: Increases
4) Coagulation: Factors 7, 8, 9, and 10 and fibrinogen increase; others remain unchanged
5) Sed rate: Elevates
6) Leukocytes: Increase (up to 18,000)
7) Blood volume: Increases; no change in RBC; dilutional "anemia" is physiologic
8) Tidal volume: Increases 40%
9) Bladder: Displaces superiorly and anteriorly
10) BUN/Cr: Decreases because of increased GFR and renal blood flow
11) GI: Gastric emptying and GI motility decrease; alkaline phosphatase increases; peritoneal signs such as rigidity and rebound are diminished or absent

○   **What kind of changes occur in the cardiovascular system of a pregnant patient?**

Cardiac output increases by 30% in the first trimester and then 50% by the second trimester, plasma volume increases 50%, pulse increases 12 to 18 bpm, systolic and diastolic blood pressure decreases by 10 – 15 mmHg in the second trimester, then gradually returns to prepregnant levels in the third trimester, stroke volume increases 25%, and hematocrit drops due to hemodilution.

○   **When does labor begin?**

Labor begins with the onset of regular, rhythmic contractions that lead to serial dilatation and effacement of the cervix. Thus, to say labor has begun, one must observe changes in the cervix. The presence of contractions alone does not qualify for the onset of labor.

○   **What are the 4 stages of labor and delivery?**

Stage I: Onset of labor to complete dilation of the cervix
Stage II: Cervical dilation to birth
Stage III: Birth to delivery of the placenta
Stage IV: Placenta delivery to stability of the mother (about 6 hours)

○   **How long is the average latent phase of labor?**

In a nullipara, the average is 6.4 hours; in the multipara, the average is 4.8 hours

○   **What is the rate of cervical dilation (active phase) in primiparous and multiparous women?**

The active phase begins when the uterus is regularly contracting and the cervix is 3-4 cm dialated. The minimal dilation is 1cm/hour for primiparous and 1.5 cm/hr for multiparous women.

○   **What are the 6 movements of delivery?**

1) Descent
2) Flexion
3) Internal rotation
4) Extension
5) External rotation
6) Expulsion

○   **How long may a patient push once fully dilated?**

Provided that the fetal heart pattern is reassuring and maternal expulsive forces remain effective, a second stage may last up to 2 hours in the nullipara; up to 3 hours is appropriate if the patient has regional analgesia/anesthesia. Beyond these time limits, one sees an increase in fetal acidosis and lower Apgar scores, as well as a greater risk of maternal postpartum hemorrhage and febrile morbidity. In a nullipara, the average second stage is approximately 40 minutes; in the multipara it is about 20 minutes

○   **What complications are seen with precipitous labors?**

There is a higher incidence of fetal trauma (intracranial hemorrhage and fractured clavicle) and long term neurologic injury. The mother is at higher risk for pelvic lacerations and postpartum hemorrhage (including, somewhat paradoxically, from uterine atony.)

○   **What is "effacement" of the cervix?**

Effacement refers to the foreshortening and thinning of cervix as it is drawn upwards (intra-abdominally). It is usually expressed in percentages by which cervical length has been reduced (from 0%, or uneffaced to 100% or fully effaced)

○   **What is oxytocin?**

Oxytocin is a decapeptide synthesized by the posterior pituitary gland. It is a powerful uterotonic agent; that is, it causes the uterus to contract. In nature, it is secreted in pulsatile fashion throughout labor. (The fetus also produces oxytocin and at least some traverses the placenta, escaping enzymatic breakdown.)

○   **Does epidural analgesia affect the course of labor?**

Studies showed that epidural analgesia does not slow the progress of labor in the first stage of labor. However, the second stage of labor appears to be prolonged an average of 20-25 minutes. There is no evidence that this prolongation is harmful to the fetus

○   **What is a "walking epidural"?**

An intrathecal opioid or epidural opioid plus an ultra-low dose of local anesthetic, followed by continuous infusion of opioid and local anesthetics, for labor analgesia. These regimens cause no or minimal motor block on the lower extremities, and allow the mother to ambulate in the early 1st stage of labor

○   **What pelvic type is the most common in women?**

Gynecoid. It is estimated that approximately 50% of women have this type of pelvis. (It should be noted that in reality most women have intermediate pelvic shapes rather than true gynecoid, anthropoid, android or platypelloid)

❍ **What is the average gestational age at delivery for twins, triplets, and quadruplets?**

Twins: 36-37 weeks
Triplets: 33-34 weeks
Quadruplets: 30-31 weeks
3 or more fetuses reduced to twins: 35-36 weeks

❍ **At term what percentage of fetuses are in vertex presentation?**

95%

❍ **What is the largest risk for breech presentation?**

Prematurity. 25% of fetuses are breech at 28 weeks, but most correct by term.

❍ **What are the three types of breech presentation?**

Frank breech: Thighs flexed, legs extended
Complete breech: At least 1 leg flexed
Incomplete (footling) breech: At least 1 foot below the buttocks with both thighs extended

❍ **What is the most common breech position?**

Frank breech.

❍ **What is the difference between high forceps, mid forceps, and low forceps deliveries?**

High forceps refers to the use of forceps when a baby is not yet in the birth canal (rarely used).

Mid forceps refers to a baby is in the birth canal and within reach (used in cases of fetal distress).

Low forceps refers to the outlet and is used when the baby's head is at the pelvic floor (most often used to shorten labor when the mother is tiring or to control normal labor).

❍ **What is the most common cause of a prolonged active phase of labor?**

Cephalopelvic disproportion caused by contraction of a narrowed midpelvis.

❍ **How can ruptured membranes be diagnosed?**

Nitrazine paper will turn blue and a ferning pattern will be seen under the microscope in the presence of amniotic fluid. Also, look for pooling of amniotic fluid in the posterior fornix.

❍ **Describe the different types of perineal tears occuring with delivery.**

First degree: Perineal skin or vaginal mucosa
Second degree: Submucosa of vagina or perineum
Third degree: Anal sphincter
Fourth degree: Rectal mucosa

❍ **What are the advantages of a mediolateral episiotomy?**

Such an episiotomy allows for greater room without lacerating the external sphincter ani or rectum. However, these episiotomies are associated with a greater blood loss and postpartum pain, greater likelihood for sub-optimal healing, and subsequent dyspareunia.

❍   **What are the advantages of a midline (median) episiotomy?**

These are easier to repair, associated with a lower blood loss, usually heal better (less postpartum discomfort and better cosmetic result), and less subsequent dyspareunia. The principal disadvantage to such an episiotomy, compared to a mediolateral one, is the greater propensity to extend into the external anal sphincter or rectum.

❍   **What are risk factors for shoulder dystocia?**

Diabetes, maternal obesity, postterm babies and mothers with excessive weight gain. Intrapartum risk factors include a prolonged second stage of labor, oxytocin use (augmentation or induction), and midforceps deliveries.

❍   **What is the difference between a classic c-section and a newer c-section?**

A classic c-section is a vertical incision in the uterus. This type of c-section predisposes women to future uterine rupture. Hence, subsequent deliveries should be made via c-section as well. The newer c-sections are low transverse incisions; they have a much lower rate of uterine rupture with subsequent deliveries.

❍   **What percentage of women can have vaginal births after low transverse incision c-sections?**

75%. Vaginal birth is contraindicated after a classic c-section.

❍   **What is the average blood loss for vaginal delivery and for cesarean section?**

Four to six hundred ml for vaginal delivery and 800 - 1000 ml for cesarean section

❍   **How can fetal lung maturity be assessed?**

The L/S ratio. If the ratio of lecithin to sphingomyelin is over 2:1, then the fetal lungs are mature.

❍   **What is the normal fetal heart rate?**

120 to 160 bpm. If bradycardia is detected, position the mother on her left side and administer oxygen and an IV fluid bolus.

❍   **Are accelerations normal?**

Yes and no. Rapid heart rate can indicate fetal distress. 2 accelerations every 20 minutes are normal. An acceleration must be at least 15 bpm above baseline and last at least 15 seconds.

❍   **What causes variable decelerations?**

Transient umbilical cord compression. These often change with maternal position.

❍   **A baby is born with a pink body, blue extremities, and a heart rate of 60. She is mildly irritable (grimaces) and has weak respirations and no muscle tone. What is this child's Apgar?**

1 + 1 + 1 + 1 + 0 = 4

Apgar points	0	1	2
Color	Blue	Extremities blue	All pink
Heart rate	Ø	< 100	> 100

Irritability	Ø	Mild grimace	Strongly irritable
Respiratory effort	None	Weak	Cry
Muscle tone	Flaccid	Weak	Strong

❍ **What is the puerperium?**

The puerperium refers to the time just after birth and lasts about 6 weeks. It is the time it takes the uterus to return to it's non-pregnant state.

❍ **How common are "postpartum" blues?**

50-70% of mothers will have postpartum blues

❍ **How common is postpartum depression?**

Only 4-10% of postpartum mothers will have true postpartum depression

❍ **What happens if some placenta or fetal membranes are left inside the uterus?**

Retained tissue or products of conception may lead to postpartum hemorrhage. It also increases the risk of postpartum endometritis.

❍ **What is lochia?**

Lochia refers to the uterine discharge that follows delivery. It consists of necrotic decidua, blood, inflammatory cells and bacteria. This discharge lasts about 5 weeks.

❍ **When does ovulation resume post-partum?**

In non-lactating women, ovulation may occur as early as 27 days postpartum. The average is ten weeks. In women exclusively breastfeeding, ovulation may be delayed for the duration of active breastfeeding, although the mean is six months.

❍ **Why is the risk of a thromboembolic event increased in the post-partum time?**

While immediate platelet count changes are variable, there is clearly an increase by two weeks. Fibrinogen levels remain elevated for at least one week; as do Factors VII, VIII, IX and X. In addition, there is clearly greater vessel trauma and less mobility.

❍ **How does colostrum differ from breast milk?**

Colostrum is more cellular and has more minerals, but is lower in calories. True milk has more fat and carbohydrate (especially lactose), but less protein

❍ **When does breast milk production typically begin?**

Colostrum secretion usually persists for 3-4 days after which the fluid begins to change in composition. Mature milk is usually present by one to two weeks postpartum.

❍ **How many extra calories above baseline does a woman need when breastfeeding?**

About 500 per day

❍ **How much daily dietary of calcium is recommended for lactating women?**

1200-1500mg per day

○　**All vitamins are found in human breast milk except which one?**

Vitamin K. This is why vitamin K is administered to newborns. Formula is also deficient in vitamin K.

○　**How does human milk differ from cow's milk?**

While the two are similar in calories, human milk has more lactose, less protein (and very different protein constitution), and slightly more fat (especially more polyunsaturated fatty acids and cholesterol which are needed for brain development.) There is significantly more calcium, phosphorus and iron in bovine milk

○　**A breast feeding mother presents to your office complaining of fever, chills, and a swollen red breast. What is the most likely causative organism?**

Staphylococcus aureus is the most common cause of mastitis. Mastitis is seldom present in the first week post partum. It is most often seen 3 to 4 weeks post partum.

○　**What is the treatment for the above patient?**

Warm compresses to breast, analgesics, dicloxacillin or a cephalosporin (penicillinase resistant)

○　**Can a nursing mother with mastitis continue to nurse?**

Yes, as long as there is no abscess formation. Nursing facilitates the drainage of the infection and the infant will not be harmed because he is already colonized.

○　**What post-partum immunizations are part of standard care?**

Rubella and Rubeola immunization-vaccinations should be administered to all susceptible postpartum women. In theory, diphtheria and tetanus toxoid boosters may also be administered if indicated. The non-isoimmunized Rh negative patient should also receive anti-D immune globulin if her child is Rh positive.

○　**When may coitus resume following delivery?**

Most physicians instruct their patients to abstain from coitus for six weeks. From a physiologic standpoint, once uterine involution and perineal healing are complete, coitus may resume.

○　**What factors predispose one to uterine atony?**

Fetal macrosomia, polyhydramnios, abnormal labor progress, amnionitis, oxytocin stimulation and multiple gestations.

○　**What are the common signs of uterine rupture?**

Fetal distress, unrelenting pain, hypotension, tachycardia, and vaginal bleeding. Fetal distress is usually the first sign of uterine rupture.

○　**What causes uterine rupture?**

Oxytocin stimulation, cephalopelvic disproportion, grand multiparity, abdominal trauma, prior hysterotomy, c-section, myotomy, curettage or manual removal of the placenta.

○　**What is the difference between placenta previa and abruptio placenta?**

Placenta previa is the implantation of the placenta in the lower uterine segment thus covering the cervical os. Presentation is painless vaginal bleeding with a soft nontender uterus. Abruptio placenta is the premature separation of the placenta from the uterine wall. Abruptio placenta causes painful uterine bleeding. Both are complications of 3rd trimester pregnancies.

○   **A patient presents in her third trimester complaining of vaginal bleeding but no pain or contractions. How should you diagnose this patient?**

With a transabdominal ultrasound. Since 95% of placenta previas can be diagnosed this way, a vaginal examination should be avoided until placenta previa has been ruled out via ultrasound. Abruptio placenta is generally accompanied by pain, shock, or an expanding uterus. It is not easily diagnosed on ultrasound.

○   **What are the risk factors for placenta previa?**

Previous cesarean section, previous placenta previa, multiparity, multiple induced abortions, maternal age over 40 and multiple gestations.

○   **What causes dependent and non-dependent edema in pregnant women?**

Compression of veins by the growing uterus causes dependent edema, whereas hypoalbuminemia can cause non-dependent edema.

○   **Name 7 risk factors for placental abruption:**

Smoking, trauma, cocaine, hypertension, alcohol, PROM, and retroplacental fibroids

○   **Why is ephedrine usually the first choice to treat maternal hypotension?**

Ephedrine does not produce significant uterine vascular constriction, therefore it does not result in decreased uterine blood flow.

○   **What viral or protozoal infections require extensive workup during pregnancy?**

TORCH

TOxoplasma gondii
Rubella
Cytomegalovirus
Herpes genitalis

○   **A patient presents 3 days post partum with a fever, malaise and lower abdominal pain. On examination, a foul lochia and tender boggy uterus are present. What is the diagnosis?**

Endometritis. This typically occurs 1 to 3 days post partum. It is felt that the mechanism of infection is from ascending cervicovaginal flora.

○   **Is endometritis more common after vaginal delivery or c-section?**

The rate of endometritis is 5 – 10 times greater after c-section.

○   **What is the treatment for endometritis?**

Admission and IV broadspectrum antibiotics

○   **What is the most common cause of post partum hemorrhage?**

Uterine atony.

○   **What is routinely done to decrease the risk of post partum hemorrhage?**

Uterine massage and oxytocin. Lacerations are sutured. In severe cases, where bleeding cannot be stopped, the hypogastric vessels are ligated or a hysterectomy is performed.

○   **What conditions are suggested by elevated maternal serum α-fetoprotein?**

Neural tube defects (anencephalopathy), ventral abdominal wall defects, fetal demise, multiple fetuses, low α-fetoprotein is indicative of Down Syndrome.

○   **What are the baseline congenital anomaly risks in the general population?**

Regardless of family history or teratogenic exposure, the background risk for major congenital anomalies is 3-5%. These include abnormalities that, if uncorrected, affect the health of the individual. Some examples are pyloric stenosis, cleft lip and palate, neural tube defects. The background rate for minor congenital anomalies is 7-10%. These include strabismus, polydactyly, misshapen ears, etc. If uncorrected, they do not significantly affect the health of the individual.

○   **Which women today are most at risk for mercury poisoning?**

Fish-eaters. The only real human exposure to organic mercury is through consumption of fish, primarily from predatory fish such as shark, swordfish, pike and bass. Fish consumption by pregnant women should be limited to 350 grams per week. Fetuses are more susceptible to toxic effects of mercury than their maternal hosts. Large exposures to methyl mercury have resulted in infants with microcephaly, mental retardation, cerebral palsy, and blindness.

○   **Is working as a medical resident harmful during pregnancy?**

Overall, residency training has not been shown to cause spontaneous abortion, preterm birth or low birth weight. However, one study when women worked more than 100 hours/week, preterm births were increased. Mild preeclampsia which was not associated with adverse pregnancy outcome was also increased in women residents.

○   **How does cocaine adversely affect pregnancy?**

Cocaine is especially toxic during pregnancy. The most common complication caused by cocaine during pregnancy is abruptio placentae, which may result in fetal death. In addition, brain anomalies, intestinal atresia and limb reduction defects have been described. Investigators have also reported increases in congenital heart defects in exposed infants. Cocaine may cause these effects by vasoconstrictions and subsequent infarction.

○   **Is methadone as bad for pregnancy as cocaine?**

Not even close. In fact, one study compared cocaine-abusing women to women being treated with methadone and found a much higher complication rate in the cocaine-abuse group. Methadone is not thought to be a teratogen.

○   **What are the signs and symptoms of fetal alcohol syndrome?**

Infants suffer from intrauterine growth restriction, mental retardation, and develop a characteristic facies which consists of short palpebral fissures, a flat midface, a thin upper lip and hypoplastic philtrum. Alcohol abuse is the most common preventable cause of mental retardation during pregnancy.

○   **At what time during gestation is the fetus most susceptible to alcohol toxicity?**

OBSTETRICS AND GYNECOLOGY PEARLS

Probably in the second and third trimesters. In a study of 60 women, those who were heavy drinkers but stopped after the first trimester had children with normal mentation and behavioral patterns.

○ **In general, during which time during pregnancy is the fetus most susceptible to teratogens?**

During the embryonic period, which lasts from 2 to 8 weeks post conception. This is the time of organogenesis.

○ **What are the major adverse effects of smoking during pregnancy?**

Smoking causes intrauterine growth restriction and increases the incidence of preterm delivery in a dose-dependent manner. The incidence of placenta previa, abruptio placentae and spontaneous abortion also appears to be increased by smokers.

○ **Folic acid deficiency is associated with what in pregnancy?**

Folate deficiency is associated with neural tube defects (i.e. spina bifida, anencephaly).

○ **What are the drug labeling categories for use during pregnancy?**

The FDA lists 5 categories of labeling:
Category A: safe for use in pregnancy.
Category B: Animal studies have demonstrated the drug's safety and human studies do not reveal any adverse fetal effects
Category C: The drug is a known animal teratogen, but no data are available about human use; or there are not data in either humans or animals
Category D: There is positive evidence of human fetal toxicity but benefits in selected situations makes use of the drug acceptable despite its risks
Category X: The drug is a definite human and animal teratogen and should not be used in pregnancy.

○ **What are the benefits of antepartum corticosteroids in premature babies?**

Increased lung compliance, increased surfactant production and less respiratory distress syndrome, less intraventricular hemorrhage, less necrotizing enterocolitis, less neonatal mortality

○ **When is the critical period of organogenesis?**

Between 15 and 56 days of gestation, or day 31 to day 71 after the first day of the last menstrual period .

○ **When is an amniocentesis performed?**

16 to 18 weeks

○ **What radiation dose increases the risk of inhibited fetal growth?**

10 rad. Typical abdominal and pelvic films deliver 100 to 350 mrad. A shielded chest x-ray should deliver under 10 mrad to the fetus. Do not withhold necessary x-rays.

○ **Can iodinated radiodiagnostic agents be used in pregnant patients?**

No. They should be avoided because concentration in the fetal thyroid can cause permanent loss of thyroid function. Nuclear medicine scans, pulmonary angiography with pelvic shielding, and impedance plethysmography are preferred.

○   **What are the indications for cardio-tocographic monitoring in a pregnant trauma patient?**

All women past 20 weeks gestation with indirect or direct abdominal trauma require 4 hours of monitoring. Loss of beat-to-beat variability, uterine contractions, or fetal bradycardia or tachycardia demands immediate obstetrical consultation.

○   **What is the most common medical complication of pregnancy?**

Urinary tract infections.

○   **What percentage of pregnant women get "morning sickness"?**

50 – 70%. It generally occurs in the first trimester.

○   **How should morning sickness be treated?**

Frequent small meals, carbohydrates, IV hydration and antiemetics.

○   **What is hyperemesis gravidum?**

Excessive vomiting durring pregnancy that results in starvation (ketonuria), dehydration and acidosis.

○   **What is the treatment for gestational diabetes?**

Diet, insulin, and exercise. Do not give patients oral hypoglycemics because these cross the blood-brain barrier.

○   **When should you be most concerned about a pregnant patient with heart disease?**

During weeks 18 to 24, when the female body experiences a maximal increase in cardiac output (40%).

○   **Define pregnancy induced hypertension.**

An increase in the systolic pressure > 30 mm Hg or an increase in diastolic pressure > 15 mm Hg over base line, measured on two separate occasions at least 6 hours apart.

○   **Define pre-eclampsia**

Hypertension and proteinuria occuring most commonly in the last trimester of pregnancy. In severe cases, patients can have edema, oliguria, headache, visual acuity changes, abdominal pain, pulmonary edema, thrombocytopenia and elevated LFT's, and intrauterine growth retardation.

○   **Who is more likely to have pre-eclampsia; primiparous or mulltiparous women?**

Primiparous. Other risk factors include pregnancies associated with a large placenta, patients with a history of HTN, renal disease, family history of pre-eclampsia, older women, women with multiple gestations, and women with prior vascular disease.

○   **What is the drug of choice for treating hypertension of pregnancy?**

Hydralazine. Antihypertensive treatment is indicated if the systolic BP is >170 or the diastolic is >110.

○   **How long should treatment continue after delivery in a woman with pre-eclampsia?**

24 hours. The cure of preeclampsia is delivery. Antihypertensives and antiseizure medication (IV magnesium sulfate) should be continued until there is no longer a risk to the mother.

○ **Define eclampsia.**

Pre-eclampsia plus grand mal seizures or coma.

○ **Can one have eclamptic seizures after delivery?**

Yes. Up to 10 days post partum.

○ **What does HELLP stand for?**

Hemolysis, **E**levated **L**iver enzymes, and **L**ow **P**latelet levels. The **HELLP** syndrome is a very severe form of pre-eclampsia. Signs and symptoms include RUQ pain/tenderness, nausea, vomiting edema, jaundice, GI bleeding and hematuria in addition to the symptoms of pre-eclampsia.

○ **What is the major cause of death in women with eclampsia?**

Intracranial hemorrhage

○ **What are the warning signs of impending seizure in a patient with pre-eclampsia?**

Headache, visual disturbances, hyperreflexia and abdominal pain.

○ **What is the treatment for eclampsia?**

Delivery!!! Until you are able to deliver you can use Magnesium sulfate, valium and hydralazine. Phenytoin or diazepam can be used for seizures resistant to magnesium therapy.

○ **At what point does magnesium become toxic?**

Respiratory arrest occurs at levels > 12 mEq/L. Loss of reflexes occurs at levels > 8 mEq/L and can therefor be used as a guide for treatment.

○ **What is the antedote for magnesium toxicity?**

Calcium gluconate (1gm IV push) Magnesium should be stopped if the DTR's disappear.

○ **What are the risk factors for abruptio placentae?**

Smoking, hypertension, multiparity, trauma, and previous abruptio placentae.

○ **What are the presenting signs and symptoms of abruptio placentae?**

Placental separation before delivery is associated with vaginal bleeding (78%) and abdominal pain (66%), as well as with tetanic uterine contractions, uterine irritability, and fetal death.

○ **What is the most likely diagnosis in a patient whose uterus is larger than expected from the history of gestation, has vaginal bleeding, and passes grape-like tissue from the vagina?**

Hydatidiform mole.

○ **A patient presents to your office for a regular prenatal check up. She is in her first trimester. You note that she has a blood pressure of 160/94. Probable diagnosis?**

Hypertension in the first half of pregnancy indicates hydatidiform mole. Patients most commonly complain of painless vaginal bleeding. The uterus is enlarged; no fetal heart tones are present. Theca lutein cysts are visible on ultrasound. The growths should be removed by suction curettage. The patient should be treated weekly with ß-hCG titers to assure there is no remaining tissue or distant metastasis.

O   **Is the hCG level high or low in a molar pregnancy?**

High.

O   **Describe the characteristics of an invasive mole.**

Invasive moles are pathologically similar to complete hydatidiform moles but invade beyond the normal placentation site into the myometrium. Penetration into the venous system can result in venous metastases to the lower genital tract and lungs.

O   **How is human chorionic gonadotropin (β-hCG) useful in the study of gestational trophoblastic disease?**

Both molar pregnancies and gestational choreocarcinomas produce β-hCG due to their trophoblastic origin. The tumor marker correlates well with the volume of disease and can be followed as a marker during therapy.

O   **How does age influence the incidence of hydatidiform moles?**

Compared to women 25 to 29 years of age, women over the age of 50 have a 300 to 400 fold increase in risk, and women under the age of 15 have a sixfold increase. Similarly, increased paternal age (above 45 years of age) also confers an increased risk of a complete molar pregnancy, although the increase in only 4.9 times (2.9 when adjusted for maternal age).

O   **What is the leading type of cancer in women?**

Breast cancer (32%).

O   **What is the leading cause of cancer deaths in women?**

Lung cancer. Breast cancer is second.

O   **What is the most common type of benign breast tumor?**

Fibroadenomas. These are usually solitary, mobile masses with distinct borders. They are more prevalent in women under age 30.

O   **A 53 year old female presents with a hard, barely palpable lump in the upper, outer quadrant of her left breast. The lump is mobile and causes no pain. The patient has noted blood oozing from her nipple. Probable diagnosis?**

Benign intraductal papilloma. Intraductal papillomas are the most common cause of bleeding from the nipple. Growths usually develop just before or during menopause, and they are rarely palpable.

O   **Are the majority of breast cancers in the ducts or in the lobes?**

Invasive ductal tumors account for 90% of all breast cancers. Only 10% are lobular.

O   **What is the most common invasive ductal tumor?**

Nonspecific infiltrating ductal carcinoma.

○ **What are the American Cancer Society's 1996 recommendations for mammography?**

Every 1 to 2 years after age 40. Annually after age 50.

○ **What are the risk factors for breast cancer, and how do they compare with the risk factors for endometrial cancer?**

Risk factors for both cancers include nulliparity, early menarche, late menopause, significant amounts of unopposed estrogen, and prior ovarian, endometrial, or breast cancer. Unopposed estrogen is a much greater risk in endometrial cancer than in breast cancer. Risk factors specific to breast cancer include family history, age over 40, high fat intake, radiation of the breast, or cellular atypia in fibrocystic disease.

○ **Geographically, where is breast cancer most common?**

North America and northern Europe have an incidence and mortality rate 5 times that of most Asian and African countries. However, while Asians and Africans who immigrate to North America or northern Europe maintain a lower rate of incidence, their offspring quickly assume a higher one. This points to environmental and dietary factors.

○ **Who have higher incidences of estrogen receptor positive tumors, premenopausal or postmenopausal women?**

Postmenopausal (60%). If the tumors are both estrogen and progesterone sensitive, then the antiestrogen drug tamoxifen is 80% effective. Otherwise, it is 40 to 50% effective.

○ **What is the most accurate prognostic indicator of breast cancer?**

Axillary node involvement, which is related to the size of the tumor, not the location. 40 to 50% of patients have axillary node involvement when diagnosed.

○ **A patient presents with crusty erosion of the nipple and no discharge. Possible diagnosis?**

Paget's disease. This rare cancer occurs in 3% of breast cancer patients. It involves the excretory ducts of the breast.

○ **What is Peau d'orange?**

French for skin of the orange, it is the dimpling and thickening of the breast in breast cancer.

○ **What are the American Cancer Society's recommendations for Pap smears?**

Pap smears should be done annually for 3 years starting at age 18 or when the patient becomes sexually active, and every 1 to 3 years thereafter.

○ **Is there an increased risk of breast cancer associated with estrogen replacement therapy?**

There may be a slightly increased risk of breast cancer especially with long duration of use (10 or more years).

○ **What marker is associated with ovarian cancer?**

CA-125

○ **If a woman has ascites, what is the most likely tumor to be found?**

An ovarian carcinoma. This is part of Meigs' syndrome.

○   **What is Meigs' syndrome?**

Ascites and hydrothorax in the presence of an ovarian tumor.

○   **What are the risk factors for carcinoma of the cervix?**

1) Multiple sexual partners
2) Early age at first intercourse
3) Early first pregnancy

○   **Most cervical cancers are of what type?**

80% are squamous cell and arise from the squamocolumnar junction of the cervix.

○   **How effective have Pap smears been in reducing the incidence of cervical cancer?**

Since the development of cytological screening in the 1940's, the incidence of cervical cancer in the United States has fallen by almost 80%. In contrast, cervical cancer remains the major cause of cancer related deaths among women in many third world countries where Pap smears are not routinely performed

○   **What is the most common presenting symptom for patients with cervical cancer?**

Up to 80% of patients present with abnormal vaginal bleeding, most commonly postmenopausal. Only 10% note postcoital bleeding. Less frequent symptoms include vaginal discharge and pain.

○   **A colposcopically directed cervical biopsy from a 25 year old G0P0 reveals a small focus of invasive squamous cell carcinoma. What is the next step in this patient's management?**

Cervical cone biopsy to establish the full extent of invasion.

○   **What clinical triad is strongly indicative of cervical cancer extension to the pelvic wall?**

1.   Unilateral leg edema
2.   Sciatic pain
3.   Ureteral obstruction

○   **A 66 year old woman presents with vaginal bleeding. What is your provisional diagnosis?**

Endometrial cancer. 15% of women with postmenopausal bleeding have endometrial cancer. 30% of these tumors are due to exogenous estrogens; 30% are due to atrophic endometriosis or vaginitis; 10% are due to cervical polyps; 5% are due to endometrial hyperplasia. Most tumors are caught in stage I.

○   **Describe the initial office evaluation of a woman whose history is suspicious for endometrial cancer?**

Pelvic examination, PAP smear, biopsy of any abnormal cervical or vaginal lesion, and endometrial biopsy.

○   **What percentage of women with endometrial cancer will have an abnormal Papanicolaou smear?**

Approximately 50%

○   **What is the most common symptom of endometrial cancer?**

Abnormal perimenopausal or postmenopausal bleeding.

○ **What is the risk of endometrial cancer in postmenopausal women on unopposed estrogen compared to those not on ERT?**

2 to 10 times higher, depending on dose and duration of exposure.

○ **What is the most common clinical condition associated with the development of endometrial hyperplasia?**

Polycystic ovary syndrome

○ **What is the Lynch syndrome type II?**

A hereditary predisposition to the development of colon, breast, ovarian and endometrial cancer

○ **What is the most common neoplasm in reproductive aged women?**

Benign leiomyomata. The most frequent presenting symptom for patients with leiomyosarcomas is vaginal bleeding, which occurs in over three quarters of patients.

○ **Why is it unlikely that you will find a uterine myoma in a 65 year old?**

Uterine myomas are begin smooth muscle growths that are responsive to hormones and grow primarily in the reproductive years. They are the most common type of gynecological pelvic neoplasm.

○ **What type of myoma is symptomatic?**

Submucosal myomas, though small, can cause profuse bleeding, potentially requiring a hysterectomy. Most other myomas are asymptomatic

IMAGING PEARLS

○ **What is the purpose of ultrasound gel?**

It displaces air and provides a medium for coupling the probe to the skin surface without impedance mismatching.

○ **When using doppler, what audible characteristics differentiate arterial from venous flow?**

Arterial flow is characterized by sharp, brisk changes in pitch throughout the cardiac cycle (higher pitched during peak systole and lower pitched during diastole; also termed multiphasic). Venous flow varies with the respiratory cycle, and venous signals are lower pitched and more consistent throughout the cardiac cycle (monophasic).

○ **What is the diagnostic test of choice for documenting DVT?**

Duplex ultrasound. The accuracy of physical examination for DVT is generally quoted to be 50%.

○ **List some of the advantages and disadvantages of DPL, CT, and ultrasound for assessing trauma patients.**

	Advantages	Disadvantages
DPL	Low complication rate, done at bedside	Invasive, time-consuming, can't identify retroperitoneal injury, significant false positive rate
CT	Identifies location and extent of injury, including the retroperitoneum	Expensive, time-consuming, requires travel and interpretation expertise, patient monitoring is not optimal
US	Fast, cheap, noninvasive, done at bedside, good for hemoperitoneum	Operator-dependent, not good for identifying specific organ injury

○ **Surgical repair of abdominal aortic aneurysms (AAA) is generally indicated for those measuring:**

> 4 cm. Ultrasound is extremely sensitive for detecting AAA, but it is not sensitive for the detection of ruptured AAA.

○ **What is the primary use of ultrasound in females with a positive hCG, who present with abdominal pain and/or vaginal bleeding?**

To verify intrauterine pregnancy. The incidence of simultaneous intrauterine and extrauterine pregnancies is about 1/30,000. Ultrasound may not be able to verify that an ectopic pregnancy exists.

○ **What is the only true diagnostic sign of an ectopic pregnancy with ultrasound?**

A fetus with cardiac activity outside the uterus. Complex masses and fluid in the cul-de-sac can be seen with other conditions (e.g., pelvic abscess and ruptured ovarian cysts).

○ **What is the role of ultrasound in detecting placenta previa and abruption?**

Ultrasound cannot detect abruption but can rule out placenta previa in the third trimester.

❍   What is the incidence of allergic reaction to IV contrast materials?

Severe allergic reactions occur in approximately 1/14,000 patients; fatal reactions occur in about 1/40,000 cases.

❍   **T/F : Oral contrast should be avoided in patients with marginal renal function.**

False. Little nephrotoxic iodine is absorbed with oral contrast administration. When barium is used, it is inert and not absorbed.

❍   **What contraindicates oral iodine or barium contrast?**

Barium cannot be given when complete colon obstruction exists or intestinal perforation is suspected. Severe allergy to iodine is the only contraindication to oral iodine containing preparations.

❍   **T/F : IV contrast material is contraindicated in chronic renal failure.**

False. The contrast material can be dialyzed, and the kidney is already maximally impaired.

❍   **Describe the typical shape and vessel origin of a subdural hematoma (SDH) and an epidural hematoma (EDH) on CT.**

An SDH is typically crescent-shaped. It can be arterial in origin but is most often caused by the tearing of bridging veins. An acute SDH is hyperdense relative to the brain and becomes isodense to the brain in 1 to 3 weeks. An EDH is biconvex (lenticular) and usually arterial in origin. An EDH does not cross intact skull sutures but can cross the tentorium and the midline.

❍   **What percentage of subdural hematomas are bilateral?**

About 25%.

❍   **Why does the performance of a DPL make the evaluation of a subsequent CT more difficult?**

Air and fluid are introduced during the DPL.

❍   **What is the test of choice for evaluating and staging renal trauma?**

IV contrast enhanced CT. CT is more accurate then IVP because IVP is not sensitive for renal injuries.

❍   **The magnetic fields of an MRI can be detrimental to patients with what?**

Ferrous metal in their body or electrical equipment whose function can be disrupted by strong magnetic fields. Examples include pacemakers, metal foreign bodies in the eye (e.g., welders), ferromagnetic cerebral aneurysm clips (unless they are made of nonmagnetic steel), and cochlear implants. Relative contraindications for an MRI include certain prosthetic heart valves, implantable defibrillators, bone growth, and neurostimulators. One might also include patients who are claustrophobic.

❍   **Although bone scans are useful for detecting subtle fractures missed on x-ray, why is it not always useful in the setting for recent fractures?**

Bone scans may not pick up the increased bone turnover until hours or days after trauma, because skeletal uptake is dependent on blood flow and osteoblastic activity. A positive scan demonstrates asymmetric skeletal uptake.

○   **Are radionucleotide studies most helpful in determining the bleeding site in upper or lower GI bleeds?**

Lower.

○   **What 2 studies can detect testicular torsion and differentiate it from epididymitis, orchitis, or torsion of the appendix testis?**

Technetium 99m nuclear studies and duplex ultrasound.

PREVENTIVE PEARLS AND STATISTICS

○ **When is screening the population for a disease appropriate?**

When the disease is prevalent, when failure to catch the disease results in significant morbidity, when appropriate screening tests exist, or when therapy initiated due to the early detection will significantly alter the pattern of the disease.

○ **Matching:**

1) Sensitive	a) Actual positives/total number of positive test results
2) Specific	b) Actual positives/total number with the disease
3) Positive predictive value	c) Actual negatives/total number without the disease
4) Negative predictive value	d) Actual negatives/total number of negative test results

Answers: (1) b, (2) c, (3) a, and (4) d.

○ **Give the equation for prevalence of a disease.**

Incidence of a disease multiplied by its duration.

○ **Differentiate between type I and type II errors.**

Type I errors reject the null hypothesis when it is true. Type II errors accept the null hypothesis when it is false.

○ **Define alternative hypothesis.**

The assumption that a real difference (not due to chance) exists. This is the hypothesis accepted when the null hypothesis is rejected.

○ **What is variance, and how does it relate to standard deviation (SD)?**

Variance is the sum of the squares of the distances from the mean. SD equals the square root of the variance.

m **Give the equation for standard deviation.**

○ **If your results on the boards are 2 standard deviations above the mean, you will have done better than what percentage of physicians/residents taking the test with you?**

97.5%. If your results are 1 standard deviation above the mean, you will have done better than 84% of your fellow medical students. 64.26% of all values lie within 1 standard deviation. 95.44% of all values lie within 2 standard deviations from the mean, and 99.72% of all values lie within three standard deviations of the mean.

○ **What is the difference between standard error of the mean (SEM) and standard deviation (SD)?**

SEM measures the uncertainty in the estimation of the mean. It represents the mean value of a collection of several sample means and is thus closer to the true mean of a population. SD measures the variability in a given population.

○   **What test should be used to determine whether smokers are more likely to develop lung cancer than non-smokers?**

Chi-square. This test is used to test qualitative data and tells how the frequencies of each group differ from the frequencies that we would expect to find if there were no relationship between the groups. The greater the difference between 2 groups, the lower the chi-square number.

○   **What is the equation for chi-square?**

$$\chi^2 = \sum \frac{(O - E)^2}{E}$$

where O = observed number and E = expected number.

○   **300 hypertensive patients are randomly assigned to three groups. Each group is given a separate treatment plan, and the results are recorded. What statistical analysis method is appropriate?**

Analysis of variance (appropriate for comparing 2 or more sample means).

○   **50 obese individuals are randomly divided into 2 groups. One group follows diet A for 3 months; the other group follows diet B. What statistical method would you use to compare the results?**

The t test is the appropriate method to use when comparing group means of 2 separate samples. It is also appropriate when dealing with small sample sizes.

○   **Why would you use a correlation coefficient?**

To measure the degree of linear relationship between 2 variables.

○   **Match the prevention with the example that fits.**

1) Primary prevention   a) Tetanus booster shots every 10 years
2) Secondary prevention   b) Controlling blood sugar with appropriate diet and insulin
3) Tertiary prevention   c) Identifying and treating a patient with asymptomatic diabetes mellitus

Answers: (1) a, (2) c, and (3) b.

Primary prevention prevents a disease from ever occurring.
Secondary prevention prevents future problems if actions are taken during an asymptomatic period.
Tertiary prevention prevents further complications in a disease that is already present.

○   **What percentage of the population is homeless?**

0.5% (250,000 to 3,000,000 people, according to a 1993 poll).

○   **What is the difference between Medicaid and Medicare?**

Medicaid: Need-based governmental entitlement that includes food stamps, aid to families with dependent children, Medicaid (financial assistance for medical bills), Medicare, Social Security, Disability, Supplemental Security Income, and Workers Compensation.

Medicare: The division of Medicaid based solely on age.

O   **What immunizations are recommended for patients with HIV?**

1) IPV and Td every 10 years
2) Influenza vaccine yearly
3) Pneumococcal vaccine once
4) Hepatitis B vaccine for at risk patients
5) Hib and MMR are optional

O   **What percentage of untreated group A ß-hemolytic streptococcal infections will progress to rheumatic fever?**

3%. Increased incidence of the disease is noted in lower socioeconomic areas.

O   **What medication is the best treatment for preventing nephropathy in diabetic patients?**

ACE inhibitors. They are found to reduce endpoint renal disease, dialysis, and transplantation by 50%.

O   **T/F: Patients with hypertension are at a greater risk for CAD and stroke than the normal population.**

True. Hypertensive patients have a 3 to 4 times greater risk of CAD and a 7 times greater risk of stroke.

O   **What is the routine health screening for an asymptomatic 56 year old male with no significant risk factors?**

History and physical, stool test for occult blood, serum cholesterol test, syphilis test, and a flexible sigmoidoscopy every 3 to 5 years.

O   **People with elevated serum cholesterol have a greater risk for cardiovascular disease. Decreasing one's cholesterol by 1% reduces the risk of death due to heart disease by what percentage?**

2%.

O   **Death rates from CAD are down 40% from 15 years ago. What is the major cause of this reduction?**

Changes in eating and exercise habits.

O   **Match the poison with the antidote.**

1) Acetaminophen	a) Deferoxamine
2) Anticholinergics	b) Digoxin antibody
3) Arsenic	c) Dimercaptosuccinic acid or penicillamine
4) Carbon monoxide	d) Acetylcysteine (Mucomyst)
5) Digoxin	e) Oxygen
6) Iron	f) Atropine
7) Lead	g) Physostigmine
8) Mercury	h) Calcium EDTA or penicillamine
9) Methanol or ethylene glycol	i) Naloxone (Narcan)

10) Narcotics   j) Ethanol
11) Organophosphates   k) Penicillamine

Answers: (1) d, (2) g, (3) k, (4) e, (5) b, (6) a, (7) h, (8) c, (9) j, (10) i, and (11) f.

○   **What percentage of poisons have specific antidotes?**

5%.

○   **What percentage of deaths due to CHD can be attributed to smoking?**

25%. Smokers with CHD have a 70% higher incidence of MI and death than non-smokers with CHD.

○   **Is a nonsmoker who has lived with a smoker for 25 years at greater risk of lung cancer than a nonsmoker who has not lived with a smoker?**

Of course. The risk is 1.34 times as great as a person living in a smoke-free environment.

○   **What percentage of smokers who quit lapse back into their smoking habits?**

85%.

○   **What percentage of people over 65 live independently?**

80%. By age 85, only 54% of men and 38% of women still live independently at home.

○   **What is appropriate preventive immunization for a child with the sickle cell trait?**

All required immunizations plus Haemophilus B conjugate, hepatitis B immunization, and a pneumococcal vaccine. These children should also take folic acid supplements and prophylactic penicillin V until age 3.

○   **When should you first check a child's blood lead level?**

1 to 2 years old. By this age, children are mobile and can easily find tasty paint chips and other lead based objects.

○   **How much does the average teenager grow during adolescence?**

Teenagers generally increase their height by 15 to 20% and double their weight.

○   **At what age do most people first have intercourse?**

Males: 16.1 years. Females: 16.9 years.

○   **According to the CDC, what are 6 health behaviors in adolescents that are modifiable and will decrease their risk of morbidity and mortality?**

1) Using seatbelts   4) Not smoking
2) Not drinking and driving   5) Eating low fat diets
3) Using condoms if having sex   6) Aerobic exercise

○   **What percentage of teenage girls have eating disorders?**

20%.

○   **What is used to control outbreaks of meningococcal meningitis?**

Rifampin and ceftriaxone are used as chemoprophylaxis for contacts.

○   **How many prescriptions does the average 65 year old have?**

3 to 5. Over 80% of senior citizens have at least 1 chronic illness.

○   **What can elderly patients do to prevent falls?**

Remove clutter from house; remove throw rugs; insure good lighting; put non-slip patches in bathtub.

○   **At what age can routine Pap smears be discontinued?**

Age 70, if the patient has had several negative examinations. Cervical cancer reaches a plateau, so further screening is not necessary.

○   **Geographically, where is multiple sclerosis most prevalent?**

In the northern US. Migration to warmer climates does not seem to affect the disease. People born in the north will still have a higher incidence of the disease.

○   **What preventive measures would you recommend to a patient planning a trip to Mexico?**

Avoidance of water, ice, foods prepared in water, and raw or pre-peeled fruits and vegetables. Prophylactic antibiotics are not routinely recommended. However, if they are a necessity, Ciprofloxacin is the drug of choice. Otherwise, treatment with antibiotics should begin with the onset of symptoms, as should rehydration.

○   **Should pregnant women abstain from intercourse?**

There is no risk to mother or fetus if mother engages in sex with orgasm in the first 2 trimesters. In the third trimester, anorgasmic intercourse is safe until the 34th week. Intercourse should be avoided if there is bleeding.

○   **What percentage of lung cancer is related to smoking?**

80%.

○   **What types of cancer are more common in farmers?**

Cancer of the lip, Hodgkin's disease, leukemia, malignant melanoma, multiple myeloma, and prostate cancer.

○   **What cancer causes the most deaths in women?**

1) Lung cancer
2) Breast cancer
3) Colorectal cancer

○   **What are the three most common cancers in men?**

1) Skin cancer
2) Lung cancer
3) Colorectal cancer
4) Prostate cancer

○   **What cancer causes the most deaths in men?**

1) Lung cancer
2) Colorectal cancer
3) Prostate cancer

○   **Overall, cancer deaths have increased 7% between 1971 and 1991. What cancers have actually shown a decrease in death rates?**

Cancer of the bladder, colon, cervix, larynx, mouth, pharynx, stomach, testes, thyroid, uterus, and Hodgkin's disease.

○   **Why is it important to identify food service workers with furunculosis?**

Furunculosis is most commonly caused by coagulase-positive staphylococcus. Staphylococcal enterotoxin is a leading cause of food poisoning.

○   **What is the biggest risk factor for prostate cancer?**

Age. The median age for diagnosis of prostate cancer is 72.

○   **Name 7 risk factors for malignant melanoma.**

1) Fair skin
2) Sensitivity to sunlight
3) Excessive exposure to the sun
4) Dysplastic moles
5) 6 or more moles > 0.5 cm
6) Prior basal or squamous cell carcinoma
7) Parental history of skin cancer

○   **What percentage of melanomas occur in sun-exposed areas?**

Only 65%. A good screen of all surface area is important. In African American, Hispanic, and Asian patients, acral lentiginous melanomas are more common. Careful examination of subungual, palmar, and plantar surfaces is important in these populations.

○   **What percentage of American adults are obese?**

30 to 40%.

○   **What percentage of obesity can be attributed to genetics?**

25 to 30%.

○   **What percentage of obesity can be attributed to organic causes?**

1%.

○   **Which malignancies are more common in obese individuals?**

Endometrial cancer, breast cancer (postmenopausal), gallbladder cancer, biliary cancer, prostate cancer, and colorectal cancer.

○   **Obesity is a risk factor for what common diseases?**

CAD, NIDDM, HTN, left ventricular hypertrophy, sleep apnea, cholelithiasis, pulmonary emboli, and osteoarthritis.

○ **What is the risk of sudden death in morbidly obese patients compared to patients with normal body mass index (BMI)?**

15 to 30 times higher.

○ **How much blood must be lost to the GI system in order to be detected on hemoccult?**

20 mL/day. Healthy patients normally lose 0.5 to 2.0 mL/day.

○ **Why does moderate alcohol consumption decrease the risk of MIs?**

Moderate drinking (< 3 drinks a day) increases HDL.

○ **What is a 26 year old's target heart rate during exercise?**

Between 126 and 175. The target heart rate is 65 to 90% of the maximal heart rate. Maximal heart rate is 220 minus age.

○ **Which immunizations do healthy senior citizens need?**

Tetanus booster every 10 years, influenza vaccination every year, and a pneumococcal vaccination.

○ **How much aspirin should patients with known CHD take as a prophylactic measure?**

75 to 325 mg/day. In addition, men over the age of 40 with at least 1 risk factor for CHD should also take 75 to 325 mg/day. Patients with histories of TIAs require higher doses: 975 to 1500 mg/day.

○ **Besides aspirin, what actions can be taken to prevent stroke in patients with increased risk factors?**

Good control of the blood pressure and anticoagulation with warfarin in patients who have atrial fibrillation.

○ **Immunocompromised patients can safely be given which vaccines?**

Killed or inactivated vaccines:

1) Diphtheria   5) Enhanced inactivated polio
2) *H. influenzae*   6) Hepatitis
3) Influenza   7) Pertussis
4) Pneumococcal   8) Tetanus

It may be easier to remember the vaccines that should be avoided. The following are live, attenuated vaccines:

1) Oral polio   2) MMR

○ **Other than immunocompromised patients, who should not receive live vaccines?**

Pregnant women. Oral polio vaccine should be avoided in anyone in close contact with an immunocompromised person because of the virus's ability to spread.

❍   **A patient comes in for vaccinations and has a URI and a fever of 37.5°C. Can you administer vaccines to this patient?**

Yes. URI or gastrointestinal illness are not contraindications to vaccination. Fever may be as high as 38°C and the vaccine still administered. Likewise, use of antibiotics or recent exposure to illness is not a reason to delay vaccination.

❍   **When administering the Mantoux skin test to a person with HIV, what induration indicates a positive reaction?**

> 5 mm. In individuals with risk factors for TB, induration must be > 10 mm. For those with no risk factors, induration must be > 15 mm to be positive.

❍   **Influenza epidemics and pandemics are generally associated with which strain of influenza?**

Influenza A.

❍   **Amantadine is 70 to 90% effective in preventing which strain of influenza?**

Influenza A. Amantadine should be prescribed as chemoprophylaxis in immunocompromised patients who are not vaccinated or as a supplement to vaccination. It can also be given to healthy unvaccinated people who want to avoid the flu.

❍   **When should the influenza vaccine be given?**

In September or October, about 1 to 2 months before the influenza season begins. The vaccine, unlike amantadine, is protective against influenza A and B.

❍   **What is a contraindication to the administration of the influenza vaccine?**

A history of anaphylactic hypersensitivity to eggs or their products.

❍   **Which routine screenings should be performed on pregnant women?**

Hepatitis B, syphilis, rubella, gonorrhea, and other STDs. Women in high-risk categories should also be screened for HIV.

❍   **Diabetes is most common in which ethnic group?**

Hispanics. The prevalence in Hispanics is 1.7 to 2.4 times higher than in non-Hispanics; the death rate is also twice as high. Reasons for the high rate of disease in this group is attributed to increased incidence of obesity and hyperinsulinemia.

❍   **What is recommended in the prevention of hemorrhoids?**

Fiber supplements and stool softeners.

❍   **What is the diet recommended to reduce the risk of colon cancer?**

Decrease fat (especially saturated fat), increase fiber, increase cruciferous vegetables, decrease ETOH, and decrease smoked, salted, or nitrate-based foods.

❍   **What are the risk factors for colon cancer?**

Age over 50, familial polyposis (100%), ulcerative colitis, Crohn's disease, radiation exposure, benign adenomas, and previous history of colon cancer.

○ **What percentage of patients with gonococcal genital infections have concomitant *Chlamydia trichomatous* infections?**

45%. This is why treatment for gonorrhea includes ceftriaxone and doxycycline to cover both infections.

○ **A woman with condyloma acuminatum is how many times more likely to develop cervical cancer than a woman without this lesion?**

4 times more likely. These women should have yearly Pap smears and be screened for other STDs.

○ **Patients with cirrhosis or chronic active hepatitis should have what routine testing to screen for hepatomas?**

α-Fetoprotein should be measured every 6 months, and an ultrasound should be performed at the same time. These patients are at a higher risk for developing liver cancer.

○ **What are the risk factors for hernias?**

Obesity, heavy lifting, chronic cough, constipation, tumors, pregnancy, ascites, and other conditions which chronically increase intra-abdominal pressure.

○ **What medications are likely to exacerbate angle closure glaucoma?**

Anticholinergics, antihistamines, antidepressants, benzodiazepine, carbonic anhydrase inhibitors, CNS stimulants, phenothiazine, sympathomimetics, theophylline, and vasodilators.

○ **Which medications put patients at risk for hearing loss?**

Aminoglycoside, antineoplastic agents, loop diuretics, and salicylates.

○ **What nutritional deficiencies may lead to aphthous ulcers?**

B12, folate, and iron deficiencies.

○ **A 22 year old male, who has no significant medical history and is taking no medication, has of a creamy white coat on his tongue. The substance easily rubs off, revealing an erythematous base. What should you be concerned about?**

HIV. In a patient who has no obvious reason for having an overgrowth of oral candida, HIV should be suspected. Other causes for oral thrush overgrowth include cancer, systemic illness, neutropenia, diabetes, adrenal insufficiency, nutritional deficiencies, or an immunocompromised state.

○ **According to Holmes and Rahe, what are life's top 10 most stressful events?**

1) Death of spouse or child
2) Divorce
3) Separation
4) Institutional detention
5) Death of close family member
6) Major personal injury or illness
7) Marriage
8) Job loss
9) Marital reconciliation
10) Retirement

○ **When should RhoGAM (anti-Rh immunoglobulin) be used?**

Within 3 days of the birth of an Rh+ child (if the mother is Rh-). It should also be used in the event of any mixing of fetal and maternal blood (e.g., trauma). RhoGAM is safe because it does not pass the placenta barrier.

○   **What is the number one cause of death for African American males between the ages of 10 and 24?**

Firearm injury. The overall homicide rate for young men in the US is over 7 times that of the next developed country.

○   **Do intentional or unintentional causes account for more firearm-related deaths?**

Intentional causes account for 94% of firearm deaths, suicide for 48%, and homicide for 46%. Unintentional firearm injuries account for about 4%. Only 1% of firearm deaths occur as a result of legal intervention. The number of firearm related fatalities has more than doubled in the last 30 years.

○   **What are risk factors for homicide?**

Most homicide victims are killed by someone they know, someone of the same race, and usually during an argument or fight. Drugs and alcohol are important co-factors, as is the presence of a handgun.

○   **What are the relative risks for suicide and homicide if a gun is kept in the home?**

Suicide is 5 times more likely. Homicide is 3 times more likely. The victim is 43% more likely to be a member of the family than an intruder. In the case of domestic violence, a gun at home increases the risk of homicide 20 fold.

○   **In addition to the history, physical examination, laboratory tests, and collection of physical evidence, what needs to be done in cases of child sexual abuse?**

File a report with child protective services and law enforcement agencies. Provide emotional support to the child and family. Give a return appointment for follow up of STD cultures and testing for pregnancy, HIV, or syphilis as indicated. Assure follow up for psychological counseling by connecting the child/family to the appropriate services in your area.

MEDICAL MNEMONICS

Achondroplasia

Autosomal dominant
Cervical spine stenosis
Hydrocephalus
Orthopedic (tibial bowing)
Nasal bridge (low/flat)
Developmental delay (hypotonia)
Respiratory distress (b/c small chest or airway obstruction due to bony anomaly)
Old paternal age usually are related to it

Acne (causes or irritants)

Androgen
Bacteria
Cosmetics
Drugs
Emotional stress
Free fatty acid (in the skin)

Acute lymphoblastic leukemia

(poor prognostic factors)
Lymphoblast high
Younger than one year old
Male
Philadelphia marker
Hgb>10
Older than ten
Blood cells > 50,000
Lymph node enlarged
Anterior mediastinum masses
Spleen enlarged
T-cells
Induction > 4 weeks
Chromosome < 46

Addison's disease (clinical features)

Anorexia
Diarrhea
Dehydration
Increased K+
Skin pigmentation
Orthostatic hypotension
Na level is abnormal

ADHD (causes or associations)

Diet (malnutrition)
Exposed to toxin (lead poisoning)
Fetal alcohol syndrome
Iron deficiency
Congenital (genetics or metabolic)
Infection (brain or ears)
Traumatic brain injuries

Alcohol Withdrawal

(clinical features)
Epileptic activity
Tremors
Hallucination
Anxiety/anorexia
Nausea/vomiting
Organic brain changes (delirium)
Loss of memory/orientation

Allergic Rhinitis (complications)

Adenoidal hypertrophy
Loss of hearing
Loss of smell sensation
Ear infection
Red eyes
Gum/teeth anomaly
Itching
Chronic sinusitis
Speech delay

Allergy to milk protein

(clinical features)
Albumin is low
Blood loss (bloody stool)
Chronic diarrhea
Distended abdomen
Emesis
Failure to thrive

Angelman syndrome

Abnormal EEG
Neural-seizure d/o
Gait anomaly (puppet-like)
Epidermal hypopigmentation
Laughter
MR
Absent speech
Nystagmus
Sleep disorder

Apert syndrome

Apnea (choanal stenosis)
Premature closure of cranial sutures
(craniosynostosis)
Extremity (syndactyly, thumb anomalies)
Retarded
Tall forehead

Atherosclerosis (risk factors)

Smoking
Cholesterol
Low HDL
Elevated blood pressure
Relatives (positive family history)
Obesity
Stress/sex (male >female)
Inactivity
Sugar (diabetes)

Beckwith-Wiedemann syndrome

Weight >90th% at birth
Insulin-like growth factor-2 involved
Ear creases or dysplasia
Defected Umbilicus (omphalocele)
Enlarged liver
Macroglossia
Asymmetric extremities
Neonatal hypoglycemia
Neoplasm (Wilms tumor or hepatoblastoma)

Beta-blockers (contraindications for use)

Bradycardia
Low blood pressure
Obstructive lung diseases
CHF
Ketoacidosis (DKA)
Edema of lung
RAD/Raynaud phenomenon

Bloom syndrome

Breakage of chromosomes
Low birth weight
Over-pigmented (café-au-lait spots)
Ocular/otic/odontic anomalies
Malignancy potential
Skin erythema of face

Carpenter syndrome

Craniosynostosis
Acrocephaly
Retarded
Poly/syndactyly
Epicanthal folds
Narrow palate
Thorax (CHD)
Extremity anomaly
Renal/genital anomalies

Cat-eye syndrome

Coloboma of iris
Anal atresia
TAPVR
Emotional retardation with mild MR
Yellow(Jaundice) due to biliary atresia
Ear anomalies

Chaga's disease (clinical features)

Cardiomyopathy
Hepatosplenomegaly
Adenopathy
Gastrointestinal
Anemia

Cholestasis (medication etiologies)

Cimetidine
Hyperalimentation
OCP
L-asparaginase
Erythromycin
Sulfonamides
Tetracycline
Acetaminophen
Salicylates
INH, Iron
Seizure medications

Contraception

(absolute contraindication to use)

Coronary disease
Obesity/Hyperlipidemia Type II
Neoplasm of liver
Cerebrovascular disease
Estrogen-dependent tumors
Pregnancy
Thrombophlebitis
IDDM
Vaginal bleeding undiagnosed
Enzymes of liver increasing

Dehydration (assessment)

Decreased weight
Eyes sunken
Heart rate increased
Yucky skin (tenting, doughy)
Dry mucous membranes
Refill of capillary slow
Appearance (alert, awake, active)
Tears
Intake
Output (urine/diarrhea/emesis)
Na level

Ectopic pregnancy (risk factors)

Endometriosis
Congenital anomaly of tubes
Tubal surgery
Old abdominal scar
PID
In votro fertilization
Contraceptive pills

Fetal alcohol syndrome

Microcephaly
Abnormal facies (short fissures, smooth philtrum)
Thorax (murmur, TOF, coarctation, ribs)
Extremity (joint laxity, palmar creases, clinodactyly)
Retarded growth
Neural-MR
ADHD
Learning disorder

Fetal Rubella syndrome

(German measles-clinical features)

Mental retardation
Eyes (cataract)
Aortic coarctation or PDA
Skin rash (petechiae)
Liver (hepatitis)
Ears (deafness)
Small for gestational age

Fetal varicella syndrome

(clinical features)

Hypoplastic limbs
Epidermal scars
Retarded (MR)
Prenatal growth deficiency (IUGR)
Eye (retinitis)
Seizure

Fragile X syndrome

Fragile site
Retarded
Autistic/ADHD
Genital anomaly (macro-orchidism)
Increased mandible
Language problem
Ears (enlarged)

Gaucher's disease

Glucosidase (beta) deficiency
Autosomal recessive (Accumulation of lipid)
Urologic (renal involvement)
CNS (not for type I)
Hematologic (anemia/bleeding)
Enlarged spleen/liver (hepatosplenomegaly)
Respiratory (lung involvement)
Skeletal (osteoporosis/osteopenia)

Goiter (etiologies)

Grave's disease
Oral contraceptives
Infection
Tumors
Environmental
Receptor defects (Resistance to thyroxin)

Heart sounds
(conditions with increased S2 split)

Septal defect (ASD)
Pulmonary embolus
Left ventricular paced beats
Incomplete pulmonic stenosis
Total right BBB

Henoch-Schönlein Purpura (HSP) (clinical features)

Hematuria/hematemesis
Skin rashes
Pain of joints/abdomen

Hypercalcemic crisis
(clinical features)

Anorexia
Belly pain
Coma
Delirium
Emesis
Fatigue/weakness

Hyper Ig E syndrome
(clinical features)

Infection
Growth retardation
Eczema

Hyperkalemia (etiologies)

Kidney
Adrenal dysfunction
Lysis of cells (transfusion, tumors)
Excessive intake
Medications (Digoxin, Heparin, PVK)
Insufficient renin
Acidosis

Hyperkalemia (treatment)

Albuterol (hypokalemia is one of the side
   effects of this drug)
Bicarbonate
Calcium
Dialysis
Exchanger (Kayexalate resin)
Flow of urine (diuretics)
Glucose/insulin
Hyperventilation

Hypokalemia (medication etiologies)

Aminoglycoside
B-amphotericin
Corticosteroids/cisplatin
Diuretics
Epinephrine

Intracranial hemorrhage
(etiologies)

Infection (herpes)
Newborn prematurity
Trauma
Recent thrombosis (venous sinus)
AVM (arterial-venous malformation)
Coagulopathy
Renal arterial anomalies (hypertension)
Aneurysm
Neoplasm of CNS
Infarction (cerebral)
Abuse of cocaine
L-Asparaginase

Lead poisoning (clinical features)

Learning disability
Encephalopathy
Anemia
Developmental

Marfan syndrome

Myopia
Aortic dilatation/insufficiency
Ratio reduction of upper/lower segment
Familial (autosomal dominant)
Arachnodactyly
Narrow face/palate
Stature (thin tall); scoliosis

Maternal serum AFP
(elevated MSAFP)

Multiple gestations
Spina bifida (NTDs)
Abdominal wall defects (Omphalocele, gastroschisis)
Fetal death
Placental anomalies

Metabolic acidosis
(with abnormal anion gap)

Alcohol
Non-ketotic coma
Iron/INH
Organic acid
Nephritic (renal) failure
Glycolates
Aspirin
Penicillin/paraldehyde

Metabolic acidosis
(with normal anion gap)

Meds (nephrotoxins)
Extra chloride from TPN
Tubular acidosis
Adrenal insufficiency
Bowel fistula
Ostomy (ureteroenterostomy)
Loose stool (diarrhea)
Intake of chloride
Carbonic anhydrase inhibitors

Mumps (parotitis) (complications)

Pancreatitis
Arthritis
Renal (nephritis)
Orchitis/Oophoritis
Thyroiditis
Intracranial (meningitis)
Thrombocytopenia
Intrauterine infection
Sensorineural hearing loss

Myocardial Infarction (management)

Tissue plasminogen activator
Heparin
Rest in bed
Oxygen
Morphine
Beta-blocker
Urinokinase/streptokinase
Salicylate (aspirin)

Nephrotic syndrome (clinical features)

Nail whitening
Edema
Proteinuria
Hyperlipidemia
Reduction of albumin
Organomegaly
Thrombosis
Infection (peritonitis)
Calcium loss

Neurofibromatosis type-1
(diagnostic criteria)

Cafe-au-lait spots
Axillary freckling
Fibroma (Neurofibroma)
Eye (Lisch nodules)
Skeletal (scoliosis, bowing legs)
Pedigree (positive family Hx)
Optic
Tumors (optic tumor = optic pathway Glioma)

Parrot fever (clinical features)

Pneumonitis
Adenopathy
Rashes
Rigid neck (meningismus)
Organomegaly
Throat (pharyngitis)

Pneumothorax (risk factors)

Tall stature
Thin body mass
Twenties of age
Tobacco smoking
Trauma
Tumors

Poisoning (contraindications for charcoal use)

Cyanide
Hydrocarbon
Acid/alkali
Relative small compounds
Charged (iron, heavy metals)
Organophosphate
Alcohol
Lithium

Polycystic ovarian syndrome
(clinical features)

Obesity
Virilization
Anovulation
Resistance to insulin (diabetes)
Increased hair
Androgen increase
No period

Primary adrenal insufficiency
(etiologies)

Addison's disease
ACTH resistance
Adrenoleukodystrophy
Adrenal hypoplasia

Psoriasis (medication triggers)

Steroids
Chloroquine
Aspirin (NSAIDs)
Lithium
Esmolol (beta-blockers)

Pyelonephritis
(clinical features in newborn)

Poor feeding
Yellow (Jaundice)
Emesis
Lethargy
Odorous urine

Rhabdomyolysis (evaluation)

Myoglobinuria
Urinalysis
Serum potassium
Creatinine
Lysis sign on CBC (hemolysis)
Enzyme (CPK) increase

Sarcoidosis (clinical features)

Granuloma
Rashes
Adenopathy
Noncaseating
Uveitis
Lung infiltration
Organomegaly
Malaise
Arthritis

Scleroderma (pathogenesis)

Skin as major target
Collagen glycosylation anomaly
Laminin auto-antibodies
Endothelin anomaly
Raynaud phenomenon
Organ involvement

Splenomegaly (etiologies)

Sickle Cell Anemia
Portal Hypertension
Lupus
Enzyme Deficiencies (Metabolic)
EBV Infection
Neoplastic (Leukemia/Lymphoma)

Sturge-Weber syndrome

Seizure
Trigeminal hemangioma
Unilateral eye involvement
Retarded (MR)
Glaucoma
Ear anomalies

Supraventricular tachycardia
(management)

Adenosine
Beta-blockers
Calcium blockers
Digoxin
Electrocardioversion

Trisomy 18

Extra chromosome 18
IQ low (MR)
Growth retardation (IUGR)
Hypertonia
Thorax (small chest/heart defects)
Eye/ear/extremities
Eating problem (always requires NGF)
Ninety percent die within first year

Turner syndrome

Thoracic aortic stenosis/coarctation
Underdeveloped gonads
Residual lymphedema
Neck webbing
Endocrine (GH and TSH deficiency)
Renal anomaly
Sexuality (delayed puberty)

Viral hepatitis (clinical features)
Hepatomegaly
Encephalopathy
Prodromic fever
Ascites
Thrive failure
Obstruction
Coagulopathy
Yellow (jaundice)
Tumor potential
Edema
Splenomegaly

Von Hippel-Lindau syndrome
Vision loss
Ocular (retinal angioma)
Nephritic (renal cell carcinoma)
Hemangioblastoma of brain (cerebella)
Increased ICP
Pheochromocytoma
Pancreas cyst
Ectopic erythropoietin
Liver cyst

RANDOM PEARLS

O   **What organ is most commonly injured as a result of a blunt trauma?**

The spleen. Generalized abdominal pain with radiation to the left shoulder subsequent to blunt trauma indicates splenic rupture (Kehr's sign). Splenic rupture can also occur following infectious mononucleosis.

O   **When performing a neurological examination on a patient with a suspected anterior dislocation of the shoulder, what sign should be monitored and documented?**

Sensation over the lateral deltoid. In anterior dislocations of the shoulder, the radial nerve may be easily torn. Intact sensation to the lateral deltoid will indicate an intact radial nerve.

O   **Boggy blue turbinates and eosinophils indicate what condition?**

Allergic rhinitis.

O   **What are the major sequelae of untreated streptococcal infections?**

Acute glomerulonephritis unrelated to treatment and rheumatic heart disease.

O   **Which type of rhinitis is associated with anxious patients?**

Vasomotor rhinitis. This is a non-allergic rhinitis of unknown etiology that involves nasal vascular congestion.

O   **A patient treated with cyclophosphamide should be monitored every two to four weeks for what condition?**

Bone marrow toxicity—most commonly leukopenia. CBCs should be obtained every 2 to 4 weeks. Urinalysis is also important for screening for hemorrhagic cystitis. Cyclophosphamide should be administered in the morning to reduce the amount present in the bladder over night.

O   **ß-Blockers, calcium channel blockers, and Digoxin are all used as prophylactic treatment for preventing paroxysmal SVTs. These drugs slow conduction through the AV node. This treatment is contraindicated in patients with which type of arrhythmia?**

Tachyarrhythmia because of accessory pathways. Digoxin is also contraindicated in multifocal atrial tachycardia.

O   **What are the two main causes of atrial fibrillation?**

CAD (40 to 50%) and hyperthyroidism (15%).

O   **What percentage of the population will display a PVC within a 24 hour period?**

50 to 80%. However, the PVCs are generally singular and benign. An individual can have 100 PVCs per day or 5 per hour and still be considered healthy.

O   **What substances increase PVCs?**

Caffeine, alcohol, and tobacco.

○   **What are the three possible schedules from which to choose when deciding the set of polio vaccines a child needs?**

1) 2 doses of IPV followed by 2 doses of OPV
2) 4 doses of IPV
3) 4 doses of OPV

○   **A child is born to an HBsAg-negative mother. Which vaccine should he receive?**

Recombivax (2.5) or Engerix-B (10). The second dose should be given at least one month after the first, and the third dose at least two months later (but not before the age of 6 months).

○   **An unvaccinated 13-year-old comes to your office. Should he receive a hepatitis vaccine if there are no known carriers in his family?**

Yes.

○   **When is the MMR vaccine given?**

The first is given at 12 to 15 months of age and the second at 4 to 6 years. Children who have not yet received the second dose should not receive it after they are 11 or 12 years old.

○   **How common is vaccine-associated paralytic polio?**

1/2.4 million cases.

○   **Which polio vaccine can induce secondary transmission of vaccine virus?**

OPV.

○   **How long do sperm stay in the vagina postcoitus?**

At least 72 hours; however, sperm are only motile for 6 hours. When performing a rape kit, it is important to test for acid phosphatase. This enzyme is present for 24 hours and confirms that ejaculation has occurred.

○   **A 44-year-old man has lost sensorineural hearing in his left ear. Better hearing will be displayed by which ear in the Weber test?**

The right. The damaged ear is less prone to detect sound waves via any route.

○   **What antibiotic most commonly produces diarrhea secondary to *Clostridium difficile*?**

Ampicillin. Vancomycin or Metronidazole are the antibiotics of choice.

○   **What is the most common anatomical abnormality associated with chronic urinary tract infections?**

Vesicoureteral reflux.

○   **Which malignant neoplasm has the highest rate of spontaneous regression?**

Neuroblastoma. This neoplasm occurs predominantly before the age of 6. Although the rate of spontaneous regression is high, the overall survival rate is only 30%, because of the spread of the disease before it is detected.

○   **What is the first line of therapy for a migraine headache with prodromal symptoms?**

Ergotamine derivatives. Second-line therapies include Sumatriptan (Imitrex), phenothiazine, NSAIDs, anti-inflammatories, and opiates.

○   **Patients with exercise-induced asthma will most likely trigger their asthma with what kind of exercise?**

High intensity exercise for more than 5 to 6 minutes.

○   **A patient who was recently hit in the eye during a bar room brawl complains of diplopia when looking up. The injured eye does not appear able to look up. What is the diagnosis?**

Orbital blowout fracture with entrapment of inferior rectus or inferior oblique. Always test extraocular movements in patients with blunt trauma to the eye.

○   **What agent usually causes anaphylactic reactions?**

Contrast media. Other causative agents include NSAIDs, thiamine, and codeine. Conversely, parenteral penicillin and hymenoptera stings are the most common causes of anaphylactic reactions. Anaphylactic reactions are IgE-mediated reactions in previously sensitized people, while anaphylactoid reactions are due to direct release of mediators, including histamine and leukotriene.

○   **What is the most common joint dislocation?**

Anterior shoulder dislocations account for half of all joint dislocations. They occur with abduction and external rotation.

○   **15 to 20% of pregnancies result in natural abortions. What is the number one cause of natural abortions?**

Genetic defects (50%), usually the result of an abnormal number of chromosomes.

○   **In spontaneous abortions, pain is most often midline and crampy. In ectopic pregnancies, it is acute, unilateral, and severe. Does pain caused by a threatened abortion occur before or after bleeding has begun?**

After.

○   **What organism is commonly found in infected wounds caused by animal bites?**

Pasteurella multocida. The second most common organism is *Staphylococcus aureus.*

○   **What organism is typically associated with CNS involvement in an AIDS patient?**

Toxoplasmosis.

○   **Meningitis in AIDS patients is frequently caused by what organisms?**

Cryptococcus.

〇   **What life-threatening infection is most commonly associated with AIDS patients?**

Pneumocystis carinii pneumonia (PCP).

〇   **What often causes a change in visual acuity in AIDS patients?**

Cytomegalovirus.

〇   **Which type of malignancy is most commonly associated with AIDS?**

Kaposi's sarcoma, followed by non-Hodgkin's lymphoma.

〇   **Where are Kaposi's sarcoma lesions found?**

Everywhere—inside and out. They typically occur on the face, neck, arms, back, thighs, and in the lungs, lymphatic system, and GI system.

〇   **How many years does a patient usually live after being diagnosed with HIV?**

8 to 10 years. Most patients eventually die from PCP.

〇   **A patient with AIDS presents with a grayish-white plaque on the lateral borders of her tongue that do not scrape off. Diagnosis?**

Hairy leukoplakia.

〇   **How is jaundice diagnosed in African American patients?**

By examining the edges of the cornea and the posterior hard palate. Darkly pigmented patients often have subconjunctival fat that results in yellowing the sclera.

〇   **How does pallor appear in a black patient?**

The skin is yellow brown or gray due to the loss of the underlying red tones. The conjunctiva appears pale.

〇   **What parts of the pulmonary system are affected by asbestosis?**

The pleura and peritoneum. Asbestosis increases the risk of mesotheliomata. It also causes pneumoconioses that invade the lungs.

〇   **What is Spanierman's sign?**

Blood under the nails. This indicates nose bleeds due to nose picking. Bleeding in such cases is generally from the Kiesselbach's plexus.

〇   **What is the most common cause of hypercalcemia?**

Hyperparathyroidism. This condition accounts for 60% of ambulatory hypercalcemics.

〇   **What are the most common causes of nongonococcal urethritis?**

Chlamydia trachomatis. Ureaplasma urealyticum is another common cause.

〇   **What is the most common clinical manifestation of disseminated gonococcal infection?**

Gonococcal arthritis-dermatitis syndrome. Arthritis, a pustular or papular rash, and tenosynovitis are exhibited with this syndrome.

○   **What is the most common cause of epididymitis?**

Chlamydia trachomatis in men under 35 years old. E. Coli in prepubertal and older patients.

○   **What is the Jarisch-Herxheimer reaction?**

Headache, fever, myalgia, hypotension, and an increased severity of syphilis symptoms that occurs after taking benzathine penicillin G for the treatment of syphilis. The reaction may result in neurological, auditory, or visual changes.

○   **What strain of influenza is more common in adults? In children?**

Adults: Influenza A. Children: Influenza B.

○   **What strain of influenza is most virulent?**

Influenza A.

○   **What are the 4 degrees of frostbite?**

First degree: Erythema and edema
Second degree: Blister formation
Third degree: Necrosis
Fourth degree: Gangrene

○   **A patient with polyuria, a low urine osmolality, and a high serum osmolality is given vasopressin but no change in osmolality is noted. Which type of diabetic insipidus does she have?**

Nephrogenic. Vasopressin will not help because the distal renal tubules are refractory to antidiuretic hormone. In central DI, the pathology involves a problem with the production of ADH in the posterior pituitary. An increase in urine osmolality of at least 50% will occur with vasopressin administration if the problem is central DI.

○   **What organisms are usually implicated in the development of diverticulitis?**

E. coli and B. fragilis.

○   **What organisms are typically responsible for causing bacterial conjunctivitis?**

Staphylococcal. The second most common are Streptococcal.

○   **A patient presents with a painful eye, blurred vision, and conjunctivitis. Upon slitlamp examination, you detect a dendritic ulcer. What is the most likely cause of this patient's symptoms?**

Herpes. This type of infection probably occurs secondary to corneal abrasions or corticosteroid eye drops. Treat with idoxuridine. If the eye has a bacterial superinfection, prescribe topical antibiotics.

○   **What is Hampton's hump?**

A chest x-ray finding associated with pulmonary embolisms. It is an infiltrate with a "hump" pointed toward the hilus and a clearing with a vascular distribution.

○   **What is the most common cause of portal hypertension in adults? In children?**

Adults: Cirrhosis of the liver. Children: Extrahepatic portal vein occlusion. (This is also the second most common cause of portal hypertension in adults.)

○   **The portal vein receives blood from what 2 tributaries?**

The splenic vein and the superior mesenteric vein.

○   **Herpangina is caused by what virus?**

Coxsackievirus group A. A sore throat, fever, malaise, and vesicular lesions on the posterior pharynx or the soft palate are prevalent with this disease.

○   **What percentage of elderly have sleep apnea?**

40%.

○   **What is the most common cause of sleep apnea in adults?**

An upper airway obstruction, generally by the tongue or enlarged tonsils. A medulla that is not responsive to CO_2 buildup is the most common cause in children. Obstruction by the tongue or enlarged tonsils also induces sleep apnea.

○   **What is a complication of central sleep apnea in children?**

SIDS. Affected children develop morning cyanosis. However, children can be treated with theophylline.

○   **A patient presents with arms extended and fingers spread apart. Her extremities are flexing and extending in a static-kinetic tremor. This tremor can be associated with what disease?**

Hyperthyroidism.

○   **A patient presents with a resting tremor, decreased range of motion, bradykinesia, and a mask-like face. What is the diagnosis?**

Parkinsonism.

○   **What are the adverse side effects of phenylthiazine therapy?**

Parkinsonism, dystonia, and akathisia (i.e., the neuroleptic triad). These side effects can be treated with antiparkinsonian medication.

○   **Hyperglycemia can cause osmotic hyponatremia because glucose draws water into the intravascular space which thereby dilutes sodium levels. What formula should be used to correct the sodium level?**

Add 1.6 mEq for every 100 mg/dL of glucose above normal.

○   **Hypovolemia is a major concern when treating a patient with hypernatremia. What is the calculation for determining water deficit?**

Water deficit = $\dfrac{(0.6 \times weight) \times (Na - 140)}{140}$

○   **What is the acid base disorder in the following situation?**

pH = 7.29, pCO2 = 30, HCO3- = 15, Na = 131, and Cl = 94

This is a primary metabolic acidosis with an elevated ion gap.

○   **What is the most common cause of secondary lymphedema?**

Malignant metastases to the lymph nodes. Lymphatic fibrosis secondary to surgery is another cause.

○   **What organisms most often induce lymphedema?**
Staphylococcal or ß-hemolytic Streptococcal.

○   **Cricothyroidotomy is not recommended in children under what age?**

10 years.

○   **Is succinylcholine a depolarizing or a non-depolarizing neuromuscu-lar block-ing agent?**

Depolarizing. Succinylcholine is the only commonly used depolarizing agent. It binds to postsynaptic acetylcholine receptors, thereby causing depolarization. The material is enzymatically degraded by pseudocholinesterase (serum cholinesterase). Onset is within 1 minute; paralysis last 7 to 10 minutes.

○   **What is the rationale for pre-treating a patient with a subpolarizing (defasciculating) dose of a non-depolarizing agent prior to treatment with succinyl-choline?**

Attenuates fasciculations from succinylcholine-induced depolarization. This may de-crease subsequent muscle pain. Increased intragastric and intraocular pressure is associated with the administration of succinylcholine.

○   **What dosage of midazolam (Versed) causes a loss of consciousness and amnesia during rapid sequence induction?**

0.1 mg/kg. 5 mg is effective for most people.

○   **What dosage of thiopental should be prescribed during rapid sequence induction?**

~ 4 mg/kg.

○   **Loss of consciousness usually occurs within 15 seconds after thiopental is administered. What is the usual duration of action?**

2 to 30 minutes, depending on the source. Under 5 minutes is commonly referenced.

○   **What is the "defasciculating" or the "priming" dose of vecuronium?**

~ 0.01 mg/kg.

○   **What dose of vecuronium should be administered for paralysis (no "prim-ing")?**

0.15 to 0.20 mg/kg.

○   **What is the "defasciculating" or the "priming" dose of pancuronium (Pavulon)?**

0.015 mg/kg. About 1 mg is a common adult dose.

❍   *Dermacentor andersoni* (wood tick) **is a pesky arthropod associated with 4 tick-borne illnesses! Name these illnesses and the cause of each.**

Rocky Mountain spotted fever is caused by *Rickettsia rickettsii*; *Dermacentor andersoni* is a vector.

Tick paralysis is caused by a neurotoxin. The symptoms, consisting of ascending paralysis with decrease or loss of DTRs, are similar to those associated with Guillain-Barré syndrome.

Q fever is caused by *Coxiella burnetii* (a Rickettsiae).

Colorado tick fever is caused by an arbovirus.

❍   **Describe the AIDS dementia complex, which is also known as HIV-I encephalopathy.**

A progressive disease caused directly by HIV-I. It is present in one-third of AIDS patients and is character-ized by recent memory impairment, concentration deficit, elevated DTRs, seizures, and frontal release signs.

❍   **What is the most common cause of focal encephalitis in AIDS patients?**

Toxoplasma gondii.

❍   **Ethylene glycol is the alcohol that is present with hypocalcemia in one-third of the cases. Where does the calcium go?**

Oxalic acid is one of the metabolites of ethylene glycol. Calcium precipitates with oxalate and forms calcium oxalate crystals. The positive birefringent calcium oxalate dihydrate crystals are pathognomonic of this inges-tion.

❍   **What is the LD50 for falling in adults?**

48 feet.

❍   **A laryngeal fracture is suggested by noting the hyoid bone elevated above what cervical level on an x-ray?**

C3.

❍   **Describe the action and side effects of diazoxide.**

Action begins within 1 to 2 minutes and lasts up to 12 hours. Side effects may include nausea, vomiting, fluid retention, and hy-perglycemia. Diazoxide is a direct arterial vasodilator. It is contraindicated in patients with aortic dissection or angina.

❍   **What species of *Plasmodium* is resistant to chloroquine?**

Falciparum.

❍   **Where in the airway are foreign bodies usually lodged in children older than 1 year?**

In the lower airway.

❍   **At what age do most children most commonly present with intestinal malrotation? Also, what are common complications, signs, and symptoms?**

Malrotation usually occurs in children under 12 months old. Volvulus is a common complication. Signs and symptoms include vomiting, blood-streaked stools, and abdominal pain.

○ **Name two causes of toxic epidermal necrolysis (TEN).**

1) Drugs or chemicals typically cause TEN in adults. It is characterized by cleavage at the derma-epidermal junction.

2) SSSS usually causes TEN in children under age 5. It results in intraepidermal cleavage beneath the stratum granulosum.

○ **Describe the presentation of SSSS.**

It begins after URI or purulent conjunctivitis. Initially, the lesions are tender, erythematous, and scarlatiniform. They are usually found on the face, neck, axillae, and groin. Later, the skin peels off in sheets with lateral pressure (Nikolsky's sign).

○ **What is appropriate treatment for toxic epidermal necrolysis?**

Treat skin loss as you would a partial thickness burn. However, do not use silver sulfadiazine. Because adults can have large fluid loss, admit patients with over 10% BSA to a burn unit. Treat SSSS patients with IV penicillinase-resistant penicillin.

○ **Which of the following drugs may not be effec-tive for treating bullous impetigo: erythromycin, amoxicillin, cefaclor, or doxycycline?**

Amoxicillin.

○ **Methanol intoxication causes early death as a result of:**

Respiratory arrest. The pathophysiology is unknown.

○ **What nerve is usually injured in glenohumeral dislocation?**

Axillary nerve.

○ **Permanent pacemakers have a coding system of five letters. The first let-ter signi-fies the chamber paced. What does the second letter signify?**

Chamber sensed.

○ **Describe the mechanism and cause of a boutonniere deformity.**

Secondary to rupture of the extensor apparatus of the PIP joint. The cause of the injury is a PIP joint which is flexed, and a DIP joint which is hyperextended. Treated by splinting the PIP joint in full extension.

○ **What type of cyanosis is present in a patient who, according to ABG results, has a low oxygen saturation?**

Central.

○ **What is peripheral cyanosis?**

The extremities are discolored but ABG reveals normal oxygen saturation, i.e., shunting or increased O2 extraction is occurring.

○   **Name the four causes of central cyanosis with decreased SaO2?**

1) Decreased PaO2 or decreased O2 diffusion
2) Hypoventilation
3) V-Q mismatch, pulmonary shunting
4) Dysfunctional hemoglobin, including sickle cell crisis and drug-induced hemoglobinopathies

Note: Hb-CO does not cause cyanosis, although a cherry red appearance of skin and mucous membranes can suggest cyanosis.

○   **A pulmonary embolism causes which type of cyanosis?**

Central cyanosis. However, secondary shock and right-heart failure can lead to periph-eral cyanosis.

○   **What is a positive Chvostek's sign?**

A twitch in the corner of the mouth which occurs when the facial nerve, in front of the ear, is tapped.   It is present in approximately 10 to 30% of normal individuals. Eyelid muscle contraction resulting from the Chvostek's maneuver generally indicates hypocalcemia.

○   **What is Trousseau's sign and when is it exhibited?**

A carpal spasm induced when a blood pressure cuff on the upper arm maintains an above-systolic pressure for approximately 3 minutes. Fingers become spastically extended at the interphalangeal joints and flexed at the metacarpophalangeal joints. Trousseau's sign is a more reliable indicator of hypocalcemia than is Chvostek's sign. It is also indicative of hypomagnesemia, severe alkalosis, and strychnine poisoning.

○   **Activated charcoal is not an effective treatment for which poisonous substances?**

Alcohols, ions, acids, and bases.

○   **What is the most common conduction disturbance in acute myocardial infarction?**

First degree AV block.

○   **What is the most common foot fracture?**

Calcaneus (60%). Talus comes in at a distant second.

○   **Where does a metatarsal fracture most commonly occur?**

At the base of the fifth metatarsal and is called a Jones' fracture.

○   **What tendons are involved in de Quervain's tenosynovitis?**

The abductor pollicis and the extensor pollicis brevis. Diagnosis is confirmed with a positive Finkelstein's test.

○   **Describe Dupuytren's contracture.**

A contraction of the longitudinal bands of the palmar aponeurosis.

○   **What is the most common form of anorectal abscess?**

Perianal abscess. Anorectal abscesses are usually mixed infections (i.e., both gram-negative and anaerobic organisms). Fistula formation is a frequent complication.

○   **What is the most common rhythm disturbance in a pediatric arrest?**

Bradycardia.

○   **How long does it take to prepare type-specific saline cross-matched blood?**

10 minutes.

○   **Describe the common features of a slipped femoral capital epiphysis.**

Injury usually occurs in adolescence. The rupture typically presents with knee or thigh pain and a painful limp. Frequently hip motion is limited, particularly internal rotation. Evaluation is aided by anteroposterior and frogleg lateral films of both hips.

○   **How should you treat torsade de pointes?**

Accelerate the heart rate and shorten the duration of ventricular repolarization. This may be accomplished with isoproterenol, magnesium sulfate, and temporary pacing. Avoid IA antiarrythmics (quinidine, procainamide and disopyramide), tricyclic antidepressants, and phenothiazine as they will increase or prolong repolarization and thereby exacerbate torsade de pointes.

○   **Dobutamine administered in moderate doses induces what cardiovascular effects?**

Decreased peripheral resistance, pulmonary occlusive pressure, and inotropic stimulation of the heart.

○   **What concerns are associated with anterior dislocation of the shoulder?**

Axillary nerve injury, axillary artery injury (geriatric patients), compression fracture of the humeral head (Hillsack's deformity), a rotator cuff tear, fractures of the anterior glenoid lip, and fractures of the greater tuberosity.

○   **Describe Galeazzi's fracture/dislocation.**

A radial shaft fracture with dislocation of the distal radioulnar joint.

○   **Describe the clinical characteristics of carboxyhemoglobin concentrations, specifically for ranges of 10 to 70%.**

10%: Frontal headache
20%: Headache and dyspnea
30%: Nausea, dizziness, visual disturbance, fatigue, and impaired judgment
40%: Syncope and confusion
50%: Coma and seizures
60%: Respiratory failure and hypotension
70%: May be lethal

○   **What is the appropriate treatment for cyanide poisoning?**

Amyl nitrite and sodium nitrite IV, followed by sodium thiosulfate IV.

○   **Which organisms produce focal nervous system pathology via an exotoxin?**

Clostridium diphtheriae, *Clostridium botulinum*, *Clostridium tetani*, *Staphylococcus aureus* plus wood and dog ticks (*Dermacentor* A and B).

○   **What are the signs and symptoms of diphtheria?**

Acute onset of exudative pharyngitis, high fever, and malaise. A pseudomembrane may form in the oropharynx with possible respiratory compromise. Powerful exotoxins directly affect the heart, kidneys, and nervous system. Diphtheria infection may lead to paralysis of the intrinsic and extrinsic eye muscles, which may be confused with bulbar palsy caused by *Clostridium botulinum*. Botulism does not cause fever.

○   **Describe botulism intoxication.**

Acute food poisoning caused by *Clostridium botulinum*. Neurologic symptoms usually occur within 24 to 48 hours of ingestion of contaminated foods. Muscle paralysis and weakness typically spread rapidly, involving all muscles of the trunk and extremities.

○   **Describe Guillain-Barré syndrome?**

A lower motor neuron disease which commonly affects people in their thirties and forties. Symptoms include ascending weakness in the legs and arms. A sensory component may be present. Bulbar muscles are usually involved late in the course of the disease. Reflexes are affected early. Paralysis can progress rapidly; recovery is usually slow, but it is almost always complete.

○   **What formula should be used to calculate the fluid requirements for resuscitation of a burn victim?**

The Parkland formula: 2 to 4 mL/kg/% area burned/day. One half of this is given in the first 8 hours, and the second half is given over the next 16 hours.

○   **Poor prognostic signs upon admission for a patient with pancreatitis include:**

1) Age over 55 years
2) Glucose levels greater than 200 mg/dL
3) LDH level greater than 700 IU/L
4) WBC count greater than 16,000
5) SGOT level greater than 250 U/L

Note: No amylase involvement!

○   **Poor prognostic signs 48 hours after admission for a patient with pancreatitis include:**

1) Hematocrit down more than 10%
2) Rise in BUN more than 5 mg/dL
3) Declining cal-cium level to less than 8 mg/dL
4) PaO_2 less than 60 mm Hg
5) Fluid accumulation over 6 L and base deficit greater than 4 mEq/L

Note: No amylase involvement!

○   **What is the best test for determining acute cholecystitis?**

Radionuclide scan of the biliary tree.

○   **What pain medications are theoretically contraindicated for the treatment of pain arising from acute diverticulitis?**

Codeine and morphine. Their use may increase intraluminal colonic pressure. Meperidine (Demerol) is a good substitute because it inhibits segmental contraction of the colon.

O   **What test should be performed to confirm the diagnosis of Boerhaave's syndrome?**

An esophagram. A water soluble contrast medium should be used in place of barium to confirm the diagnosis.

O   **A patient presents with Mallory-Weiss syndrome. A Sengstaken-Blakemore tube is considered to control the hemorrhage. What prior problem could a patient have had that would prevent its use?**

Hiatal hernia. Neither proper placement of the balloon not proper traction can be attained in such individuals.

O   **What are the signs and symptoms of Boerhaave's syndrome?**

Substernal and left sided chest pain with a history of forceful vomiting, leading to spontaneous esophageal rupture.

O   **What is the most common cause of intestinal obstruction?**

Adynamic ileus.

O   **What are the most common causes of small bowel obstruction?**

Adhesions, followed by hernias.

O   **What are the most common causes of large bowel obstruction?**

Carcinoma, followed by volvulus and sigmoid diverticulitis.

O   **What is the most common cause of upper GI tract hemorrhage?**

Duodenal ulcers.

O   **What layers of the bowel wall and mesentery are affected by regional enteritis?**

All layers.

O   **Which hernia is the most common in women?**

Inguinal hernia. It is also the most common in men.

O   **What are Kanavel's four cardinal signs of infectious digital flexor tenosynovitis?**

1) Tenderness along the tendon sheath
2) Finger held in flexion
3) Pain on passive extension of the finger
4) Finger swelling

O   **What symptoms are associated with regional enteritis?**

Fever, abdominal pain, weight loss, and diarrhea. Fistulas, fissures, and abscesses may also be noted. Ulcerative colitis, on the other hand, usually presents with bloody diarrhea.

○   **What organism most commonly causes subacute infectious endocarditis?**

S. viridans.

○   **Subacute bacterial endocarditis (SBE) most commonly affects which valve?**

The mitral valve. The aortic valve is the second most commonly involved valve. Rheumatic fever is the most probable cause of valvular damage associated with SBE. Mitral stenosis is a very common predisposing factor in SBE. Drug addicts tend to develop right-sided SBE, usually involving the tricuspid valve.

○   **What organism most commonly induces acute infectious endocarditis?**

Staphylococcus aureus.

○   **What antibiotic is a good choice for the empiric treatment of acute infectious endocarditis?**

Gentamycin, 1 to 1.5 mg/kg every 8 hours for normal adults, and oxacillin, 12 g/day.

○   **How should you treat a patient who has been bitten by a wild raccoon?**

Wound care, tetanus prophylaxis, RIG, 20 IU/kg (1/2 at bite site and 1/2 IM), and HDCV, 1 cc IM.

○   **Describe the skin lesions found in a patient with disseminated gonococcemia.**

Umbilicated pustules with red halos.

○   **Describe the skin lesions associated with a *Pseudomonas aeruginosa* infection.**

Pale, erythematous lesions 1 cm in size with an ulcerated necrotic center.

○   **What is the fundamental pathology of sickle cell disease?**

Valine is substituted for glutamic acid in the sixth amino acid of the ß-chain.

○   **Describe the intracorporeal dissipation of the rabies virus.**

The virus spreads centripetally up the peripheral nerve into the CNS. The incubation period for rabies is usually 30 to 60 days with a range of 10 days to 1 year. Transmission usually occurs via infected secretions, saliva, or infected tissue. Stages of the disease include upper respiratory tract infection symptomatology, followed by encephalitis. The brainstem is affected last.

○   **What animals are the most prevalent vectors of rabies in the world? In the US?**

Worldwide, the dog is the most common carrier of rabies. In the US, the skunk has become primary carrier. In descending order bats, raccoons, cows, dogs, foxes, and cats are also sources.

○   **What is the IM treatment for adult streptococcal pharyngitis?**

1.2 million units of benzathine penicillin G. Use 0.6 million units of benzathine penicillin G for children under 27 kg.

○   **Describe the signs and symptoms of spinal shock.**

Flaccid paralysis, complete sensory loss, areflexia, and loss of autonomic function. Patients are usually bradycardic, hypotensive, hypothermic, and vasodilated.

○ **Active adduction of the thumb tests which nerve?**

Ulnar nerve.

○ **Describe the rash associated with exanthem subitum (roseola).**

The rash is usually found on the trunk and the neck and is maculopapular.

○ **What is the most common cause of death among children between 1 to 12 months old?**

Sudden infant death syndrome.

○ **Alkali causes what type of necrosis?**

Liquefactive necrosis.

○ **What antibiotic is used to treat Rocky Mountain Spotted Fever in a patient allergic to tetracycline?**

Chloramphenicol.

○ **Describe the chest x-ray image of *Mycoplasma pneumoniae*.**

Patchy densities involving the entire lobe. Pneumatoceles, cavities, abscesses and pleural effusions can occur but are uncommon. Treat with erythromycin.

○ **Which type of bacterial pneumonia commonly occurs secondary to viral illness?**

Staphylococcal infection.

○ **What two types of pneumonia are often contracted during the summer months?**

Staphylococcal and *Legionella* pneumonia.

○ **Describe the chest x-ray image of *Legionella* pneumonia.**

Dense consolidation and bulging fissures. Expect elevated liver enzymes and hypophosphatemia. Relative bradycardia is evident upon physical examination.

○ **What are the classic symptoms of TB?**

Night sweats, fever, weight loss, malaise, cough, and greenish yellow sputum most commonly seen in the mornings.

○ **What do chest x-rays reveal in cases of tuberculosis?**

Cavitation of the right upper lobe. Lower lung infiltrates, hilar adenopathy, atelectasis, and pleural effusion are also common.

○ **Is GI bleeding common with a perforated ulcer?**

No.

❍   **During which trimester of pregnancy is acute appendicitis most common?**

The second trimester.

❍   **What is the most common cause of paralytic ileus?**

Surgery.

❍   **An elderly female presents with pain in the knee and medial aspect of the thigh. What GI diagnosis should be considered?**

An obturator hernia.

❍   **Where is the most common site of volvulus?**

The sigmoid colon.

❍   **Describe the location of an indirect inguinal hernia.**

Lateral to the epigastric vessels, protruding through the inguinal canal.

❍   **Describe the location of a femoral hernia.**

Protrudes through the femoral canal and below the inguinal ligament.

❍   **Describe the location of a Spigelian hernia.**

3 to 5 cm above the inguinal ligament.

❍   **What is a Pantaloon hernia?**

A hernia with both direct and indirect inguinal hernia components.

❍   **What is a sliding hernia?**

A hernia in which one wall of the hernia sac includes viscus.

❍   **Describe a Richter's hernia.**

An incarceration containing only one wall of viscus.

❍   **Which is the most common type of hernia in children?**

Indirect. Direct inguinal hernias are more common in the elderly.

❍   **What are the signs and symptoms of Crohn's disease?**

Fever, diarrhea, right lower quadrant pain with mass possible, fistulas, rectal prolapse, perianal fissures, and abscesses. Arthritis, uveitis, and liver disease are also associated with this condition.

❍   **What systemic diseases are associated with Crohn's disease?**

Pyoderma gangrenosum, uveitis, episclerosis, scleritis, arthritis, erythema nodosum, and nephrolithiasis.

❍   **What contrast x-ray findings are associated with Crohn's disease?**

The segmental involvement in the colon with an abnormal mucosal pattern and fistulas, often without involvement of the rectum. A narrowing of the small intestine may also be displayed.

○ **What are the principal signs and symptoms of ulcerative colitis?**

Fever, weight loss, tachycardia, panniculitis, and 6 bloody bowel movements per day.

○ **Does toxic megacolon commonly occur with ulcerative colitis or with Crohn's disease?**

Ulcerative colitis.

○ **Which medications may be used for Crohn's disease but not for ulcerative colitis?**

Antidiarrheal agents.

○ **Does cancer more often develop with ulcerative colitis or Crohn's disease?**

Ulcerative colitis. Think of toxic megacolon and cancer. Always avoid antidiarrheal agents in the treatment regime.

○ **What bacterial cause of diarrhea is most commonly associated with seizures?**

Shigella.

○ **What organism induces rose spots and watery diarrhea, as well as high fever and relative bradycardia?**

Salmonella.

○ **What is the treatment for individuals infected with *Salmonella*?**

Supportive care without antibiotics. However, if a severe fever is exhibited, antibiotic therapy may be warranted.

○ **What microbial agent is associated with mesenteric adenitis and pseudoappendicitis?**

Yersinia.

○ **Which type of diarrhea is profuse and bloody, but does not involve vomiting?**

Entamoeba histolytica. Diarrhea which is not necessarily bloody, but can be associated with contaminated meat could be due to *Clostridium perfringens.*

○ **What is the most common parasite in the US?**

Giardia. Infected individuals presents with foul-smelling, floating stools; abdominal pain; and perfuse diarrhea. The parasite may be identified with a positive string test or duodenal aspiration for trophozoites.

○ **What causes the type of diarrhea commonly seen in AIDS patients?**

Cryptosporidiosis. This agent is diagnosed by a positive acid fast stain. Patients with this condition present with profuse, watery diarrhea that is not bloody.

○ **What is the incubation period for hepatitis A?**

30 days. The disease is caused by a retro-virus.

○ **What does an elevated IgM anti-HBc indicate?**

Exposure to hepatitis B with antibody to the core antigen. High titers indicate the contagious disease, low titers suggest chronic hepatitis B.

○ **Which type of hepatitis is caused by a DNA virus?**

Hepatitis B. The incubation period is 90 days.

○ **What does an anti-HB indicate?**

Prior infection and immunity.

○ **What defects cause left-to-right shunt murmurs?**

ASD, VSD, and PDA.

○ **What cardiovascular defects produce diminished pulses in the lower extremities of a pediatric patient?**

Coarctation of the aorta.

○ **What conditions produce cardiac syncope in pediatric patients?**

Aortic stenosis, does not cause cyanosis, and Tetralogy of Fallot, which does cause cyanosis.

○ **What are two unique clinical findings of Tetralogy of Fallot?**

A boot-shaped heart on x-ray and exercise intolerance that is relieved by squatting. Treat shortness of breath by placing patient in the knee-chest position and administering morphine.

○ **What are the signs of left-sided heart failure in an infant?**

Increased respiratory rate, shortness of breath, and sweating during feeding.

○ **What is the most common cause of CHF in the second week of life?**

Coarctation of the aorta.

○ **What is the most common cause of otitis media?**

Streptococcus pneumoniae.

○ **What is the most common cause of impetigo?**

Group A ß-hemolytic *Streptococcus.*

○ **What is the most common cause of orbital infections?**

Staphylococcus aureus. Periorbital infections are usually caused by *H. influenzae.*

○ **What is the most common cause of pediatric bacteremia?**

Streptococcus pneumoniae.

○ **A patient has a staccato cough and a history of conjunctivitis in the first few weeks after birth. What type of pneumonia?**

Chlamydia.

○ **How do steroids function in the treatment of asthma?**

Steroids increase cAMP, decrease inflammation, and aid in restoring the function of ß-adren-ergic responsiveness to adrenergic drugs.

○ **What two viral illnesses are prodromes for Reye's syndrome?**

Varicella (chickenpox) and influenzae B.

○ **What are the signs and symptoms of Reye's syndrome?**

Irritability, combativeness, lethargy, right upper quadrant tenderness, history of influenzae B or recent chicken pox, papilledema, hypoglycemia, and seizures. Lab results reveal hypoglycemia, an ammonia level 20 times greater than normal, and a normal bilirubin level.

○ **Describe the 5 stages of Reye's syndrome.**

Stage I: Vomiting, lethargy, and liver dysfunction

Stage II: Disorientation, combativeness, delirium, hyperventilation, increased deep tendon reflexes, liver dysfunction, hyperexcitable, tachypnea, fever, tachycardia, sweating, and pupillary dilatation

Stage III: Coma, decorticate rigidity, increased respiratory rate, and a mortality rate of 50%

Stage IV: Coma, decerebrate posturing, no ocular reflexes, loss of corneal reflexes, and liver damage

Stage V: Loss of deep tendon reflexes, seizures, flaccidity, respiratory arrest, and 95% mortal-ity

○ **What are the first, second, and third drugs of choice for the treatment of seizures in children?**

Phenobarbital, phenytoin, and carbamazepine, respectively.

○ **What is the drug of choice for the treatment of a febrile seizure?**

Phenobarbital.

○ **Why is diazepam (Valium) avoided in neonatal seizures?**

It may cause hyperbilirubinemia by uncoupling the bilirubin-albumin complex.

○ **What serious complication may arise from the use of valproic acid?**

Hepatic failure.

○ **What complications may occur with phenytoin use?**

Folate deficiency, osteomalacia, neutropenia, neuropathies, lupus, and myasthenia.

○ **What is the most common cause of painless lower GI bleeding in an infant or child?**

Meckel's diverticulum.

❍   **A 16 month old presents with bilious vomiting, a distended abdomen, and blood in the stool. Diagnosis?**

Malrotation of the mid-gut.

❍   **A child presents with periodic abdominal cramps, currant jelly stools, and a sausage-like tumor mass in the right lower quadrant. A contrast x-ray shows a coil spring sign. Diagnosis?**

Intussusception.

❍   **What are some possible complications of sodium bicarbonate therapy?**

Hypokalemia, paradoxical CSF acidosis, impaired O2 dissociation, and sodium overload.

❍   **Differentiate between non-ketotic hyperosmolar coma and DKA.**

Non-ketotic hyperosmolar coma: Glucose is high (often > 800); serum osmolality is high (average about 380); and nitroprusside test is negative.

DKA: Glucose is often in the range of 600; serum osmolality is approximately 350; and nitroprusside test is positive.

❍   **What focal signs may be present in a patient with non-ketotic hyperosmolar coma?**

Hemisensory deficits or perhaps hemiparesis. 10 to 15% of these patients will have a seizure.

❍   **What is the most common precipitating cause of thyroid storm?**

Pulmonary infection.

❍   **What is another name for life-threatening hypothyroidism?**

Myxedema coma. This condition occurs in elderly women during the winter months and is stim-ulated by infection and stress.

❍   **What is the second most common cause of hypothyroidism?**

Autoimmune Hashimoto's thyroiditis.

❍   **How can primary hypothyroidism be distinguished from secondary hypothyroidism?**

Primary hypothyroidism: The TSH levels are high, patients often have a history of thyroid surgery, and they may have a goiter.

Secondary hypothyroidism: the TSH levels are low or normal, there is no history of surgery, and no goiter is evident.

❍   **What drugs may worsen myxedema?**

Propranolol and phenothiazine.

❍   **What common surgical problem encountered with myxedema should be treated conservatively?**

Acquired megacolon.

○   **What is the cause of primary adrenal insufficiency?**

Failure of the adrenal cortex (also known as Addison's disease).

○   **What hormones are produced by the adrenal cortex?**

Mineralocorticoids, glucocorticoids, and androgenic steroids. (Remember: Salt, sugar, sex.)

○   **What is the major mineralocorticoid?**

Aldosterone. Regulated by the renin angiotensin system, it increases sodium reabsorption and H+ and K+ excretion.

○   **What is the major glucocorticoid?**

Cortisol.

○   **What hormones are produced by the medulla of the adrenal gland?**

Epinephrine and norepinephrine.

○   **Two weeks after a myocardial infarction, a patient takes warfarin and has sudden onset of hypotension, right flank pain, right CVA pain, epigastric pain, fever, nausea, and vomiting. Diagnosis?**

Adrenal gland hemorrhage (adrenal apoplexy).

○   **Define Waterhouse-Friderichsen syndrome?**

Septicemia secondary to meningococcemia with associated bilateral adrenal gland hemorrhage. The patient will have a petechial rash, purpura, shaking, chills, and a severe headache.

○   **What effect does Addison's disease have on cortisol and aldosterone levels?**

It lowers them. Low cortisol levels induce nausea, vomiting, anorexia, lethargy, hypoglycemia, water intoxication, and the inability to withstand even minor stress without shock. Low aldosterone levels cause sodium depletion, dehydration, hypotension, and syncope.

○   **What are the signs and symptoms of Addison's disease?**

Hyperpigmentation, hyperkalemia, alopecia, and ascending paralysis secondary to hyperkalemia. Lab findings in Addison's disease indicate hypoglycemia, hyponatremia, hyperkalemia, and azotemia.

○   **What are the principal signs and symptoms of adrenal crisis?**

Abdominal pain, hypotension, and shock. The most common cause is withdrawal of steroids. Treat by administering hydrocortisone; 100 mg IV bolus and 100 mg added to the first liter of D5 0.9 NS.

○   **Does cyanide evoke cyanosis?**

No (except secondarily, when bradycardia and apnea precede asystolic arrest). If hypoxia is not present according to ABG results; consider administering cyanide to an acidotic, non-cyanotic, comatose patient.

O   **What key lab results are expected with SIADH?**

Low serum sodium levels and high urine sodium levels (i.e., > 30).

O   **What is the typical anatomic source of an epidural hematoma?**

The middle meningeal artery.

O   **What is the most common anatomic source of a subdural hematoma?**

Bridging veins.

O   **What is the most common source of a subarachnoid bleed?**

A saccular aneurysm.

O   **If a lesion is in the right hemisphere, which way will the eyes deviate?**

Toward the lesion.

O   **If a lesion is in the brain stem, which way will the eyes deviate?**

Away from the lesion in the brain stem.

O   **Where is the most common intraparenchymal site of intracranial bleeding?**

The putamen.

O   **In the pediatric esophagus, where is a foreign body most commonly lodged?**

The cricopharyngeal narrowing.

O   **Do household pets transmit *Yersinia*?**

Yes.

O   **What is the most common cause of intrinsic renal failure?**

Acute tubular necrosis.

O   **What is the most common cause of cardiac arrest in an uremic patient?**

Hyperkalemia.

O   **What is the first cardiac finding in a cyclic antidepressant overdose?**

Sinus tachycardia.

O   **What is the most common cause of chronic heavy metal poisoning?**

Lead. Arsenic is the most common cause of acute heavy metal poisoning.

O   **What is the most commonly injured area of the mandible?**

The angle.

○   **Erythema nodosa is associated with which type of gastroenteritis?**

Yersinia.

○   **What is the most reliable method of diagnosing a posterior shoulder dislocation?**

Performing a physical examination. Order a Y-view x-ray; it may be helpful.

○   **The mortise view of the ankle is important in the diagnosis of:**

Medial (deltoid) ligament disruption of the ankle.

○   **What is the best x-ray view for diagnosing lunate and perilunate dislocations?**

Lateral x-ray views of the wrist.

○   **What are the common anticholinergic compounds?**

Atropine, tricyclic antidepressants, antihistamines, phenothiazine, antiparkinsonian drugs, belladonna alkaloids, and some Solanaceae plants (i.e., deadly nightshade and jimson weed).

○   **How long should a tricyclic antidepressant overdose patient, demonstrating tachycardia and conduction disturbances, be monitored?**

24 hours.

○   **A baby is brought to the emergency department because of vomiting and persistent crying. On examination, a testicle is tender and enlarged. Diagnosis?**

Testicular torsion.

○   **A child presents with bluish discoloration of the gingiva. Probable diagnosis?**

Chronic lead poisoning. Expect the erythrocyte protoporphyrin level to be el-evated with this condition.

○   **In a humeral shaft fracture, what nerve is most commonly injured?**

The radial nerve.

○   **Which type of hip dislocation is most common: anterior, posterior, lateral, or medial?**

Posterior.

○   **What disorder is most likely to be confused with erythema nodosum?**

Cellulitis.

○   **What is the most common dysrhythmia in a child?**

Paroxysmal atrial tachycardia.

○   **What is the most common cause of hyponatremia?**

Dilution.

○   **Of the following, which is not a common cause of large bowel obstruction: diverticulitis, adhesions, sigmoid volvulus, or neoplasms?**

Adhesions.

○   **A fracture of the acetabulum may be associated with damage to what nerve?**

The sciatic nerve.

○   **What are some common causes of increased anion gap?**

Aspirin, methanol, uremia, diabetes, idiopathic (lactic), ethylene glycol, and alcohol.

○   **What are the causes of normal anion gap metabolic acidosis?**

Diarrhea, ammonium chloride, renal tubular acidosis, renal interstitial disease, hypoadrenalism, ureterosigmoidostomy, and acetazolamide.

○   **What are some common causes of respiratory alkalosis?**

Respiratory alkalosis is defined as a pH above 7.45 and a pCO2 less than 35. Common causes of respiratory alkalosis include any process that may induce hyperventilation: shock, sepsis, trauma, asthma, PE, anemia, hepatic failure, heat stroke, exhaustion, emotion, salicylate poisoning, hypoxemia, pregnancy, and inadequate mechanical ventilation.

○   **How should a patient with hypertrophic cardiomyopathy, chest pain, and normal vital signs, except for a heart rate of 140, be treated?**

Treat with ß-antagonists. Calcium channel blockers are second-line therapeutics.

○   **What is the adult dose of epinephrine for acute anaphylactic shock?**

0.3 to 0.5 mg of 1:10,000 IV.

○   **How should neurogenic shock be managed?**

With replacement of the volume deficit, followed by vasopressors.

○   **What medication is most appropriate for hypertensive patients with acute aortic dissections?**

Nitroprusside and Beta-blockers.

○   **An elderly male presents with ataxia, confusion, amnesia, and ocular paralysis. He is apathetic to his situation and his neurologic examination is normal. Probable diagnosis?**

Vitamin B deficiency associated with Wernicke-Korsakoff's syndrome.

○   **What is the most common cause of sporadic encephalitis?**

Herpes simplex virus.

○   **What are the classic ECG results associated with posterior MI?**

A large R wave and ST depression in V1 and V2.

○ **What are the classic ECG finding for Wolff-Parkinson-White syndrome?**

A change in the upstroke of QRS, the delta wave.

○ **What agent is usually responsible for the onset of endemic encephalitis?**

Arbovirus.

○ **What are the most common dysrhythmias associated with digitalis?**

PVCs. AV block and PSVT with block are next.

○ **What is the most common cause of pelvic pain in an adolescent female?**

Ovarian cysts.

○ **What is the most common cause of valvular-induced syncope in the elderly?**

Aortic stenosis.

○ **Describe the signs, symptoms, and ECG findings associated with lithium toxicity.**

Tremor, weakness, and flattening of the T waves, respectively.

○ **How many days after a measles vaccine does a fever and rash usually develop?**

7 to 10 days.

○ **What is the most common complication of acute otitis media?**

Tympanic membrane perforation. Other complications include mastoiditis, cholesteatoma, and intracranial infections.

○ **Compare and contrast the rashes and the corresponding symptoms and signs of roseola and measles.**

Roseola usually causes a fever as high as 40°C (104°F), which lasts 3 to 5 days. The child does not appear particularly ill, although adenopathy may be noted. As the fever falls, the child may develop a maculopapular rash, which will last from a few hours to a few days.

Measles usually begins with 3 to 4 days of fever, con-junctivitis, and upper respiratory tract symptoms. The characteristic rash is also maculopapular and confluent, but it distinctively begins on the face and moves down the body. Koplik's spots are diagnostic.

○ **What is the appropriate treatment for a non-immunized individual exposed to hepatitis B?**

Immune globulin, specifically HBIG. Consider vaccination.

○ **What is the most common cause of sigmoid volvulus in the elderly?**

Constipation.

○ **The anterior drawer test of the ankle is used to test what ligament?**

The anterior talofibular ligament.

O   **Which type of injury should be suspected in a patient with a shortened, internally rotated right leg as the result of an accident?**

Posterior hip dislocation.

O   **Describe a mallet finger deformity.**

Deformity produced by forced flexion of the DIP joint when finger is in full extension. It is a result of either a rupture of the distal extensor tendon or an avulsion fraction of the tendon insertion on the distal phalanx with a dorsal plate avulsion.

O   **What viral agent most commonly induces laryngotracheitis?**

Parainfluenza virus type I. Staphylococcus aureus is the most common bacterial pathogen.

O   **A patient has a fracture of the proximal third of the ulna. Which type injury should be ruled out?**

The dislocation of the radial head, also known as a Monteggia fracture. An anterior dislocation is most common.

O   **What gynecological infection presents with a malodorous, itchy, white to gray and sometimes frothy vaginal discharge?**

Trichomoniasis.

O   **What are the signs of an upper motor neuron lesion?**

Upper motor neuron lesion involves the corticospinal tract. The lesion usually induces paralysis with:

1) The initial loss of muscle tone and then increased tone, resulting in spasticity
2) Babinski sign
3) The loss of superficial reflexes
4) Increased deep tendon reflexes

A lower motor neuron lesion is associated with the anterior horn cells' axons. These lesions cause paralysis with decreased muscle tone and prompt atrophy.

O   **What condition frequently presents with ocular bulbar deficits?**

Botulism. Patients with myasthenia gravis may present similarly. The diphtheria toxin rarely produces ocular bulbar deficits.

O   **Describe the initial symptoms and signs of myasthenia gravis.**

Weakness and fatigue with ptosis, diplopia, and blurred vision. Bulbar muscle weakness is also prevalent with dysarthria and dysphagia.

O   **Describe the symptoms of botulism poisoning.**

Botulism poisoning often presents with ocular bulbar deficits. Symmetrical descending weakness, usually with no sensory abnormalities, also develops. Other classical symptoms include dysphagia, dry mouth, diplopia, and dysarthria. The deep tendon re-flexes may be decreased or absent.

O   **Describe the signs and symptoms of Guillain-Barré disease.**

Guillain-Barré disease classically presents with symmetrical weakness in the leg, which ascends to include the arms or trunk. Distal weakness is usually greater than proxi-mal. The onset of the disease rarely involves the cranial nerves.

○ **What nerve provides sensations to both the dorsum and volar aspects of the hand?**

Ulnar. Radial is primarily dorsum, and median is primarily volar.

○ **Describe the key features of Ménière's disease, also known as endolymphatic hydrops.**

Vertigo, hearing loss, and tinnitus. Ménière's disease typically presents with the rapid onset of vertigo, nausea, and vomiting that lasts for hours to 1 day. Nystagmus may be spontaneous during the critical stage. Tinnitus may be present and is louder during attacks, and sensorineural hearing loss may occur. There also may be an aura with a sensation of fullness in the ear during an attack. Symptoms are unilateral in over 90% of patients, and recurring attacks are typical.

○ **What are the distinguishing characteristics of benign positional vertigo?**

Positional vertigo is usually provoked by certain head positions or movement. Nystagmus is always positional, of brief duration, and with fatigability.

○ **What are the key features of viral labyrinthitis or vestibular neuritis?**

Severe vertigo (usually lasting 3 to 5 days), with nausea and vomiting. Symptoms generally regress over 3 to 6 weeks. Nystagmus may be spontaneous dur-ing the severe stage.

○ **What is a major concern for a patient with unilateral Parkinsonian features?**

Intracranial tumor.

○ **Describe signs and symptoms of acoustic neuroma.**

Unilateral high tone sensorineural hearing loss and tinnitus. Decreased corneal sensitivity, diplopia, headache, facial weakness, and positive radiographic findings may also be displayed. Vertigo usually appears late, is more often exhibited as a progressive feeling of imbalance, and can be provoked by changes in head movement. Nystagmus is frequently present and is usually spontaneous. The CSF may have elevated protein.

○ **Describe the key features of vertebrobasilar insufficiency.**
Vertigo (nearly always positional accompanied by nystagmus). Other signs of arteriosclerosis may be found. Vertebrobasilar insufficiency is typically prevalent in older persons and may occur with other symptoms of brainstem ischemia.

○ **What's the little bone seen behind the tympanic membrane?**

The malleus.

○ **What is the mortality rate of Wernicke's encephalopathy?**

10 to 20%.

○ **What is the treatment of Wernicke's encephalopathy?**

Thiamine IV.

○   **What are the symptoms of Wernicke's encephalopathy?**

Ocular palsies, nystagmus, confusion, and ataxia.

○   **Deep tendon reflexes are usually maintained in which of the following diseases: myasthenia gravis, Guillain-Barré, or Eaton-Lambert syndrome?**

Myasthenia gravis. Reflexes are usually depressed in Eaton-Lambert syndrome and absent in Guillain-Barré.

○   **What major tranquilizer displays the most hypotensive tendency?**

Thorazine.

○   **What is the most common cause of odontogenic pain?**

Dental caries.

○   **What factors and substances decrease theophylline metabolism and increase theophylline levels?**

Factors: Age greater than 50, prematurity, liver and renal disease, pulmonary edema, CHF, pneumonia, obesity, and viral illness in children.

Substances: Drugs that increase theophylline levels include cimetidine, erythromycin, allopurinol, troleandomycin, BCPs, and quinolone antibiotics.

In smokers, the theophylline half-life is decreased, which causes the levels of serum theophylline to decrease. Phenobarbital, phenytoin, rifampin, carbamazepine, marijuana smoking, exposure to environmental pollutants, and the consumption of charcoal-broiled foods can also decrease serum theophylline levels.

○   **What therapy should be used for a patient with hemophilia A who is suffering from a head injury?**

Cryoprecipitate. Maintain a low total volume, if possible. Cryoprecipitate has a higher concentration of factor VIII complex than fresh frozen plasma.

○   **What therapy should be initiated for a bleeding patient who is on warfarin and has a high PT?**

D/C warfarin, followed by a water soluble form of vitamin K. Prescribe SQ and consider a test dose. If the bleeding is severe or in a dangerous location (i.e., the brain), fresh frozen plasma containing active factors X, IX, VII, and II should be given. (Remember: 1972)

○   **What electrolyte abnormality is commonly associated with the transfusion of packed RBCs?**

Hypocalcemia secondary to citrate toxicity. Citrate, when rapidly infused, binds ionized calcium and therefore decreases the calcium level. Hyperkalemia may also develop, especially if the patient is in renal failure or if the blood products are old.

○   **What invasive procedure should be performed to evaluate a patient whose face, neck, and arms are swollen?**

CVP. Swelling of the face, neck and arms suggests superior venacava syndrome. To confirm, an increased CVP pressure in the upper body and abnormal pressure in the lower extremities must be documented. A chest x-ray will detect only about 10% of the masses causing this syndrome.

❍   **Describe Leriche's syndrome.**

Impotence with buttock, calf, and back pain. It usually occurs with aortoiliac disease.

❍   **What condition should be suspected in a patient with vision loss and a pale fundus?**

Central retinal artery occlusion. Vision loss is usually acute and painless.

❍   **Describe a patient with sigmoid volvulus.**

Sigmoid volvulus usually affects psychiatric patients and elderly patients suffering from severe chronic constipation. Symptoms include intermittent cramping, lower abdominal pain, and progressive abdominal distention.

❍   **Describe a typical patient with intussusception.**

It usually occurs in children ages 3 months to 2 years, although the majority are 5 to 10 months old. It is more common in boys.

❍   **What are the signs and symptoms of hyperthyroidism?**

Signs: Fever, tachycardia, wide pulse pressure, CHF, shock, thyromegaly, tremor, liver tenderness, jaundice, stare, hyperkinesis, and pretibial myxedema. Mental status changes include somnolence, obtundation, coma, or psychosis.

Symptoms: Weight loss, palpitations, dyspnea, edema, chest pain, nervousness, weakness, tremor, psychosis, diarrhea, hyperdefecation, abdominal pain, myalgias, and disorientation.

❍   **A patient suffers a rotational knee injury and hears a pop. Within 90 minutes a hemarthrosis develops. Where is the suspected location of injury?**

The anterior cruciate.

❍   **What are the radiological and laboratory results of duodenal injury?**

Retroperitoneal air and increased serum amylase.

❍   **What drugs should be avoided in G-6-PD deficiency?**

ASA, phenacetin, primaquine, quinine, quinacrine, nitrofurans, sulfamethoxazole, sulfacetamide, and methylene blue.

❍   **What is the current therapeutic regimen for treatment of meningitis in a neonate?**

Ampicillin and cefotaxime. A combination of these 2 antibiotics should be used in infants up to 2 months of age to cover coliform, group B streptococci, *Listeria*, and *Enterococcus*. In children aged 2 months to 6 years, cefotaxime alone is indicated.

❍   **How do pH changes affect the potassium concentration?**

For a pH increase of 0.1, expect the potassium to drop by 0.5 mmol/L.

❍   **Describe the presentation of alcoholic ketoacidosis (AKA).**

Nausea, vomiting, and abdominal pain occurring 24 to 72 hours after the cessation of drinking. No specific physical findings are evident, although abdominal pain is a common complaint. AKA is thought to be secondary to an increased mobilization of free fatty acids with lipolysis to acetoacetate and ß-hydroxybutyrate.

❍   **What is the appropriate treatment for a patient with alcoholic ketoacidosis (AKA)?**

Normal saline and glucose. As acidosis is corrected, K+ may drop. Sodium bicarbonate should not be given unless the pH drops below 7.1.

❍   **Describe the symptoms of optic neuritis.**

Variable loss of central visual acuity with a central scotoma and change in color perception. The disk margins are blurred from hemorrhage, the blind spot is increased, and the eye is painful.

❍   **Compare and contrast primary and secondary myxedema.**

	Primary	Secondary
Source	Thyroid	Pituitary
Frequency	Common (95%)	Uncommon (5%)
Heart	Big	Small
TSH	High	Low
Iodine	$< 2\mu g/dL$	$> 2\mu g/dL$
Coarse voice	Yes	No
Goiter	Yes	No
Pubic hair	Yes	No

❍   **Differentiate between radiolucent and radiopaque renal calculi.**

90% of all stones are radiopaque and are composed of calcium oxalate, cysteine, calcium phosphate, or magnesium ammonium phosphate. Radiolucent obstruction consists of uric acid stones and blood clots.

❍   **Cyanide binds to metals and disrupts the function of metal-containing enzymes. Which is the most important of these enzymes?**

Cytochrome A (also known as cytochrome oxidase) is necessary for aerobic metabolism.

❍   **Why administer nitrites for cyanide poisoning?**

Nitrites form methemoglobin and methemoglobin, which strongly bind to cyanide.

❍   **Why prescribe sodium thiosulfate for cyanide poisoning?**

Rhodanese, an intrinsic enzyme, transfers cyanide from its attachment to methemoglobin to sulfur, thereby forming thiocyanate. Thiocyanate is excreted. Sodium thiosulfate acts as a sulfur donor for this process.

❍   **What is the antidote for ethylene glycol?**

Ethanol and dialysis.

❍   **What is the antidote for gold?**

British anti-Lewisite (BAL).

❍ **What is the antidote for nitrites?**

Methylene blue 1%, 0.2 mL/kg IV over 5 minutes. Severe methemoglobinemia requires an exchange transfusion.

❍ **What are the signs and symptoms of organic brain syndrome?**

Signs: Mental status changes (such as disorientation, clouded sensorium, asterixis, or mild clonus) and focal neurologic signs. Vital signs are often within normal limits.

Symptoms: Visual hallucinations and perceptions of the unfamiliar as familiar.

Onset may occur at any age.

❍ **What is the most common cause of airway obstruction in trauma?**

CNS depression.

❍ **What wound is most commonly associated with pericardial tamponade?**

Right ventricular injury.

❍ **What are the signs and symptoms of acute pericardial tamponade?**

Triad of hypotension, elevated CVP, and tachycardia. Muffled heart tones may be auscultated.

❍ **What ECG result is pathognomonic of pericardial tamponade?**

Total electrical alternans. Pulsus paradoxus is nonspecific. Muffled heart tones are subjective findings and are difficult to appreciate.

❍ **How much lactated Ringer's solution should be infused into a child undergoing a peritoneal lavage?**

10 cc/kg of lactated Ringer's solution allows for the accurate interpretation of cell counts.

❍ **Name two retroperitoneal organs that can be injured without producing a positive DPL.**

The pancreas and the duodenum.

❍ **Name two organs that do not tend to bleed enough to produce a positive DPL when injured.**

The bladder and the small bowel.

❍ **What RBC count is considered positive in a peritoneal lavage fluid analysis in a patient who has received blunt abdominal trauma?**

RBC count > 100,000 per mm3 is considered positive for both blunt and penetrating trauma to the abdomen. If penetrating trauma has occurred to the low chest or high abdominal region and diaphramatic perforation is a possiblity, then 5000 RBCs per mm3 is also regarded as positive.

❍ **Define sensitivity and specificity.**

Sensitivity: True positives divided by true positives plus false negatives. It represents how well a test identifies people who have a condition from among all the people who have the condition.

Specificity: True negatives divided by true negatives plus false positives. It is the percentage of people who do not have a disease and are thus correctly classified as negative by the test.

○ **Identify the zones of the neck and the appropriate method of evaluation for injuries to each zone.**

Zone	Location	Evaluation
1	Below the cricoid cartilage	Angiography to evaluate major vessels
2	Between the angle of the mandible and the cricoid cartilage	Surgical (Remember "2 surgery!")
3	Above the angle of the mandible	Angiography to evaluate major vessels

○ **What cause of death is secondary to an untreated tension pneumothorax?**

Decreased cardiac output. The vena cava is compressed, which lowers the right heart blood return and severely compromises stroke volume, blood pressure and cardiac output.

Editor's note: Secondary arrhythmias can also occur. V-tach in a young, apparently healthy person is secondary to a tension pneumothorax until proven otherwise. (JNA)

○ **How does a chronic pericardial effusion appear on a chest x-ray?**

A gradual pericardial sac distention results in a "water bottle" appearance of the heart.

○ **Describe a patient with acute narrow angle closure glaucoma.**

Symptoms include nausea, vomiting, and abdominal pain. Visual acuity is markedly diminished. The pupil is semidilated and nonreactive. There is usually a glassy haze over the cornea, and the eye is red and very painful. Intraocular pressure may be as high as 50 to 60 mm Hg.

○ **Describe the treatment of acute narrow angle glaucoma.**

Use Mannitol to decrease intraocular pressure, miotics (such as pilocarpine) to open the angle, and carbonic anhydrase inhibitor to minimize aqueous humor production. An iridectomy is eventually performed to provide aqueous outflow.

○ **What is the appropriate treatment of hyphema?**

Elevate the head. Other treatments are controversial; however, most ophthalmologists recommend hospitalization for patients. Treatment may include a double eye patch, topical cortisone, and cycloplegics.

○ **What signs and symptoms are prevalent with post streptococcal glomerulonephritis?**

Facial edema and decreased urinary output. Urine may be dark. Other laboratory results include normochromic anemia because of hemodilution, increased sedimentation rate, numerous RBCs and WBCs in the urine with casts, and hyperkalemia. Hospitalization is advised.

○ **Name the five major modified Jones criteria.**

1) Erythema marginatum
2) Polyarthritis
3) Subcutaneous nodules
4) Carditis
5) Chorea

Other criteria include rheumatic fever or rheumatic heart disease, arthralgias, fever, prolonged PR interval on an ECG, C reactive protein, elevated sedimentation rate, and antistreptolysin O titer.

O **What disorder is present when two out of the five major modified Jones criteria are met?**

Rheumatic fever.

O **Describe the signs and symptoms of varicella (chicken pox).**

Onset of varicella rash 1 to 2 days after prodromal symptoms of slight malaise, anorexia, and fever. The rash begins on the trunk and scalp, appearing as faint macules and later becoming vesicles.

O **What is the standard dose of atropine for a child?**

0.02 mg/kg.

O **How is the normal systolic blood pressure (SBP) for pediatric patients (toddlers and up) calculated?**

Average SBP (mm Hg) = $\frac{\text{age x 2}}{90}$

Low normal limit SBP (mm Hg) = (age x 2) + 70
SBP for a term newborn is about 60 mm Hg.

O **How does a patient over 12 months present with sickle cell disease?**

Pain in the joints, bones, and abdomen. The child may have abdominal tenderness and even rigidity. Mild icterus and anemia may be present.

O **How does a child present with erythema infectiosum (fifth disease or "slapped-cheek" syndrome)?**

There are no prodromal symp-toms. The illness usually begins with the sudden appearance of erythema of the cheeks, followed by a maculopapular rash on the trunk and extremities that evolves into a lacy pattern.

O **What doses of epinephrine and atropine should be administered during a pediatric code?**

Epinephrine: 0.01 mg/kg/dose. Atropine: 0.02 mg/kg/dose.

O **What is the initial antibiotic treatment for a child with epiglottitis?**

Treat with a second or third generation cephalosporin. The most likely cause of this condition is *H. influenzae*.

Note: With the widespread use of the Hib vaccine, streptococci are becoming an even more common cause. The number of cases is decreasing.

O **What are the key features of anterior spinal cord syndrome?**

Compression of the anterior cord causes complete motor paralysis and loss of pain and temperature sensation distal to the lesion. Posterior columns are spared; light touch and proprioception are preserved.

O **What organism typically causes paronychia?**

Staphylococcus.

O **What visual deficit is typically associated with lesions at the optic chiasm?**

Bitemporal hemianopsia.

O   **A ring lesion is noted on a CT scan of the brain of an immunocompromised patient. The patient is confused and has a lymphadenopathy, fever, and headache. Probable diagnosis?**

Toxoplasmosis secondary to Toxoplasma gondii cyst. The disease is typically treated with pyrimethamine and sulfadiazine.

O   **What are the signs and symptoms of posterior inferior cerebellar artery syndrome?**

Cerebellar dysfunction, such as vertigo, ataxia, and dizziness.

O   **Describe the signs and symptoms of neuroleptic malignant syndrome.**

Patients present with muscle rigidity, autonomic disturbances, acute organic brain syndrome, and a fever as high as 42°C (108°F). Blood pressure and pulse fluctuation wildly. Muscle necrosis may occur with resultant myoglobinuria.

O   **Describe the presentation of placenta previa.**

Painless, bright red vaginal bleeding.

O   **Describe the presentation of abruptio placentae.**

Painful, dark red vaginal bleeding.

O   **What is the most common growth plate (Salter class) injury?**

A Salter II fracture.

O   **Signs of tension pneumothorax on a physical examination include:**

Tachypnea, unilateral absent breath sounds, tachycardia, pallor, diaphoresis, cyanosis, tracheal deviation, hypotension, and neck vein distention.

O   **What is the most common cause of abdominal pain in children?**

Constipation.

O   **What is the most frequent carpal fracture?**

Navicular fracture.

O   **In the wrist, what bone is dislocated most often?**

Lunate. It is also the second most commonly fractured bone in the wrist.

O   **What medications should be used to treat preeclampsia and eclampsia?**

Magnesium and hydralazine.

O   **Do local anesthetics freely cross the blood brain barrier?**

Yes. Most systemic toxic reactions to local anesthetics involve the CNS or cardiovascular system.

O   **What are the most common causes of hemoptysis in the US?**

Bronchitis and bronchiectasis.

○ **Where is the most common site of thrombophlebitis?**

The deep muscles of the calves, particularly the soleus muscle.

○ **What is the most common cause of acute aortic regurgitation?**

Infectious endocarditis.

○ **What are the most common causes of aortic stenosis?**

Rheumatic fever and congenital bicuspid valve disease.

○ **What is the most common cause of acute mitral regurgitation?**

Inferior wall infarcts.

○ **What is pulsus paradoxus?**

A change in measured systolic BP of > 10 mm Hg from expiratory to inspiratory phases.

○ **What are the most common causes of pulsus paradoxus?**

COPD and asthma.

○ **What is the worst way to confirm diagnosis of a delayed pericardial injury after blunt trauma?**

By an autopsy.

○ **What are the signs and symptoms of aortic stenosis?**

Exertional dyspnea, angina, and syncope. Narrowed pulse pressure with decreased SBP, slow carotid upstroke, prominent S4 are also present.

○ **What metabolic disorder is associated with hypercalcemia?**

Hypokalemia.

○ **Which is the most common type of hepatitis transmitted through blood transfusions?**

Hepatitis C.

○ **Which gender is more apt to develop symptomatic gallstones?**

Females.

○ **What is the differential diagnosis of a red eye with decreased visual acuity?**

Iritis, glaucoma, and central corneal lesions.

○ **What disease is associated with retrobulbar optic neuritis?**

MS.

○   **How can mydriasis caused by third cranial nerve compression be distinguished from mydriasis induced by anticholinergic drugs or mydriatics?**

Mydriasis caused by third cranial nerve compression is reversible with pilocarpine; other causes are not.

○   **What is the best method to open an airway while maintaining C-spine precautions?**

Jaw thrust.

○   **What is the absolute contraindication to MAST?**

Pulmonary edema.

○   **T/F: Increased blood pressure in hypovolemic patients associated with MAST application is primarily because of autotransfusion.**

False. The primary mechanism of MAST appears to be because of increased peripheral vascular resistance. Autotransfusion of a few hundred mL of blood may occur but is not of great significance.

○   **What is the formula for determining the appropriate ET tube size for children older than 1?**

ET size = (age + 16) / 4.

○   **What is the correct ET tube size for a 1- to 2-year-old child?**

4.0 to 4.5 mm.

○   **What is the correct ET tube size for a 6 month old?**

3.5 to 4.5 mm.

○   **What is the correct ET tube size for a newborn?**

3.0 to 3.5 mm. For a premature newborn, use a 2.5 to 3.0 mm ET tube.

○   **What is the average distance from the mouth to 2 cm above the carina in men and in women?**

Men: 23 cm. Women: 21 cm.

○   **What is the treatment for hyperkalemia?**

1) Diurese with loop diuretic (i.e., furosemide or ethacrynic acid).

2) Sodium polystyrene sulfonate ion exchange resin (Kayexalate) enema (associated Na load can cause failure). It may be hours before an effect is seen.

3) 1 ampule of D50, insulin, 5 to 10 units IV for redistribution, followed by 50 g glucose and 20 U insulin over 1 hour. It takes about 30 minutes for an effect to occur.

4) Sodium bicarbonate, 50 to 100 mEq IV over 10 to 20 minutes. It takes 5 to 10 minutes to be effective.

5) Calcium. Calcium chloride has more Ca per ampule (13.4 mEq) than gluconate (4.6 mEq) and acts faster. Administer 1 ampule (10 mL) of 10% solution over 10 to 20 min-utes. Be careful if prescribing to a patient on digitalis—it will potentiate toxicity and the onset is rapid.

6) 3% sodium chloride IV may serve as a temporary antagonist.

7) Peritoneal or hemodialysis.

8) Digoxin specific Fab (Digibind) if secondary to digitalis overdose.

○ **How should hypercalcemia be treated?**

Administer furosemide and normal saline. IV Pamidronate is very effective in reducing serum calcium levels to normal for extended periods of time. Oral or IV steroids are also an effective alternative.

○ **What is the most common cause of multifocal atrial tachycardia?**

COPD.

○ **What is the treatment for multifocal atrial tachycardia?**

1) Treat underlying disorder.
2) Administer magnesium sulfate, 2 grams over 60 seconds, with supplemental potassium to maintain serum K+ above 4 mEq/L.
3) Consider verapamil, 10 mg IV, as a second treatment.

○ **What is the treatment for ectopic SVT because of digitalis toxicity?**

1) Stop digitalis
2) Correct hypokalemia
3) Consider digoxin specific Fab, magnesium IV, lidocaine IV, or phenytoin IV

○ **What is the treatment for ectopic SVT that is not because of digitalis toxicity?**

1) Digitalis, verapamil, or ß-blocker to slow rate
2) Quinidine, procainamide, or magnesium to decrease ectopy

○ **What is the treatment for verapamil-induced hypotension?**

Calcium gluconate, 1 gram IV over several minutes.

○ **Which type of drug is contraindicated for the treatment of Torsade de pointes?**

Any drug that prolongs repolarization (QT interval). For example, class Ia antiarrhythmics, such as quinidine and procainamide, are contraindicated for treating Torsade de pointes. Other drugs that share this effect include TCAs, disopyramide, and phenothiazine.

○ **What is the treatment for Torsade de pointes?**

The goal is to accelerate the heart rate and shorten ventricular repolarization.

1) Crank pacemaker to 90 to 120 bpm ("overdrive").
2) Administer isoproterenol.
3) Administer magnesium sulfate, 2 grams IV.

○ **What "hypos" can lower the seizure threshold?**

Hypoglycemia, hyponatremia, and hypocarbia.

○ **What motor function is spared in locked-in syndrome?**

Upward gaze.

○   **What are the signs and symptoms of a middle cerebral artery lesion?**

Hemiplegia or hemiparesthesia, homonymous hemianopsia, and speech disturbance.

○   **Which is the most common cause of cerebral artery occlusion, embolic or thrombotic?**

Thrombotic.

○   **What symptoms present with an anterior cerebral artery lesion?**

Paralysis of the contralateral leg with a sensory loss in the leg only and incontinence. No aphasia will be evident.

○   **What deficits can result from ocular motor nerve paralysis?**

Ptosis, which result from a levator palpebrae superioris/cranial nerve III injury. Lateral nerve gaze is controlled by the cranial nerve VI, and the corneal reflex is controlled by the cranial nerve V. The superior oblique muscle moves the gaze downward and laterally. It is controlled by CN IV.

(LR6SO4)3

○   **Describe the signs and symptoms of pressure on the first sacral root (S1).**

Symptoms of S1 injury include pain radiating to the mid-gluteal region, posterior thigh, posterior calf, and down to the heel and sole of the foot. Sensory signs are localized to the lateral toes. S1 root compression typically involves the plantar flexor muscles of the foot and toes. The ankle reflex is decreased or absent.

○   **What drug should be used to treat a patient in cardiac arrest secondary to**
hyper-kalemia?

Calcium chloride—IV acts fastest. Also provide $NaHCO_3$.

○   **What are the potential complications of excess sodium bicarbonate?**

Cerebral acidosis, hypokalemia, hyperosmolality, and an increased binding of hemoglobin to oxygen.

○   **What are the effects of dopamine at various doses?**

1 to 10 mg/kg: Renal, mesenteric, coronary, and cerebral vasodilation.
10 to 20 mg/kg: Both α- and ß-adrenergic.
20 mg/kg: Primarily α-adrenergic.

○   **What are common entities in the differential diagnosis of pinpoint pupils?**

Narcotic overdose, clonidine overdose, and sedative hypnotic overdose, including alcohol, cerebellar pontine angle infarct, and subarachnoid hemorrhage.

○   **What medications are appropriate in the treatment of a patient with tachycardia resulting from cocaine abuse?**

Benzodiazepines may sedate the patient and decrease tachycardia. Nitroprusside may be administered to treat hypertension. Caution must be used with ß-adrenergic antagonist agents alone because these medications may leave α-adrenergic stimulation unopposed thereby increasing the patient's risk for intracranial hemorrhage or aortic dissection.

○ **When should blood products be supplemented with fresh frozen plasma for a trauma patient receiving multiple units of transfused blood?**

For each 5 units of transfused blood, fresh frozen plasma should be given.

○ **What is the universal type of blood donor?**

Type Rh negative blood with anti-A and anti-B titers of less than 1:200 in saline.

○ **What are the common presentations of a transfusion reaction?**

Myalgia, dyspnea, fever associated with hypocalcemia, hemolysis, allergic reactions, hyperkalemia, citrate toxicity, hypothermia, coagulopathies, and altered hemoglobin function.

○ **What are the signs of the Cushing reflex?**

Increased systolic blood pressure and bradycardia secondary to neurological event.

○ **A woman comes to your office frantic because her husband has just received a positive VDRL result. They have been happily married for 35 years and she can't believe he has been unfaithful. Is it at all possible that he has been loyal to his wife?**

Yes. False-positive tests can occur if the patient has had a viral or mycoplasma infection in the near past, if the patient is an IV drug user, or if the patient has SLE. The presence or absence of syphilis can be confirmed with the fluorescent treponemal antibody absorption test (FTA-ABS).

○ **A 63-year-old woman asks you about the risk-benefit ratio for estrogen therapy. What do you tell her?**

Estrogen therapy is currently recommended for postmenopausal-menopausal women that are not at high risk for breast cancer. Research suggests that estrogen decreases the risk of CHD by 35%, the risk of hip fractures by 25%, and the risk of vertebral fractures by 50%. Unopposed estrogen increases the risk of endometrial cancer 8 times, yet estrogen given with progestins eliminates this risk. A minor side effect of progestin is weight gain.

○ **How is hepatitis A transmitted?**

By the oral-fecal route. No carrier state exists.

○ **Which type of gastroenteritis involves diarrhea and is associated with the consumption of seafood?**

Vibrio parahaemolyticus.

○ **Which type of hypersensitivity reaction is responsible for anaphy-laxis?**

Type I (IgE mediated).

Hypersensitivity	Reaction	Mediator	Examples
Type 1:	Immediate	IgE binds allergen, includes cells and basophils	Food allergies, mast pediatric asthma
Type 2:	Cytotoxic	IgG and IgM antibody reactions to antigen on cell surface activates complement and killers	Blood transfusion rxn, ITP, hemolytic anemia, ITP
Type 3:	Immune complex, Arthrus	Complexes activate complement	Tetanus toxoid in sensitized persons, poststreptococcal glomerulonephritis

| Type 4: | Cell mediated, delayed hypersensitivity | Activated T-lympho-cytes | Skin tests |

○   **A core temperature of less than 32°C is commonly associated with what complications?**

Arrhythmias that are resistant to treatment and the loss of the shivering reflex. The prognosis is poor.

○   **What are some common causes of polyhydramnios?**

Maternal causes include diabetes, Rh incompatibility, and other hematological diseases. Fetal causes are anencephaly, duodenal atresia, tracheoesophageal fistula, and pulmonary disorders.

○   **What clinical findings will there be in a 7-year-old with an ovarian granulosa cell tumor?**

Pseudoprecocious puberty. She may have vaginal bleeding, axillary hair, and early breast budding.

○   **What two drugs are used to treat eclampsia?**

Magnesium sulfate, 4 to 6 g bolus IV followed by a 2 g/hour infusion, and Hydralazine, 10 to 20 mg IV. Labetalol may also be used.

○   **Endometriosis is responsible for what percentage of infertility in women?**

25 to 50%.

○   **Where is the most common site of endometriosis?**

The ovaries (60%). Other sites include the cul-du-sac, uterosacral ligaments, broad ligaments, fallopian tubes, uterovesical fold, round ligaments, vermiform appendix, vagina, rectosigmoid colon, cecum, and ileum.

○   **Surgery is curative for liver cancer in what percentage of resectable, asymptomatic tumors?**

> 70% of children without cirrhosis and > 40% of adults without cirrhosis. If patients have cirrhosis and a tumor under 2 cm, then surgery is curative 70% of the time. The cure rate for patients with cirrhosis and a tumor under 3 cm is only 10%.

○   **What is the most common anatomical abnormality in the arterial blood supply to the liver?**

The right hepatic artery branches from the superior mesenteric instead of the common hepatic, which arises from the proper hepatic in 15 to 20% of the population.

○   **What is Kehr's sign?**

Pain in the left shoulder made worse in Trendelenburg, which indicates splenic injury. However, it is only present in 50% of such cases. In addition to the patient's history and physical examination, peritoneal lavage will determine if the spleen is bleeding.

○   **What spinal level innervates the diaphragm?**

C3, C4, C5. Remember: "3, 4, and 5 keep the diaphragm alive!"

○   **List five toxic syndromes and the hepatotoxic drugs that cause them.**

Acute hepatitis: Halothane, methyldopa, isoniazid.
Cholestatic jaundice: Anabolic steroids, oral contraceptives, oral hypoglycemics, erythromycin estolate.
Massive hepatic necrosis: Carbon tetrachloride, phosphorus, acetaminophen, *Amanita* mushrooms.
Chronic active hepatitis and cirrhosis: Vinyl chloride, arsenic.
Steatosis, hepatocellular necrosis: Ethanol.

〇   **What is the most common cause of hyperparathyroidism?**

Surgery, due to devascularization, removal, or trauma.

〇   **What are the most common causes of shock in patients who have received a blunt chest trauma?**

Pelvic or extremity fractures.

〇   **If a population doubles in 35 years, what is its annual rate of increase?**

2%. Use this easy approximation: .

The rate of population increase is the difference between the crude birth and death rates.

〇   **Technetium-99m–labeled studies of the gallbladder are viewed every 10 minutes for 1 hour. If the gallbladder is not visualized at the 1 hour interval, what does this signify?**

Either complete obstruction of the cystic duct due to inflammation and stones (acute cholecystitis) or partial obstruction with a slow filling rate because of scaring (chronic cholecystitis). Images delayed up to 4 hours are obtained to rule out the latter possibility.

〇   **What is the characteristic profile of a woman with endometriosis?**

Nulliparous over-achiever with a type A personality.

〇   **A patient who is taking oral contraceptives is concerned about the added risk of gynecological cancers. What should you tell her?**

Combined (estrogen and progesterone) oral contraceptives are not associated with a significant risk for breast cancer. In fact, they decrease the risk of ovarian and endometrial cancer. Oral contraceptives do increase the risk for thromboembolism, MIs, CVAs, hypertension, amenorrhea, cholelithiasis, and benign hepatic tumors, but they help regulate the menstrual cycle, decrease cramping, and curb the progression of endometriosis, ovarian cysts, and benign breast disease. They also decrease the incidence of ectopic pregnancy, salpingitis, and anemia, and they are therapeutic against rheumatoid arthritis.

〇   **What percentage of distal tibial (medial malleolus) fractures that are treated closed result in non-union?**

10 to 15%.

〇   **Why is needle aspiration preferred over incision and drainage for a fluctuant, acute cervical lymphadenitis?**

Development of a fistula tract is possible if the patient has atypical mycobacterium or cat scratch fever instead of bacterial lymphadenitis.

〇   **What is the most common thoracolumbar wedge fracture in the elderly?**

L1.

❍   What is the significance of the fat pad sign with an elbow injury?

Indicates effusion or hemarthrosis of the elbow joint. This suggests an occult fracture of the radial head.

❍   Which test is more sensitive when used to determine an anterior cruciate ligament tear in the knee: the anterior drawer test or the Lachman test?

Lachman test. While the knee is held at 20° flexion and the distal femur is stabilized, the lower leg is pulled forward. More than 5 mm anterior laxity compared to the other knee is evidence of an anterior cruciate ligament tear.

❍   Where are the most common sites of the hematologic spread of breast cancer?

Lungs and liver. Other sites include bone, adrenals, ovaries, brain, and pleura.

❍   What characteristics are associated with the best prognosis in breast cancer?

No nodal involvement, increased age, and positive estrogen receptor tumors.

❍   What is the most common cause of hyperthyroidism?

Graves' disease (toxic diffuse goiter).

❍   What is the most common cause of hypothyroidism?

Over-treatment of Graves' disease with iodine or subtotal thyroidectomy.

❍   How should cholesterol be monitored in patients with a history of CHD? Without a history of CHD?

A baseline total cholesterol and HDL-C should be obtained for all adults over 20. If the cholesterol is less than 200 mg/dL and the HDL is greater than 35 mg/DL, then repeat monitoring can be done every 5 years. For patients with CHD, a full lipoprotein analysis should be done as a base line. If LDL-C is less than 100 mg/dL, then annual lipoprotein monitoring is sufficient. If the patient's LDL-C is greater than 100 mg/dL, then diet and/or drug intervention is required with more frequent testing.

❍   What is the difference between a malingering and a factitious disorder?

A malingerer's incentive is external, such as workman's compensation. The goal of someone with a factitious disorder is to enter into the sick role. Both involve feigning illness.

❍   A patient has a fracture of the proximal third of the ulna. Which type of injury should be ruled out?

A dislocation of the radial head, also known as a Monteggia fracture. An anterior dislocation is most common.

Little known fact: This fracture/dislocation is named after the now world-famous quarterback, Joe Monteggia, who suffered this injury during a scuffle with the Michigan University Police Department.

MUPD

Michigan University Police Department
Monteggia, Ulnar fracture, Proximal Dislocation

❍   What are the only reliable indicators of a potentially violent patient?

Male gender, history of violence, and history of substance abuse. Cultural, educational, economic, and language barriers to effective patient/staff communication can increase the patient's frustration and lower his or her threshold for violence; as can trivialization of the patient or the family's concerns.

○   **What should you do when handling intoxicated, violent, psychotic, or threatening patients?**

Conduct careful histories and physicals with attention to mental status. Look for evidence of trauma, toxic ingestion, or metabolic derangement. Historical sources (e.g., family, paramedics, mental health workers, police, or medical records) may need to be accessed. Patients may need to be physically or chemically restrained in order to obtain an adequate examination and to ensure the safety of the patient and hospital staff.

○   **Define the following.**

Akathisia: Internal restlessness. Patient feels as if she is "jumping out of her skin."

Echolalia: Meaningless automatic repetition of someone else's words. This may occur immediately or even months after hearing the words.

Catalepsy: Patient maintains the same posture over a long period of time.

Waxy flexibility: Patient resists changing position, then gradually allows himself to be moved, much like a clay figure.

Stereotypy: Patient goes through repetitive motions that have no purpose.

Verbigeration: Verbal stereotypy. The patient repeats words over and over.

Gegenhalten: The patient resists external manipulation with the same force as is applied.

○   **What is respiratory alkalosis?**

A pH above 7.45 and a pCO2 less than 35. Alkalosis shifts the O2 disassociation curve to the left. It also causes cerebrovascular constriction. The kidneys compensate for respiratory alkalosis by excreting HCO_3.

○   **What is the most commonly injured nerve during parotidectomies?**

Injury to the ramus marginalis mandibularis that innervates the depressor muscles of the lower lip. The facial nerve should always be dissected when performing a parotidectomy.

○   **If medical management fails to relieve symptoms of gastroesophageal reflux after a 1 year trial period, what surgical methods might be attempted?**

The Hill gastropexy, the Nissen fundoplication, the Angelchik antireflux preostesis placement, or the Belsey IV operation. Surgical correction provides a 90% cure rate.

○   **In the Glasgow coma scale, a dead person rates a three. How many points are possible by measuring eye-opening response?**

4. (Remember: "I've got an eye 4 U.")

○   **How many points equal the best verbal response in the Glasgow coma scale?**

5.

❍   **How many points is the best motor response in the Glasgow coma scale?**

6.

❍   **What results are normal in the oculocephalic reflex?**

Conjugate eye movement is opposite to the direction of head rotation.

❍   **When testing a patient's oculovestibular reflex, which direction of nystagmus is anticipated in response to cold water irrigation: toward or away from the irrigated ear?**

Away from the irrigated ear. Recall that nystagmus is defined as the direction of the fast component of saccadic eye movement. (Remember: COWS = Cold Opposite, Warm Same.)

❍   **What does tonic eye movement towards an irrigated ear in response to warm caloric testing in a comatose patient signify?**

Life.

❍   **What affect do ß-blockers have on Prinzmetal's variant angina?**

They worsen the syndrome by allowing unopposed a-adrenergic stimulation of the coronary arteries.

❍   **What are the signs and symptoms of an ophthalmoplegic migraine?**

Diplopia. Mydriasis and exotropia may be noted. Palsies of the muscles served by cranial nerves III, IV, and VI may also occur. Typical duration of the migraine is 3 to 5 days.

❍   **Define strabismus.**

Strabismus: Lack of parallelism of the visual axis of the eyes.
Esotropia: Medial deviation.
Exotropia: Lateral deviation.

❍   **What drugs commonly cause bradycardia?**

ß-Blockers, cardiac glycosides, pilocarpine, and cholinesterase inhibitors, such as organophosphates, are all responsible for bradycardia.

Sympathomimetics, such as amphetamines and cocaine, and anticholinergics, such as atropine and cyclic antidepressants, commonly cause tachycardia.

❍   **Which street drug commonly causes both horizontal and vertical nystagmus?**

Phencyclidine (PCP).

❍   **What mnemonic may assist in recalling the signs of life-threatening cholinergic poisoning?**

DUELS.

Diaphoresis
Urination
Eye changes (miosis)
Lacrimation
Salivation

❍ **How long should sutures remain in the face? In the scalp or trunk? In the extremities? In the joints?**

Facial sutures: 3 to 5 days.
Scalp or trunk: 7 to 10 days.
Extremities: 10 to 14 days.
Joints: 14 days.

❍ **What are the signs and symptoms of uncal herniation?**
An uncal herniation typically compresses the ipsilateral third cranial nerve, resulting in ipsilateral pupil dilation. Contralateral weakness occurs because the pyramidal track decussates below this level. Occasionally, a shift will be great enough to cause compression of both sides, leading to a combination of ipsilateral or contralateral pupillary dilatation and weakness.

❍ **What common finding on a sinus x-ray suggests a basilar skull fracture?**

Blood in the sphenoid sinus.

❍ **The best view of the zygomatic arch on a face x-ray is:**

The modified basal view. This is also called jug-handle, submentaloccipital, or submental-vertical view.

❍ **What x-ray view should be ordered to evaluate the maxilla, maxillary sinus, orbital floor, inferior orbital rim, or zygomatic bones?**

Water's view.

❍ **Name five drugs or conditions that cause hypertension or tachycardia.**

SWAMP

Sympathomimetics
Withdrawal
Anticholinergics
MAO Inhibitors
Phencyclidine (PCP)

❍ **Name six common drugs that can cause hyperthermia.**

SANDS-PCP.

Salicylates
Anticholinergics
Neuroleptics
Dinitrophenols
Sympathomimetics
Phencyclidine (PCP)

❍ **What drugs and/or environmental exposures can induce bullous lesions?**

Sedative hypnotics, carbon monoxide, snake bite, spider bite, caustic agents, and hydrocarbons.

❍ **What drugs cause an acetone odor on the breath?**

Ethanol, isopropanol, and salicylates. Ketosis is often accompanied by the same odor.

❍   **What substances induce an odor of almonds on the breath?**

Cyanide, Laetrile, and apricot pits (latter two contain amygdalin).

❍   **What drugs induce a garlic odor on the breath?**

DMSO, organophosphates, phosphorus, arsenic, arsine gas, and thallium.

❍   **What drug induces a peanut odor on the breath?**

Vacor (RH-787).

❍   **What drugs induce a pear odor on the breath?**

Chloral hydrate and paraldehyde.

❍   **What compounds induce a rotten eggs odor on the breath?**

Hydrogen sulfide, mercaptans, and sewer gas.

❍   **What is the medical term for "bad breath"?**

Halitosis.

❍   **What mnemonic can be used for remembering what drugs or conditions commonly cause seizures?**

SHAKE WITH eL SPOC.

Salicylates
Hypoxia
Anticholinergics
Karbon monoxide (CO)
EtOH withdrawal

Withdrawal
Isoniazid
Theophylline and tricyclics
Hypoglycemia

Lead, lithium, and local anesthetics

Strychnine and sympathomimetics
PCP, phenothiazine, and propoxyphene
Organophosphates
Camphor, cholinergics, carbon monoxide, and cyanide

❍   **What is a mnemonic for remembering the drugs that cause nystagmus?**

MALES TIP.

Methanol
Alcohol
Lithium
Ethylene glycol
Sedative hypnotics and solvents

Thiamine depletion and Tegretol (carbamazepine)
Isopropanol
PCP and phenytoin

O   **What is a mnemonic for remembering drugs that are radiopaque?**

BAT CHIPS.

Barium
Antihistamines
Tricyclic antidepressants

Chloral hydrate, calcium, cocaine
Heavy metals
Iodine
Phenothiazine, potassium
Slow-release (enteric coated)

O   **What is the antidote for ß-blockers?**

Glucagon.

O   **What three toxicologic emergencies require immediate dialysis?**

Ethylene glycol, methyl alcohol, and *Amanita phalloides*.

O   **What is the antidote for isoniazid?**

Pyridoxine.

O   **What drugs are commonly excreted by using alkaline diuresis?**

Long-acting barbiturates, INH, tricyclic antidepressants, salicylates, and less commonly, lithium.

O   **Name some side effects of alkalization of the urine.**

Hypernatremia and hyperosmolality.

O   **Can theophylline be dialyzed?**

Yes.

O   **What four mechanisms induce tricyclic toxicity?**

1) Anticholinergic atropine-like effects secondary to competitive antagonism of acetylcholine.
2) Reuptake blockage of norepinephrine.
3) A quinidine-like action on the myocardium.
4) An a-blocking action.

O   **When does acetaminophen become toxic?**

When there is no glutathione to detoxify its toxic intermediate.

O   **Would you like to have four Aces?**

Of course! So check ACEtaminophen levels 4 hours after ingestion.

○ **Which type of acid-base disturbance initially occurs with a salicylate overdose?**

Respiratory alkalosis. Approximately 12 hours later, an anion gap metabolic acidosis or mixed acid base picture may occur.

○ **Is hyperglycemia or is hypoglycemia expected with a salicylate overdose?**

Expect either hyperglycemia or hypoglycemia.

○ **What are the common signs and symptoms of chronic salicylism?**

Fever, tachypnea, CNS alterations, acid base abnormalities, electrolyte abnormalities, chronic pain, ketonuria, and noncariogenic pulmonary edema.

○ **A patient presents with an acute salicylate ingestion. What symptoms are expected with a mild, moderate, and severe overdose?**

Mild: Lethargy, vomiting, hyperventilation, and hyperthermia.
Moderate: Severe hyperventilation and compensated metabolic acidosis.
Severe: Coma, seizures, and uncompensated metabolic acidosis.

○ **What is the treatment for a salicylate overdose?**

Decontaminate, lavage and charcoal, replace fluids, supplement with potassium, alkalize the urine with bicarbonate, cool for hyperthermia, administer glucose for hypoglycemia, place on oxygen and PEEP for pulmonary edema, prescribe multiple dose activated charcoal, and initiate dialysis.

○ **What are the signs and symptoms of a cyanide overdose?**

Dryness and burning in the throat, air hunger and hyperventilation. If the individual is not removed from the toxic environment, loss of consciousness, seizures, bradycardia and apnea will occur followed by asystole.

○ **What drugs can cause methemoglobinemia?**

Nitrites, local anesthetics, silver nitrate, amyl nitrite and nitrites, benzocaine, commercial marking crayons, aniline dyes, sulfonamides, and phenacetin.

○ **For which type of overdoses is atropine used?**

Organophosphate and carbamate.

○ **For which type of an overdose may the drug pralidoxime (2-PAM) be used?**

Organophosphate.

○ **Chronic bromism is treated with what drug?**

Sodium Chloride.

○ **Vitamin K is used to treat:**

Warfarin overdose.

○   **Methylene blue is used to treat:**

Methemoglobinemia.

○   **Isoniazid and Gyromitra mushroom poisoning is best treated with what drug?**

Pyridoxine.

○   **Name two selective cardioselective ß-blockers.**

Metoprolol and Atenolol. (Remember: "Look MA! I'm cardioselective!")

○   **An overdose of ß-blockers produces what signs and symptoms?**

Nausea, vomiting, bradycardia, hypotension, respiratory depression, seizure, CHF, bronchospasm, hypoglycemia, and hyperkalemia.

○   **When evaluating a pediatric C-spine film, what are the normal values?**

The predental space in a child is < 5 mm; in an adult, it is < 3 mm. The posterior cervical line attaching the base of the spinous process of C1 to C3 should be considered. If the base of C2 spinous process lies > 2 mm behind the posterior cervical line, a hangman's fracture should be suspected. The anterior border of C2 to the posterior wall of the fornix distance is < 7 mm. Finally, the anterior border of C6 to the posterior wall of the trachea distance is 14 mm in children younger than 15 years of age; it is < 22 mm in an adult.

○   **Describe a hangman's fracture.**

It is a C2 bilateral pedicle fracture.

○   **Injury to what cervical area results in Horner's syndrome (ptosis, miosis, and anhidrosis)?**

Disruption of the cervical sympathetic chain at C7 to T2.

○   **What spinal level corresponds to the dermatomal innervation of the perianal region? The nipple line? The index finger? The knee? The lateral foot?**

Perianal region: S2–S4.
Nipple line: T4.
Index finger: C7.
Knee: L4.
Lateral foot: S1.

○   **Describe central cord syndrome.**

An injury to the ligamentum flavum and to the cord, which causes an upper extremity neurologic deficit that is greater than the lower extremity deficit.

○   **Describe the presentation of a patient with Brown-Séquard syndrome.**

Ipsilateral motor paralysis, ipsilateral loss of proprioception, and a vibratory sensation. Contralateral loss of pain and a temperature sensation are also exhibited.

○   **Describe the presentation of a patient with anterior cord syndrome.**

Complete motor paralysis and loss of pain/temperature sensations distal to the lesion. Posterior column sparing results in intact proprioception and vibration sense. The cause is attributed to the occlusion of the anterior spinal artery or the protrusion of fracture fragments into the anterior canal.

○   **Under what conditions does trench (immersion) foot develop?**

Trench foot occurs when the extremity is exposed for several days to wet or cold conditions at temperatures that are above freezing. The extremity develops superficial damage resembling partial thickness burns.

○   **Describe pernio (chilblain).**

Exposure of an extremity for a prolonged period of time to dry, cold but above freezing temperatures. Patients develop superficial, small, painful ulcerations over the chronically exposed areas. Sensitivity of the surrounding skin, erythema, and pruritus may also develop.

○   **Describe frostnip.**

The skin becomes numb and blanched and then cessation of discomfort occurs. A sudden loss of the "cold" sensation at the location of injury is a reliable sign of precipitant frostbite. Frostnip will proceed to frostbite if treatment is not initiated.

○   **How is frostnip treated?**

It is treated by warming the affected area(s) by using the hands, breathing on the skin, or by placing the exposed extremities under the armpit. The affected part should not be rubbed because this treatment does not thaw the tissues completely. Frostnip is the only form of frostbite that can be treated at the scene.

○   **What is appropriate treatment for frostbite?**

Do not use dry heat! The exposed extremity should be rewarmed rapidly by immersing the affected area in 42°C circulating water for 20 minutes or until flushing is observed. Refreezing thawed tissue greatly increases damage. Remember to provide tetanus prophylaxis. Debride white or clear blisters as toxic mediators (prostaglandin and thromboxanes) may be present. However, leave hemorrhagic blisters intact. Topical antibiotics, such as silver sulfadiazine, may be used. After admission, the patient should undergo whirlpool treatments with a warm antibiotic solution at least twice a day.

○   **What are some common complications of frostbite?**

Rhabdomyolysis, permanent depigmentation of the extremity, and an increased probability of a subsequent injury caused by cold conditions. An x-ray, approximately 3 to 6 months after a frostbite injury, will reveal irregular, fine, punched-out lytic lesions which may appear on the MTP, PIP, and DIP joints.

○   **Where do endoscopic perforations of the esophagus typically occur?**

Near the distal esophagus or at the site of a pre-existing disease, such as a caustic burn.

○   **Where are the three most common sites of foreign body perforation of the esophagus?**

The levels of the cricopharyngeus muscle, the left mainstem bronchus, and the gastroesophageal junction.

○   **Where is the most common site of penetrating ureteral injuries?**

In the upper third of the ureter.

○   **What is the most common cause of a coagulopathy in patients who require massive transfusions?**

Thrombocytopenia.

○   **What percentage of individuals with ureteral injuries present without hematuria?**

33%.

○   **How is a posterior urethral tear diagnosed in males?**

A high-riding, boggy prostate is indicative of this injury.

○   **What signs and symptoms are associated with an anterior urethral tear?**

Severe perineal pain with blood usually found at the meatus. A good urinary stream will be maintained.

○   **A patient has a pelvic fracture with probable bladder or ureteral injury. Which test should be performed first, a cystogram or an IVP?**

The cystogram. This is done so that distal ureteral dye from the IVP will not mimic extravasation from the bladder.

○   **What is the half-life of carboxyhemoglobin?**

6 hours for 21% FIO_2, 1.5 hours for 100% FIO_2, and 0.5 hours in 3 atmospheres for hyperbaric 100% FIO_2.

○   **What is the most common cause of Ludwig's angina?**

An odontogenic abscess of a lower molar. The most common pathogen is hemolytic Streptococcus.

○   **The most common adverse effects of AZT is:**

Granulocytopenia and anemia.

○   **Isopropyl alcohol, glycerol, and a polyethylene glycol mixture are useful when treating which type of chemical burn?**

Phenol (carbolic acid).

○   **What is the best method for transporting an amputated extremity?**

Wrap the extremity in sterile gauze moistened with saline. Place it in waterproof plastic bag then immerse in ice water.

○   **What is the antidote for phosphorus poisoning?**

Copper sulfate, 1% solution. Remove phosphorus within 30 minutes of exposure. Phosphorus may be identified by the formation of an insoluble black precipitate when swabbing with copper sulfate.

○   **What dose of SQ/intradermal 10% calcium gluconate should be used to treat a hydrofluoric acid skin burn?**

0.5 cc per cm2 of the area burned.

○   **Explain the significant features of each axis in the DSM-IV official diagnostic criteria and the nomenclature for psychiatric illnesses.**

Axis I: Organic brain syndromes that are caused by intoxication or a physical illness. The major psychiatric disorders include psychosis, affective disorders, and disorders of substance use.
Axis II: Personality disorders, including antisocial, schizoid, and histrionic types.
Axis III: Medical problems, such as heart disease and infections.
Axis IV: Life events that contribute to the patient's problems.
Axis V: Patient's adaptation to these problems.

○ **What local anesthetics may cause anaphylaxis?**

The ester derivatives containing para-aminobenzoic acid (PABA) are known to stimulate IgE antibody formation and thereby cause anaphylaxis. Such anesthetics include procaine and tetracaine.

○ **What neighboring structures may be injured with a supracondylar distal humeral fracture?**

The anterior interosseous nerve (a branch of the median nerve) and the brachial artery.

○ **What test best discriminates between functional and organic blindness?**

Optokinetic drum. Black and white lines will produce nystagmus in patients with intact vision.

○ **What ligament is commonly injured after an inversion ankle sprain?**

The anterior talofibular ligament.

○ **How is a perilunate dislocation diagnosed?**

By AP and lateral x-rays. The lunate remains in alignment with the radial fossa, while the other carpal bones appear displaced.

○ **What is the cause of granuloma inguinale?**

The bacterium *Donovania granulomatis*, recently renamed *Calymmatobacterium granulomatis*.

○ **What is the best diluent for treating the ingestion of solid lye?**

Milk.

○ **What is the cause of condylomata acuminata?**

Papilloma virus.

○ **What organ is most severely affected in a blast injury?**

The lungs.

○ **What organ is most commonly affected in a blast injury?**

The ears.

○ **A patient has previous focal deficits from CVAs. Is it true that such a patient can present with confusion when afflicted with a new focal lesion?**

Yes. The presentation of a new focal lesion may be displayed with generalized or non-focal symptoms in the context of previous insults.

❍ **A patient with a dementia contracts a wound infection. Is it true that such a patient can present with a severe decrease in mental status?**

Yes. Normal minor insults can cause drastic changes in the neurologic functioning of patients with pre-existing deficits.

❍ **A patient had right arm and hand paralysis from a previous CVA; however, only residual weakness remains. If the patient has a subsequent episode of hyponatremia, can right arm and hand paralysis reoccur?**

Sure. Formerly compensated deficits may return in response to a generalized neurological insult.

❍ **RBC basophilic stippling occurs with what 2 disorders?**

Thalassemia and lead poisoning.

❍ **What triad is associated with Reiter's syndrome?**

Non-gonococcal urethritis, polyarthritis, and conjunctivitis. Conjunctivitis is the least common and occurs in only 30% of the patients. Acute attacks respond well to NSAIDs.

❍ **What are the most common causes of immediate post partum hemorrhage?**

Uterine atony, followed by vaginal/cervical lacerations and retained placenta or placental fragments.

❍ **What complication of rheumatoid arthritis requires emergency treatment?**

Vasculitis. This condition should be treated promptly with systemic steroids. If treatment is delayed, irreversible neuropathy may occur.

❍ **What is Felty's syndrome?**

Rheumatoid arthritis with splenomegaly and neutropenia. It is a late complication of rheumatoid arthritis.

❍ **What drugs can induce a lupus reaction?**

Procainamide, hydralazine, isoniazid, and phenytoin.

❍ **What is the most serious complication associated with dental infections (besides possible respiratory compromise, from Ludwig's angina)?**

Septic cavernous sinus thrombosis.

❍ **What joint is most commonly affected with gout?**

The great toe MCP joint.

❍ **What joint is most commonly affected with pseudogout?**

The knee. The causative agent is calcium pyrophosphate crystals.

❍ **What are the complications of impetigo?**

Streptococcal-induced impetigo can result in post streptococcal glomerulonephritis. However, it has not been shown to be associated with rheumatic fever. Treat with erythromycin, dicloxacillin, or cephalexin to help eliminate the skin lesions. There is no conclusive proof that treatment prevents glomerulonephritis.

○   **What is the most effective method for decontaminating the skin following radiation exposure?**

Wash with soap and water after removing all clothes.

○   **What is the most probable cause of a unilateral transient loss of vision in a patient's eye (amaurosis fugax)?**

Carotid artery disease. This usually is the result of platelet emboli from plaques in the arterial system.

○   **What is the most common cause of a transudative pleural effusion?**

Congestive heart failure.

○   **Where does botulism toxin exert its effects?**

At the myoneural junction. The toxin prevents the release of acetylcholine.

○   **A patient with a sickle cell trait most commonly presents with:**

Hematuria and decreased urine concentrating ability.

○   **What is the pathophysiology of myasthenia gravis?**

Circulatory antibody against ACh receptor which binds at the motor end plate. In myasthenics, ACh receptors are in short supply, resulting in fatigable weakness.

○   **What is the most serious transfusion reaction?**

Hemolytic. Treat with aggressive fluid replacement and Lasix.

○   **What is the most common transfusion reaction?**

Febrile.

○   **What diseases are associated with myasthenia gravis?**

Rheumatoid arthritis, pernicious anemia, SLE, sarcoidosis, and thyroiditis. 10 to 25% of patients with this condition are also afflicted with thymoma.

○   **A patient presents with ocular, bulbar, and limb weakness which worsens during the day and decreases with rest. What is the diagnosis?**

Myasthenia gravis.

○   **What is the best emergency treatment of an Ellis III dental fracture in an adult?**

Cover tooth with moist cotton and then dry aluminum foil and refer immediately to an orthodontist.

○   **What are some factors commonly associated with meningitis?**

Age less than 5 years or greater than 60 years, low socioeconomic status, male sex, crowding, black race, sickle cell disease, splenectomy, alcoholism, diabetes, cir-rhosis, immunologic defects, dural defect from congenital, surgical or traumatic source, contiguous infections such as sinusitis, household contacts, malignancy, bacterial endocarditis, IV drug abuse, and thalassemia major.

○   **A patient has xanthochromic CSF with a low protein count. What is the most likely cause?**

Subarachnoid hemorrhage.

○   **A patient has xanthochromic CSF with a high protein count (> 150 mg/dL). What is the most likely cause?**

Traumatic tap.

○   **What disease is associated with periaqueductal petechial hemorrhages?**

Wernicke's disease.

○   **What disorders are associated with cerebrocortical neuronal degenera-tion?**

Anoxic, hypoglycemic, and hepatic encephalopathies.

○   **What is the most commonly abused volatile substance?**

Toluene.

○   **A patient presents with hypokalemia of 2.0, hyperchloremia, and acido-sis. What is the most likely toxicologic cause?**

Chronic toluene abuse.

○   **A patient has been abusing nitrous oxide for a long time. What symptoms might be expected?**

Paresthesias and motor weakness may be present in chronic abusers. Such symptoms are often mistaken for symptoms of multiple sclerosis.

○   **Describe the features of the three stages of PCP intoxication.**

Stage I: Agitation or violence, normal vital signs.
Stage II: Tachycardia, hypertension, no response to pain.
Stage III: Unresponsive, depressed respirations, seizures, death.

○   **Should the urine be acidified in the treatment of PCP intoxication?**

Although acidification of the urine is theoretically advantageous, clinical experience has not shown this to be efficacious. Let's call that a "no."

○   **A patient presents with belladonna alkaloid poisoning resulting in anticholinergic effects. Explain the dangers of treating this patient with physostigmine.**

Physostigmine acts to increase acetylcholine levels. In doing so, it can precipitate a cholinergic crisis resulting in heart block and asystole. As a result, it is recommended to reserve physostigmine for life-threatening anticholinergic complications.

○   **Does botulism produce fever?**

No. This can be important in differentiating neurologic symptoms in a sick patient who could have diphtheria.

O   **Describe a patient with Chlamydial pneumonia.**

Chlamydial pneumonia is usually seen in children 2 to 6 weeks of age. The patient is afebrile and does not appear toxic.

O   **A patient has had three days of diarrhea which was abrupt in onset. The patient reports slimy green, malodorous stools that contain blood. In addition, the patient is febrile. What is the most likely cause?**

Salmonella. Treat with the antibiotics Ampicillin, TMP/SMX or Chloramphenicol.

O   **What is the treatment for *Campylobacter*?**

Erythromycin or tetracycline.

O   **In a child, does coarctation of the aorta typically cause cyanosis?**

No.

O   **How much elemental iron will 100 mg of deferoxamine bind?**

About 8.5 mg of elemental iron is bound by 100 mg of deferoxamine.

O   **What is the treatment for persistent E. coli?**

Trimethoprim with sulfamethoxazole (TMP-SMX).

O   **What is the treatment for *Giardia lamblia*?**

Quinacrine or metronidazole or furazolidone.

O   **What is the pharmacological treatment for persistent salmonellosis?**

Ampicillin, TMP-SMX, Chloramphenicol.

O   **What is the treatment for *Shigella* sp.?**

TMP-SMX or Ciprofloxacin (if resistant).

O   **What is the treatment for *Yersinia* sp.?**

TMP-SMX, tetracycline, third generation cephalosporin.

O   **What are the eight common clinical presentations of pediatric heart dis-ease?**

1) Cyanosis
2) Pathologic murmur
3) Abnormal pulses
4) CHF
5) HTN
6) Cardiogenic shock
7) Syncope
8) Tachyarrhythmias

○   **What is the function of aldosterone?**

Aldosterone causes sodium conservation and K+ excretion. As a result, it causes increased resorption of sodium and fluid.

○   **What drug will most rapidly decrease K+?**

Calcium chloride IV (1 to 3 minutes). Contraindicated in patients with Digoxin toxicity.

○   **What is a potential side effect of the use of Kayexalate?**

Kayexalate exchanges sodium for K+. As a result, sodium overload and CHF may oc-cur.

○   **What vital sign might be affected with hypermagnesemia?**

Hypermagnesemia causes hypotension because it relaxes vascular smooth muscle. Deep tendon reflexes may disappear.

○   **Common causes of hypercalcemia:**

PAM P. SCHMIDT

Parathyroid hormone
Addison's
Multiple myeloma

Paget's

Sarcoidosis
Cancer
Hyperthyroidism
Milk - alkali syndrome
Immobilization
D vitamin excess
Thiazides

○   **In whom does alcoholic ketoacidosis commonly occur? When?**

It usually occurs in chronic alcoholics after an interval of binge drinking followed by 1 to 3 days of protracted vomiting, abstinence, and decreased food intake.

○   **What dose of ASA will cause mild to moderate toxicity?**

200 to 300 mg/kg. Greater than 500 mg/kg is potentially lethal.

○   **What is the ferric chloride test and what toxic ingestion does it detect?**

Add a few drops of 10% ferric chloride solution to a few drops of urine. A purple color indicates presence of salicylic acid. Ketones or phenothiazine can lead to falsely positive results.

○   **What is the treatment of lithium overdose?**

Saline diuresis and hemodialysis.

○   **What is the treatment for chloral hydrate overdose?**

Hemodialysis and/or charcoal hemoperfusion will clear the active metabolite, trichloroethanol.

〇   **What are the common effects of barbiturate overdose?**

Hypothermia, hyperventilation, venodilation with hypotension, and negative inotropic effect on the myocardium. Clear vesicles and bullae may also be seen.

〇   **What is the pediatric dose of naloxone?**

0.01 mg/kg to 0.8 mg/kg, may repeat.

〇   **What are some signs and symptoms of thrombotic thrombocytopenic purpura (TTP)?**

Thrombocytopenia, purpura, and microangiopathic hemolytic anemia. Patient with TTP presents with fever, fluctuating neurologic signs, and renal complications. If the disease goes untreated, it is almost uniformly fatal. Therapy includes steroids, splenectomy, plasmapheresis and exchange, and antiplatelet agents, such as dipyridamole and aspirin.

〇   **How does a patient present with Boerhaave's syndrome?**

Boerhaave's syndrome is spontaneous esophageal perforation. It usually occurs after forceful vomiting. The patient suffers an acute collapse with chest and abdominal pain. A left pleural effusion is seen on chest x-ray in 90% of patients; most have mediastinal emphysema.

〇   **In which type of patients is staphylococcal pneumonia likely?**

Patients who are hospitalized, debilitated, or abusing drugs.

〇   **What are the five key lab findings in DIC?**

1) Increased PT.
2) Increased PTT.
3) Increased fibrin degradation products.
4) Decreased fibrinogen.
5) Decreased platelet levels.

〇   **In the thrombocytopenic patient, one unit of platelets will raise the platelet count by about how much?**

One unit raises the platelet count by about 10,000/mm3.

〇   **What are the classic findings of shaken baby syndrome?**

1) Failure to thrive.
2) Lethargy.
3) Seizures.
4) Retinal hemorrhages.
5) CT may show subarachnoid hemorrhage or subdural hematoma from torn bridging veins.

〇   **Define spondylolysis.**

A defect in the pars interarticularis.

〇   **Define spondylolisthesis.**

The forward movement of one vertebral body on the vertebra below it.

○ **T/F: High fever in neonates with bacterial pneumonia usually follows a period of general fussiness and decreased feeding.**

True.

○ **Conjunctivitis is an associated finding in about what percentage of neonates with *Chlamydia* pneumonia?**

About 50%.

○ **What is the immediate treatment for cord prolapse?**

Displace the head cephalad.

○ **What nerve may be injured in a distal femoral fracture?**

Peroneal nerve.

○ **How many days after birth should newborns stop losing weight?**

About 6 days.

○ **T/F: A neonate's stool color can be an important sign.**

False. Unless blood is evident, stool color is insignificant.

○ **What is the difference between vomiting and regurgitation?**

Very little once it's on you! Vomiting is caused by forceful diaphragmatic and abdominal muscle contraction. Regurgitation occurs without effort.

○ **Is regurgitation dangerous in an otherwise thriving neonate?**

No. However, it can be dangerous for newborns with failure to thrive or respiratory problems, and it may be associated with chronic aspiration.

○ **Projectile vomiting in the neonate is often associated with pyloric stenosis. When this is the case, such vomiting becomes a prominent sign at what age?**

2 to 3 weeks.

○ **What is the name for diarrhea associated with sepsis, otitis media, UTI or any other systemic disease?**

Parenteral diarrhea.

○ **Infectious diarrhea is usually viral. What are the two most common agents?**

Rotavirus and Norwalk agent.

○ **T/F: Bacterial and parasitic etiologies of diarrhea in the neonate are rare.**

True.

○ **What are some entities in the differential diagnosis of bloody diarrhea in the neonate?**

Necrotizing enterocolitis, bacterial enteritis, allergic reactions to milk , and iatrogenic causes secondary to antibiotics.

❍   **What are some of the signs of sepsis to look for in babies with necrotizing enterocolitis?**

Poor feeding, lethargy, fever, jaundice, abdominal distention, and poor color.

❍   **What should be considered in the case of a neonate who has never passed stool?**

Meconium ileus or plug, Hirschsprung's disease, intestinal stenosis, or atresia.

❍   **Anal stenosis, hypothyroidism, and Hirschsprung's disease can all present with what clinical sign?**

Constipation that was not present at birth but which began before the infant was 1 month old.

❍   **Describe the signs and symptoms of a patient with chondromalacia patellae.**

Chondromalacia patellae typically occurs in young, active females. The pain is localized to the knee. There is no effusion and no history of trauma. Patella compression tests are usually positive.

❍   **Describe the signs and symptoms of tarsal tunnel syndrome.**

Insidious onset of paresthesia, as well as burning pain and numbness on the plantar surface of the foot. Pain radiates superiorly along the medial side of the calf. Rest decreases pain.

❍   **What causes swimmer's itch (Schistosome dermatitis)?**

An invading cercariae.

❍   **What is the vector of malaria?**

Anopheles mosquito.

❍   **What is the vector of trypanosomiasis?**

Tsetse fly.

❍   **What is the infectious agent of elephantiasis?**

Nematode microfilaria.

❍   **What vector transmits Chagas' disease (*Trypanosoma cruzi*)?**

Reduviid (assassin or kissing bug).

❍   **Cysticercosis is associated with:**

 New onset seizure.

❍   **Hookworm is associated with what sort of anemia?**

Iron deficiency anemia.

❍   **Fish tapeworm (*Diphyllobothrium latum*) is associated with what type of anemia?**

Pernicious anemia.

O   **Onchocerciasis (from Onchocerca volvulus) is associated with what visual deficit?**

Blindness.

O   **Chagas' disease is associated with:**

Acute myocarditis. *Trypanosoma cruzi* invades the myocardium resulting in myocarditis. Conduction defects may occur. The vector for this parasite is the insect Reduviid.

O   **Roundworm is associated with what GI problem?**

Small bowel obstruction.

O   **What is the presentation of a patient with post extraction alveolitis?**

"Dry socket" pain occurs on the second or third day after extraction.

O   **Ludwig's angina typically involves what spaces in the head?**

The submental, sublingual, and submandibular spaces.

O   **What are the signs and symptoms of a peritonsillar abscess?**

Sore throat, dysarthria (hot potato voice), odynophagia, ipsilateral otalgia, low grade fever, trismus, and uvular displacement.

O   **What is the presentation of a patient with diphtheria?**

Sore throat, dysphagia, fever, and tachycardia. A dirty, tough gray fibrinous membrane so firmly adherent that removal causes bleeding may be present in the oropharynx. *Corynebacterium diphtheriae* exotoxin acts directly on cardiac, renal, and nervous systems. It can cause ocular bulbar paralysis that may suggest botulism or myasthenia gravis. The exotoxin may also cause flaccid limb weakness. Of note, such weakness may also include decreased or absent DTRs, a finding suggestive of Guillain-Barré or tick paralysis.

O   **How does a patient present with a retropharyngeal abscess?**

Patients typically prefer a supine position. Retropharyngeal abscesses are common under 3 years of age. On examination, the uvula and tonsil are displaced away from the abscess. Soft tissue swelling and forward displacement of the larynx are present. Soft tissue x-ray films of the neck may assist in the diagnosis.

O   **How does an adult with epiglottitis present?**

Pharyngitis and dysphagia are prominent symptoms. Adenopathy is uncommon. The patient may have a muffled voice and speak softly; however, hoarseness is rare. Pain is out of proportion to objective find-ings.

O   **What are the two common pathogens in adult acute sinusitis?**

Streptococcus pneumoniae and *H. influenzae*.

O   **What is rhinocerebral phycomycosis?**

Rhinocerebral phycomycosis, also known as mucormycosis, is a fungal infection typically seen in diabetic patients with ketoacidosis and immunocompromised patients. The disease is rapidly fatal if not recognized and treated quickly. Treatment includes antifungal drugs and surgical debridement.

○   **Magnesium containing antacids may cause:**

Diarrhea.

○   **Aluminum containing antacids may cause:**

Constipation.

○   **When does an elevation of HBsAg occur in relation to symptoms of Hepatitis B?**

HBsAg always rises before clinical symptoms of hepatitis B.

○   **Is hepatitis A associated with jaundice?**

Typically not, as more than 50% of the population has serologic evidence for hep-atitis and do not recall being symptomatic.

○   **Describe a patient with intussusception.**

Patients are most likely very young. 70% of patients have intussusception within the first year of life. In children, the cause is thought to be secondary to lymphoid tissue at the ileocecal valve; in adults, it is thought to be caused by local lesions, Meckel's diverticulum, or tumor. On examination, bowel sounds are usually normal. Intussusception typically involves the terminal ileum. Meckel's diverticulum is the single most common intrinsic bowel lesion involved.

○   **Should *Salmonella* gastroenteritis be treated with antibiotics?**

Only if symptomatic infection persists. Treat with ampicillin, TMP-SMX, or Chloramphenicol.

○   **What are the common features of *Vibrio parahaemolyticus*?**

This condition is caused by organisms associated with oysters, clams, and crabs. Symptoms include cramps, vomiting, dysentery, and explosive diarrhea. Severe infections are treated with tetracycline and chloramphenicol.

○   **Which types of anorectal abscesses can be drained in the ED?**

Perianal, submucosal, and pilonidal abscesses. Ischiorectal and supralevator abscesses need to be drained in the operating room.

○   **Painful, bright red rectal bleeding is most often due to:**

Anal fissure. External hemorrhoids present with acute painful thrombosis and are not typically associated with constant, bright red bleeding. Internal hemorrhoids present with painless bright red bleeding, usually with defecation.

○   **Where is the narrowest part of the ureter?**

The ureterovesical junction.

O **Acute testicular pain and relief of pain with elevation of the scrotum (Prehn's sign) is classically associated with:**

Epididymitis.

O **What is the drug of choice for treating urinary tract infection due to *Proteus mirabilis*?**

Ampicillin. This condition is common in young boys.

O **What is the most common organism causing epididymitis in a 20-year-old?**

Chlamydia trachomatis.

O **How should hydralazine be dosed for a preeclamptic patient?**

Hydralazine should be given in 5 mg boluses every 20 minutes until adequate BP control is achieved or a total of 20 mg is reached.

O **What is the antidote for magnesium sulfate overdose?**

Calcium gluconate infusion.

O **In an ectopic pregnancy, is an adnexal mass a common finding?**

No. An adnexal mass is actually found in less than 50% of cases. Abdominal pain is the most frequent symptom. Amenorrhea is the second most common symptom.

O **As pCO_2 increases, pH will decrease. How much is the pH expected to de-crease for every 10 mm Hg increase in pCO_2?**

pH decreases by 0.08 units for each 10 mm increase Hg in pCO_2.

O **What is the therapy of choice to neutralize heparin in a patient who was inadvertently been administered to much?**

Protamine. 1 mg of protamine will neutralize about 100 units of heparin. The maximum dose of protamine is 100 mg.

O **What are the most common symptoms of a PE?**

Chest Pain (88%) and dyspnea (84%).

O **What are the most common signs of a PE?**

Tachypnea (92%) and rales (58%).

O **What is the most common radiographic finding of a PE?**

An elevated hemidiaphragm (41%).

O **What is the most common ECG finding of a PE?**

T-wave inversion (42%). Also seen is the S, Q3T3 pattern.

O **Of patients with a PE, what percentage have a normal ECG?**

13%.

○ **Of patients with a PE, what percentage of ECGs show the classic S1Q3T3 pattern?**

12%. Incidence is 18% with a massive PE.

○ **What test is most sensitive for evaluating a PE?**

Ventilation-Perfusion scan is the most sensitive test. However, it is not as specific as a pulmonary angiogram. 5% of normal volunteers will have an abnormal scan, and virtually any pulmonary pathology will produce an abnormal scan (i.e. pneumonia).

○ **What organisms are most commonly present in a pulmonary abscess?**

Mixed anaerobes.

○ **What are some causes of thoracic outlet syndrome?**

The most common cause is a cervical rib. Additional causes include: compression of the subclavian artery by an anomalous cervical rib, compression of the neurovascular bundle as it passes through the interscalene triangle; when the arms are hyperabducted, compression of the neurovascular bundle in the retroclavicular space, anterior to the first rib. Symptoms are typically produced when the shoulders are moved backward and downward.

○ **What is the most common cause of endocarditis in IV drug abusers?**

Staphylococcus aureus, most commonly involving the tricuspid valve.

○ **What are the classic signs and symptoms of aortic stenosis?**

Left heart failure, angina, and exertional syncope.

○ **What patient position will enhance the murmur of mitral stenosis?**

Left lateral decubitus.

○ **What is the optimal patient position and maneuver for auscultation of aortic insufficiency?**

Have the patient sit up and lean forward with his or her hands tightly clasped. During exhala-tion, listen at the left sternal border.

○ **What murmurs will the Valsalva maneuver increase?**

Only IHSS. All other murmurs are diminished.

○ **What is the most common valvular disorder in the US?**

Mitral valve prolapse.

○ **What is the most common cause of endocarditis in late onset prosthetic valve endocarditis?**

Streptococcus viridans.

○ **What are the symptoms of endocarditis?**

Fever, chills, malaise, anorexia, weight loss, back pain, myalgia, arthralgia, chest pain, dyspnea, edema, headache, stiff neck, mental status changes, focal neurologic complaints, extremity pain, paresthesia, hematuria, and abdominal pain.

○ **What are the key diagnostic features of coarctation of the aorta?**

Rib notching seen on x-ray and significant differences in the blood pressure between the upper and lower extremities.

○ **What is an interesting diagnostic feature of aortic regurgitation?**

Head bobbing.

○ **What is the most common arrhythmia associated with digitalis?**

PVC (60%), ectopic SVT (25%), and AV block (20%).

○ **What effect does furosemide have on calcium excretion?**

Furosemide causes increased calcium excretion in the urine.

○ **What is the most common arrhythmia in mitral stenosis?**

Atrial fibrillation.

○ **The most common cause of CHF in an adult is:**

Hypertension.

○ **What is the differential diagnosis of pulmonary edema with a normal size heart?**

Constrictive pericarditis, massive MI, non-cardiogenic pulmonary edema, and mitral stenosis (not mitral regurgitation).

○ **How does dobutamine differ from dopamine?**

Dobutamine decreases afterload with less tendency to cause tachycardia.

○ **Describe Kerley A and B lines.**

Kerley A lines are straight, non-branching lines in the upper lung fields. Kerley B lines are horizontal, non-branching lines at the periphery of the lower lung fields.

○ **Does nifedipine typically affect preload or afterload?**

Nifedipine is a vasodilator whose primary affects are on afterload reduction.

○ **What effect does the Valsalva maneuver have on the heart?**

Valsalva decreases blood return to both the right and left ventricles. All murmurs decrease in intensity except IHSS and MVP.

○ **Does prednisone cross the placenta?**

No. Prednisone is metabolized through prednisolone, which does not cross the placenta.

❍   **How do you treat a patient with a severe, high concentration hydrofluoric acid burn?**

In addition to topical jelly and cutaneous injections of calcium gluconate, provide IV treatment with 10 cc of 10% calcium gluconate (not calcium chloride) diluted in 50 cc of D5W. This is given via a pump over 4 hours.

❍   **How should an ocular burn secondary to hydrofluoric acid be treated?**

Use calcium gluconate in a 1% solution mixed with saline to irrigate the eyes. The solution is made by diluting 1 part of standard 10% calcium glu-conate solution with 10 parts of saline which produces a 1% solution.

❍   **What electrolyte is depleted in a victim of a hydrofluoric acid burn?**

Hydrofluoric acid results in hypocalcemia. Patients may require calcium replacement. Keep in mind that normal signs and symptoms of hypocalcemia, such as Chvostek's sign, do not typically appear with hypocalcemia secondary to HF.

❍   **A 35-year-old female presents with altered mental status and a temperature of 105°F. The patient's muscles are rigid. She feels very hot in the trunk, but her extremities are cool. What diagnosis is likely?**

Neuroleptic malignant syndrome. Check the CPK.

❍   **How should a patient with neuroleptic malignant syndrome be treated?**

1) Ice packs to the groin and axilla.
2) Cooling blankets.
3) Fan.
4) Water mist evaporation.
5) Dantrolene at an IV rate of 0.8 to 3 mg/kg IV every 6 hours to a total of 10 mg/kg.

❍   **How should a patient with a black widow spider bite be treated?**

Consider antivenin, IV calcium gluconate, and IV opiates plus IV benzodiazepines.

❍   **T/F: Centruroides scorpion antivenin should be administered for all Centruroides envenomations.**

False! Scorpion antivenin is rarely necessary and is typically only used in children who have a severe (grade IV) envenomation with peripheral motor and cranial nerve involvement. It is important to use Centruroides antivenin only in severe cases, as serum sickness or rash after administration is very common. In fact, as many as 60% of patients develop a rash or serum sickness secondary to this antivenin.

❍   **What is a significant complication of scorpion envenomation?**

Rhabdomyolysis.

❍   **In what states could a scorpion bite be deadly?**

Centruroides, which is the most toxic of scorpion stings, is only found in Arizona, California, Texas, and New Mexico.

❍   **An elderly patient presents with the complaint of seeing halos around lights. What diagnosis is suspected?**

Glaucoma. Another presenting complaint of glaucoma is blurred vision. Also, consider digitalis toxicity.

○   **A patient presents with back pain and complaints of incontinence. On examination, loss of anal reflex and decreased sphincter tone is noted. What is your diagnosis?**

Cauda equina syndrome. The most consistent finding is urinary retention. On physical examination, you should expect saddle anesthesia, that is, numbness over the posterior superior thighs as well as numbness of the buttocks and perineum.

○   **Where is the most common site of lumbar disc herniations?**

98% of clinically important lumbar disc herniations are at the L4–L5 or L5–S1 intervertebral levels. Evaluate these patients by checking for weakness of ankle and great toe dorsiflexors (L5). Also check pinprick sensation over the medial aspect of the foot (L5) and the lateral portion of the feet (S1).

○   **What WBC count is expected during pregnancy?**

WBC counts of 15,000 to 20,000 are considered normal in pregnancy.

○   **When monitoring a pregnant trauma victim, whose vital signs are the most sensitive, those of the mother or those of the fetus?**

The fetal heart rate is more sensitive to inadequate resuscitation. Remember that the mother may lose 10 to 20% of her blood volume without a change in vital signs, whereas the baby's heart rate may increase or decrease above 160 or below 120, indicating significant fetal distress. The most common pitfall is failure to adequately resuscitate the mother.

○   **What two findings on physical examination are indicative of uterine rupture?**

Loss of uterine contour and palpable fetal part.

○   **What physical examination findings may be discovered in abruptio placenta?**

Rapidly increasing fundal height secondary to bleeding into the uterus or a higher than expected fundal height.

○   **What is the number one risk factor for uterine rupture?**

Previous cesarean section.

○   **How should a diagnostic peritoneal lavage be performed for a pregnant patient?**

Use an open supraumbilical approach. Always make sure an NG tube and Foley are in place.

○   **An unconscious 60-year-old patient presents to the emergency department with a head injury. An ECG shows significant ST segment elevation. What is your concern?**

Although MI should be considered, don't forget the possibility of an intracerebral hemorrhage. This may also cause significant ST segment elevation.

○   **Why should the use of atropine be considered in a pediatric patient prior to intubation?**

Many pediatric patients develop bradycardia associated with intubation, which can be prevented by pre-treatment with atropine (0.01 mg/kg).

O   **What size tracheotomy tube is appropriate for an adult female and for an adult male?**

An adult female generally requires a No. 4 tracheostomy tube, and an adult male generally requires a No. 5.

O   **What are the effects of using ketamine in a pediatric patient?**

The child's eyes will be wide open with a glassy stare. He or she will have nystagmus, hyperemic flush, and hypersalivation. There will also be a slight rise in the heart rate. A very rare complication of ketamine use is laryngospasm. Hallucinations are a common side effect in children over the age of 10; as a consequence, ketamine should be restricted to use only in patients under the age of 10.

Note: Ketamine may also cause sympathetic stimulation, which increases intracranial pres-sure and may cause random movements of the head and extremities. Thus, it is not a good sedative for children going to CT scan.

O   **Why are quinolones contraindicated for children?**

Quinolones impair cartilage growth.

O   **What is the dose of acyclovir (Zovirax) used to treat herpes zoster infections in an immunocompetent adult?**

800 mg po 5 times/day for 7 to 10 days. For herpes simplex genitalis, the dose is much lower (i.e., 200 mg po 5 times/day for 10 days).

O   **What are the indications for giving digitalis-specific Fab (Digibind)?**

1) Ventricular arrhythmias
2) K+ > 5.5 mEq/L
3) Unresponsive bradyarrhythmias

Some authors refer to an ingestion of more than 0.3 mg/kg as requiring Fab. The number of vials required is 1.33 mg ingested. You can use this formula to determine dose based on serum digoxin level, or you can give 10 vials (40 mg Fab each) if the amount ingested is unknown.

Children and adolescents have an even higher sensitivity to digoxin overdose and may need Fab therapy with ingestion of less than the recommended 0.3 mg/kg.

Remember: In an acute overdose situation, the serum level of digitalis is unreliable for evaluating toxicity. Digitalis levels typically only become accurate after 4 to 6 hours; this is too long to wait for treatment.

O   **You give digoxin specific antibody (Fab) to a digoxin-toxic patient with an elevated digoxin level. A repeat digoxin level is obtained after this treatment and it is much higher than the previous level! What gives? Didn't the Fab work?**

Digoxin assay measures free and bound digoxin; the latter increases about 15 times via binding to Fab.

O   **What electrolyte change is expected with a serious digoxin ingestion?**

Expect hyperkalemia. After Fab, the potassium level may drop quickly and the patient may become hypokalemic. Monitor carefully.

O   **A near-drowning victim is comatose and intubated. A diagnosis of severe pulmonary edema is made. What specific pulmonary treatment should be provided in the ED?**

It is important to give these patients PEEP early, in order to decrease intrapulmonary shunting and prevent terminal airway closure.

○ **There are four types of hypersensitivity reactions. Name them in order and cite an example.**

Hypersensitivity	Reaction	Mediator	Example
Type 1:	Immediate	IgE binds allergen, includes mast cells and basophils	Food allergy. Asthma in children.
Type 2:	Cytotoxic	IgG and IgM antibody reactions to antigen on cell surface activates complement and killers	Blood transfusion rxn. ITP, hemolytic anemia.
The least common rxn.			
Type 3:	Immune complex, Arthrus	Complexes activate complement	Tetanus toxoid in sensitized persons.
Poststreptococcal glomerulonephritis.			
Type 4:	Cell mediated, delayed hypersensitivity	Activated T-lymphocytes	Skin tests

○ **What distinguishes heat stroke from heat exhaustion?**

Heat exhaustion involves the progressive loss of electrolytes and body fluid. Therapy is rehydration. Heat stroke occurs when body temperature exceeds 42°C and enzyme systems cease to function normally. As a result, there is necrosis, denaturing, and organ failure. Heat stroke requires much more aggressive treatment than simple fluid rehydration.

Remember: in patients with an altered sensorium and a core temperature above 42°C, always suspect heat stroke. Only half of these patients will be diaphoretic.

○ **What lab abnormalities may be found with heat stroke?**

High elevations in SGOT, SGPT, and LDH. The BUN/CR ratio will also show dehydration in many cases.

○ **How should a patient with heat stroke be treated?**

1) Cool the patient with lukewarm water and fans.
2) Pack the axillae, neck, and groin with ice.
3) Give fluids cautiously as large boluses of fluids may precipitate pulmonary edema.
4) Treat shivering with chlorpromazine (Thorazine) 25 to 50 mg IV.

○ **What complications can result from heat stroke?**

Renal failure, rhabdomyolysis, DIC, and seizures. Remember: Antipyretics won't help.

○ **What conditions may make the end tidal CO_2 monitor inaccurate?**

Monitor may be falsely yellow due to contamination from acid dilutants and drugs, such as lidocaine-HCl and epinephrine-HCl. Contamination with vomitus or acid dilutants may also produce false readings.

○ **You are having a hard time remembering which anesthetics are amides and which anesthetics are esters. What is a fairly easy way of telling these two classifications apart?**

With the exception of the suffix -caine, only the anesthetics in the amide classification include the letter I.

Amides Esters
Lidocaine (Xylocaine)
Bupivacaine (Marcaine)
Mepivacaine (Carbocaine)

Procaine (Novocain)
Cocaine
Tetracaine (Pontocaine)
Benzocaine

O   **An elderly patient presents with sudden onset of severe abdominal pain fol-lowed by a forceful bowel movement. Probable diagnosis?**

Acute mesenteric ischemia. Keep in mind that abdominal series may be normal early in acute mesenteric ischemia. Possible late x-ray findings include: Absent bowel gas, ileus, gas in the intestinal wall, and thumb-printing of the intestinal mucosa. In most cases, films are normal or not specifically suggestive. Expect heme-positive stools. Patients especially prone to mesenteric ischemia include those with CHF and chronic heart disease.

O   **Under what conditions does neurogenic pulmonary edema occur?**

Neurogenic pulmonary edema is commonly associated with increased intracranial pressure. It is commonly seen with head trauma, subarachnoid hemorrhage, and even with seizures.

O   **A patient had a severe headache two days ago. The headache is now subsiding, and the physical examination is normal. Should the possibility of a subarachnoid hemorrhage be evaluated, and if so, how?**

Yes. CT.

Note: A significant percentage of scans will be negative 48 hours after intracranial hemorrhage. However, an LP done 2 to 3 days after a bleed should still be positive, and xanthochromia typically persists for 7 to 10 days.

O   **An elderly patient presents with an altered mental status, a history of IDDM, and hypoglycemia. Core temperature is 32°C. What endocrinologic condition is likely?**

Myxedema coma. Other clues to look for are history of thyroid surgery, hypothyroidism, and use of anti-thyroid medications.

O   **What three conditions may cause a falsely low sodium concentration?**

Pseudohyponatremia may be caused by (1) hyperglycemia, (2) hyperlipidemia, or (3) hyperproteinemia.

O   **A patient presents with very low sodium and you suspect SIADH. What lab findings would confirm the diagnosis?**

Serum osmolality should be low; urine sodium and osmolality should be high. Treatment of severe symptomatic hyponatremia includes a loop diuretic, such as furosemide, and the simultaneous infusion of small boluses of 3% saline over 4 hours or normal saline. If hyponatremia is corrected too rapidly, neurologic sequelae may result.

O   **A young competitive figure skater complains of generalized weakness following practice. What might be the cause?**

Hypokalemic "paralysis" is a cause of acute weakness.

O   **How may hyperglycemic, hyperosmolar, non-ketotic coma be differ-entiated from DKA?**

In NKHC, serum osmolality is higher and pH is usually maintained at > 7.2. $NaHCO_3$ is normal in NKHC and depleted in DKA.

○ **How should non-ketotic hyperosmolar coma be treated?**

Fluids, fluids, and more fluids! Patients can be as much as 12 liters deficient. Give normal saline until adequate blood pressure and urinary output are established. Follow with half normal saline. When blood glucose falls to 250 to 300 mg, the solution should be changed to saline and glucose to avoid cerebral edema.

It is important to note that these patient's require very little insulin. Give as little as 5 to 10 units of insulin IV. However, they are commonly deficient in potassium and will need 10 to 15 mEq/hour once urine flow has been established. This disorder has a grave prognosis with up to a 50% mortality for severe cases.

○ **T/F: Phenytoin is the drug of choice for a patient with non-ketotic hyperosmolar coma who experiences a seizure.**

False. Phenytoin is contraindicated in patients with hyperglycemic, hyperosmolar, non-ketotic coma. The drugs of choice for this seizure disorder are lorazepam (Ativan) or diazepam (Valium). Phenobarbital use is also appropriate.

○ **Activated charcoal is not indicated for which types of overdose?**

Alcohol ingestion, electrolytes, heavy metals, lithium, hydrocarbons, and caustic ingestions.

○ **Which type of blood test is used to determine if a patient needs RhoGAM therapy?**

A Kleihauer-Betke checks for fetomaternal bleeding.

○ **A young patient has a threatened abortion in the first trimester. Laboratory studies reveal she is Rh negative and her husband is Rh positive. Treatment?**

The patient will need 50 μg of Rh immunoglobulin (RhoGAM) IM. After the first trimester, the dose is increased to 300 μg IM.

○ **What are the signs and symptoms of preeclampsia?**

Upper abdominal pain, headache, visual complaints, cardiac decompensation, creatinine greater than 2, proteinuria greater than 100 mg per deciliter, and a blood pressure of greater than 160 mm Hg systolic or 110 mm Hg diastolic. Preeclampsia is most common in nulliparous women late in pregnancy, typically after 20 weeks gestation. Look for edema, hypertension, and proteinuria to diagnose these pa-tients.

The emergency department treatment for preeclampsia is IV hydralazine titrated to a blood pressure of 90 to 110 diastolic using 5 mg boluses every 20 to 30 minutes. Blood pressure must be lowered slowly to avoid compromising the uteroplacental blood flow. Patients with moderate to severe preeclampsia need IV magnesium (though its true utility is not well demon-strated).

○ **What is the most commonly missed hip fracture?**

Femoral neck fracture.

○ **Which is more common, a medial or a lateral tibial plateau fracture?**

The lateral tibial plateau is most commonly fractured. If AP and lateral films are neg-ative, follow up with oblique views if you are suspicious of a tibial plateau fracture.

○ **What is the most commonly missed fracture in the elbow region?**

A radial head fracture. Like the navicular fracture, radiographic signs of a radial head fracture may not show up for days after the injury. A positive fat pad sign may be the only finding suggestive of this injury.

O   **What are the two most common errors made in the intubation of a neonate?**

1) Placing the neck in hyperextension; this moves the cords even more anteriorly.
2) Inserting the laryngoscope too far.

O   **What is the most common cause of food-borne viral gastroenteritis?**

Norwalk virus commonly found in shell fish.

O   **What are the symptoms of "Chinese Restaurant" syndrome?**

Headache, dizziness, abdominal discomfort, facial flushing, and chest or facial burning. Symptoms typically start within an hour of eating Chinese food.

O   **A patient is in anaphylactic shock. She happens to be taking ß-blockers. She is not responding to epinephrine. What alternative agents might you consider?**

Norepinephrine, diphenhydramine, and glucagon.

O   **A young boy is presented for evaluation after suffering a coral snake bite. He appears to be fine. What is appropriate management?**

Admit to the Intensive Care Unit and be ready for respiratory arrest. Coral snake venom is neurotoxic.

O   **Describe the appearance of a coral snake.**

This is a round snake with red, yellow, and black stripes and a black spot on the head. Coral snake bites typically do not cause immediate local pain, whereas viper bites do. Remember: "Red on yellow kills a fellow."

O   **Which type of rattlesnake bite leads to most deaths?**

The diamond back rattlesnake accounts for nearly all lethal snake bites in the US. However, it accounts for only 3% of the snake bites seen. Treat with 10 to 20 vials of antivenin.

O   **How does an thrill seeker recognize a pit viper?**

If he is close enough, he will observe heat sensing pits and an elliptical pupil that looks like a football standing on end.

O   **What are some common entities in the differential diagnosis of a limp or gait abnormality in a child?**

Legg-Calvé-Perthes disease (avascular necrosis of the femoral head), Osgood-Schlatter disease, avulsion of the tibial tubercle, infection, toxic transient tenosynovitis, patellofemoral subluxation, chondromalacia patella, slipped capital femoral epiphysis, septic arthritis, metatarsal fracture, proximal stress fracture, and toddler fracture (spiral tibia fracture).

O   **What treatment is recommended for a patient with a cluster headache?**

Treat as you would a migraine except skip ß-blockers, add O_2, and try lidocaine 4% in the ipsilateral nostril.

○ **What is the treatment for trigeminal neuralgia?**

Carbamazepine (Tegretol) 100 to 200 mg tid. Obtain baseline CBC and platelet count before starting carbamazepine.

○ **What is the only absolute contraindication to IVP?**

Profound hypotension—the kidneys can't be perfused. Two relative contraindications are renal insufficiency with a creatinine greater than 1.6 and a history of allergic reactions.

○ **What signs indicate an HIV positive patient is at increased risk for opportunistic infections like PCP?**

An absolute CD-4 count of less than 200 and a CD-4 lymphocytic percentage of less than 20.

○ **What are the National Institutes of Health's recommendations for treating spinal cord injuries?**

Give high dose methylprednisolone (Solu-Medrol) 30 mg/kg bolus over 15 minutes followed by 45 minutes normal saline drip. Over the subsequent 23 hours the patient should receive an infusion of 5.4 mg/kg/h of methylprednisolone.

○ **What is the most common cause of small bowel obstruction in the sur-gically virgin abdomen?**

Incarcerated hernia.

○ **A patient with a temperature of 29°C develops ventricular fibrillation. Is defibrillation likely to be successful?**

Defibrillation should be attempted but is unlikely to be successful at temperatures less than 29°C.

○ **T/F: The presentation of infectious endocarditis in an IV drug abusing patient does not usually include a murmur.**

True. Less than half present with a murmur.

○ **A straight (Miller) blade is preferred for intubating children of less than what age?**

4 years.

○ **What is the Parkland formula for treating a pediatric burn victim?**

Ringer's lactate 4 mL/% body surface area/kg over 24 hours with half given in first 8 hours. Large burns in children less than 5 years old may require colloid (5% albumin or fresh frozen plasma) at 1 mL/ % BSA/kg/day. This same formula is used for adults.

○ **How much fluid is required for maintenance of pediatric patients?**

100 mL/kg/day for each kg up to 10 kg, 50 mL/kg/day for each kg from 10 to 20 kg, and 20 mL/kg/day for each kg thereafter.

○ **When examining a lateral adult C-spine film, the predental space looks particularly wide. What width space is normal for an adult?**

Normal is 2.5 to 3 mm. If it is greater than 3 mm, consider that the transverse ligament has ruptured or is at least lax.

○　**What disease is commonly associated with central retinal vein occlu-sion?**

Hypertension.

○　**What are common eye findings in patients with AIDS?**

Cotton wool spots and CMV retinitis.

○　**With which types of injuries is Purtscher's retinopathy associated?**

Thoracic injuries and broken bones. Findings include retinal hemorrhage and cotton wool spots.

○　**What are the common features of central vertigo?**

Symptoms are gradual and continuous. They include focal signs, nausea, and vomiting. Hearing loss is rare.

○　**What are the signs and symptoms of peripheral vertigo?**

Symptoms are usually acute and intermittent. Hearing loss is common; nausea and vomiting are severe.

○　**In the evaluation of retropharyngeal abscess, what is the usual age of the patients, how do they present, what diagnostic tests are used in their evaluation, and what treatment modalities are recommended?**

Retropharyngeal abscess is most commonly seen in children less than 4 years old. Usual presentation is with dysphagia, a muffled voice, stridor, and a sensation of a lump in the throat. Patients usually prefer to lie supine. Diagnosis is made with a soft tissue lateral neck film which may demonstrate edema and air/fluid levels. CT may be useful. Treatment includes airway, IV antibiotics, and admission to the ICU. Intubation may rupture the abscess.

○　**The causes of epiglottitis include:**

H. influenzae is by far most common. *Pneumococcus*, *Staphylococcus*, and *Branhamella* may also be causes. Presentation is most common among children around age five.

○　**What is the usual cause of facial cellulitis in children less than 3 years of age?**

H. influenzae.

○　**A trauma patient presents with a complaint of severe burning pain in the upper extremities and associated neck pain. On physical examination, the patient has good strength in his upper extremities and no obvious neurologic deficits in the lower extremities. Although the C-spine series is negative, what problem is still suspected?**

Central cord syndrome. This injury is because of hyperextension of the spinal cord. Diagnostic findings include tingling, paresthesias, burning pain, and severe weakness or paralysis in the upper extremities with few or no symptoms in the lower extremities.

○　**An asthmatic patient suddenly develops a supraventricular tachycardia. Blood pressure is normal and the QRS complex is also narrow. What therapy is most appropriate?**

Verapamil. Avoid the use of adenosine as it is relatively contraindicated and may exacerbate bronchospasm in asthmatic patients. Also avoid ß-blockers.

O   **How is a laryngeal fracture diagnosed on plain films?**

On a lateral soft tissue x-ray of the C-spine, check for retropharyngeal air, and elevation of the hyoid bone. The hyoid bone is usually at the level of C3 if there is no evidence of a laryngeal frac-ture. Elevation of the hyoid bone above C3 suggests a laryngeal fracture.

O   **Differentiate between a hypertensive emergency and a hypertensive urgency.**

Hypertensive emergency: Elevated BP with end organ damage.

Hyptertensive urgency: Elevated BP with no symptoms or signs of end organ damage. DBP usu-ally > 115 mm Hg. Requires acute treatment.

O   **What are the antibiotics of choice in a wound resulting from a skin diving in-cident?**

Ciprofloxacin or TMP-SMX.

O   **How should a jellyfish sting be treated?**

Rinse with saline. Apply 5% acetic acid (vinegar) locally to the wound for approximately 30 minutes. In addition, corticosteroid agents may be applied topically. No antibiotics are necessary. Tetanus prophylaxis. Chironex flexeri antivenin only for this coelenterate.

O   **A young man was found on the street by police and is brought to the ED. He has a temperature of 105°F, altered mental status, and muscle rigidity. You find a bottle of thioridazine (Mellaril) in his pocket. What conditions should be considered?**

Neuroleptic malignant syndrome should be considered first.   Meningitis, encephalitis, hyperthyroidism, anticholinergic, strychnine poisoning, and heat stroke also come to mind. Patients may also have hypotension, hypertension, and tachycardia.

O   **When does dysbaric air embolism (DAE) typically occur?**

DAE develops within minutes of surfacing after a dive. Symptoms are sudden and dramatic; they include loss of consciousness, focal neurologic symptoms (such as monoplegia, convulsions, blindness, and confusion), and sensory disturbances. Sudden loss of consciousness or other acute neurologic deficits immediately after sur-facing is because of DAE unless proven otherwise. Treatment includes high flow oxygen and rapid transport for hyperbaric oxygen treatment.

O   **A 2-year-old has jammed a pencil into her lateral soft palate. What complication might develop?**

Ischemic stroke is a complication of soft palate pencil injuries which result in contralateral hemiparesis.

O   **What is the appropriate paralyzing agent to use when intubation is required in a seizing patient?**

Use pancuronium (Pavulon) because succinylcholine has a greater tendency to increase serum potassium and ICP.

O   **Distinguish the key differences between strychnine and tetanus poisoning.**

Tetanus poisoning produces constant muscle tension, whereas strychnine produces tetany and convulsions with episodes of relaxation between muscle contractions.

O   **What is the common name for *Dermacentor andersoni*?**

Wood tick.

❍ **What nerve supplies taste to the anterior two-thirds of the tongue and the lacrimal and salivary glands?**

Cranial nerve VII.

❍ **What disease is associated with anti-acetylcholine receptor antibodies that affect the postsynaptic neuromuscular site and is also more common in females with a peak incidence in the third decade of life?**

Myasthenia gravis. 50% of myasthenia gravis patients have thymomas, and 75% have lymphoid hyperplasia.

❍ **What antibiotics should be avoided in myasthenia gravis patients?**

Polymyxin and aminoglycoside have curare-like properties that may cause paralysis in these patients.

❍ **What is the treatment for myasthenia gravis?**

Steroids, thymectomy, immunosuppressive drugs, plasmapheresis, and cholinergic agents such as pyridostigmine.

❍ **Eaton-Lambert syndrome is associated with which class of diseases?**

Malignancies, particularly oat-cell carcinoma. Symptoms include aching muscle pain and; cranial nerves are usually not involved. Muscle strength may increase with repeated use in Eaton-Lambert syndrome, whereas it will decrease with use in Myasthenia gravis.

❍ **What is a chalazion?**

This is a Meibomian gland granuloma.

❍ **How should a chalazion be treated?**

Surgical curettage.

❍ **A patient presents with eye pain. She has a constricted pupil, ciliary flush, and red injected sclera at the limbus. Diagnosis?**

Acute iritis.

❍ **A patient presents with loss of central vision. Likely diagnosis?**

A retrobulbar neuritis is likely. MS is associated with about 25% of retrobulbar neuritis cases. Macular degeneration and central retinal vein occlusion can also lead to loss of central vision.

❍ **I am used to treat acute angle closure glaucoma (and occasionally in vain at-tempts to treat retinal artery occlusion). I also play a role in the treatment and prevention of acute mountain sickness. I decrease aqueous humor production via talent as a carbonic anhydrase inhibitor. Who am I?**

Acetazolamide (Diamox).

O   A patient presents with fever, neck pain or neck stiffness, and trismus. Examination reveals pharyngeal edema with tonsil displacement and edema of the parotid area. Diagnosis?

Parapharyngeal abscess.

O   A patient presents with hearing loss, nystagmus, facial weakness, and diplopia. Vertigo is provoked with sudden movement. A lumbar puncture reveals ele-vated CNS protein. What diagnosis is suspected?

An acoustic neuroma.

O   Can a parapharyngeal abscess present with an associated finding of edema in the area of the parotid gland?

Yes.

O   In a trauma patient, facial dimpling of the cheek is associated with:

Zygomatic arch fracture.

O   What x-rays should be ordered to diagnose a fracture of the zygoma?

A jug handle, Water's view, or submental view.

O   Describe Stevens-Johnson syndrome?

It is a bullous form of erythema multiforme that involves mucous membranes. It may cause corneal ulcerations, an-terior uveitis, or blindness.

O   Blood is originating from a tooth after trauma. What is the Ellis classification?

3.

O   What are the most common drugs causing TEN?

Phenylbutazone, barbiturates, sulfa drugs, anti-epileptics, and antibiotics.

O   Rhomboid-shaped crystals from a joint aspiration are associated with:

Pseudogout.

O   Needle-shaped crystals are associated with:

Gout.

O   Where is the most common site of aseptic necrosis?

The hip.

O   What is the acute treatment for gout?

Colchicine, indomethacin, and other NSAIDs.

O   What is the most common presentation of a Charcot's joint?

A swollen ankle and a "bag of bones" appearance on x-ray.

❍   **What is the most common cause of a Charcot's joint?**

Diabetic peripheral neuropathy.

❍   **What is the most common tendon affected in calcified tendonitis?**

The supraspinatus.

❍   **Which epicondyle is involved in tennis elbow?**

The lateral epicondyle.

❍   **Where is the most common site of infectious arthritis?**

The knee, followed by the hip. *Staphylococcus* is the most common cause.

❍   **At what cervical level is the thyroid located?**

It's located at the level of the fourth cervical vertebra.

❍   **Where is the most common site of cervical disc herniation?**

C5–C6. Patient will complain of bilateral shoulder pain.

❍   **What nerve is located in the tarsal tunnel?**

The tibial nerve.

❍   **A patient has difficulty squatting and standing. What is the most likely spinal pathology?**

L4 root compression with involvement of quadriceps.

❍   **What STD pathogens cause painful ulcers?**

Type II Genital herpes and chancroid.

STD	Ulcer	Node
Genital herpes	Painful	Painful
Chancroid	Painful	Painful
Syphilis	Painless	Less painful
Lymphogranuloma venereum	Painless	Moderately painful

❍   **A patient presents with a complaint of pain at the site of the deltoid insertion with radiation into the back of the arm (C5 distribution). On examination, there is increased pain with active abduction from 70° to 120°. X-rays reveal calcification at the tendinous insertion of the greater tuberosity. Diagnosis?**

Supraspinatus tendonitis.

❍   **An absent knee jerk involves which spinous level?**

L4.

❍   **An absent Achilles reflex involves which spinous level?**

S1.

○ **Paresthesia of the great toe involves which spinous level?**

L5.

○ **Paresthesia of the little toe involves which spinous level?**

S1.

○ **Where is the most common site of compartment syndrome?**

The anterior compartment of the leg.

○ **Describe the leg position associated with an anterosuperior hip dislocation.**

Leg is externally rotated with a slight abduction. In the pubic type, the hip is extended; in the iliac type, it is slightly flexed.

○ **Describe the leg position associated with an obturator hip dislocation.**

External rotation, flexion, and abduction.

○ **Describe the leg position associated with posterior hip dislocation.**

Internal rotation, flexion, and adduction.

○ **A patient in the emergency department cannot recall ever having a tetanus shot. The nurse gives him a tetanus shot. Later, he develops a hypersensitivity reaction and recalls that he recently had a tetanus shot. Which type of reaction does he have?**

Type 3—an Arthus reaction caused by immune complexes or antigen-antibody complexes that activate complement and platelets forming aggregates and complexes with IgE.

○ **A positive TB test is which type of reaction?**

Type 4. Cells are mediated, hypersensitivity is delayed, and neither complements nor antibodies are involved.

○ **What drugs commonly cause erythema multiforme?**

Carbamazepine, penicillin, sulfa, pyrazolone, phenytoin, and barbiturates.

○ **What aerobe is most commonly found in cutaneous abscesses?**

Staphylococcus aureus.

○ **What is the most common gram-negative aerobe found in cutaneous ab-scesses?**

Proteus mirabilis.

○ **Describe the Gram stain appearance of Staphylococcus aureus.**

Gram-positive cocci in grape-like clusters.

○   **What is the cause of erysipelas?**

Group A ß-hemolytic streptococcus.

○   **How is erysipelas treated?**

With penicillin—or erythromycin for allergic patients.

○   **A child presents with a history of fever, conjunctival hyperemia, and erythema of the mucous membranes with desquamation. Diagnosis?**

Kawasaki's disease. Lesions may resemble erythema multiforme.

○   **What are some common causes of prerenal acute renal failure?**

Volume depletion and decreased effective volume (CHF, sepsis, cirrhosis).

○   **What are the causes of post renal failure?**

Ureteral and urethral obstruction.

○   **What findings mark the presentation of a patient with rapidly progressive glomerulonephritis?**

Hematuria (most common), edema (periorbital), HTN, ascites, pleural effusion, rales, and anuria.

○   **What arrhythmia is frequently encountered during renal dialysis?**

Hypokalemia induced ventricular fibrillation.

○   **In which trimester of pregnancy is UTI and pyelonephritis most common?**

Third.

○   **What is inflammation of the foreskin called?**

Balanitis or balanoposthitis.

○   **What is phimosis?**

A condition in which the foreskin cannot be retracted posterior to the glans. The preliminary treatment is a dorsal slit.

○   **What is paraphimosis?**

A condition in which the foreskin is retracted posterior to the glands and cannot be advanced over the glans.

○   **What causes priapism?**

Prolonged sex, leukemia, sickle cell trait and disease, blood dyscrasias, pelvic hematoma or neoplasm, syphilis, urethritis, and drugs including phenothiazine, prazosin, tolbutamide, anticoagulants, and corticosteroids.

○   **What causes a greenish gray frothy vaginal discharge with mild itching?**

Trichomonas vaginitis. On physical examination, the cervix will have a strawberry appearance 20% of the time.

O   **Describe the presentation of a patient with *Gardnerella* vaginitis?**

On physical examination, note a frothy, grayish white, fishy smelling vaginal discharge. Wet mount may show clue cells (clusters of bacilli on the surface of epithelial cells).

O   **Do you know why I hate it when my foot falls asleep during the day?**

It'll be up all night!

O   **Sulfamethoxazole may lead to hemolysis in a patient with what disorder?**

G6PD deficiency.

O   **Painless third trimester vaginal bleeding likely represents:**

Placenta previa.

O   **Painful third trimester vaginal bleeding likely represents:**

Abruptio placenta.

O   **What effect does pregnancy have on BUN and creatinine?**

Both are decreased. This is as the result of increased renal blood flow and increased glomerular filtration rate.

O   **When can one auscultate the fetal heart?**

Ultrasound: 6 weeks.
Doppler: 10 to 12 weeks.
Stethoscope: 18 to 20 weeks.

O   **Describe a Brudzinski sign.**

Flexion of the neck produces flexion of the knees.

O   **Describe Kernig's sign.**

Extension of the knees from the flexed thigh position results in strong passive resistance.

O   **What is the normal opening pressure in a spinal tap?**

15 cm H_2O.

O   **What is the normal CSF protein level?**

40 mg/dL.

O   **What does the India ink test show?**

Cryptococcus neoformans.

○   **What is the most significant pathophysiologic mechanism of death from cyclic antidepressants?**

Myocardial depression, including hypotension and conduction blocks.

○   **What are some common side effects of phenothiazine use?**

Malaise, hyperthermia, tachycardia, anticholinergic effects, and quinidine-like membrane stabilization. The most dangerous side effect is neuroleptic malignant syndrome.

○   **How should stable ventricular tachyarrhythmias associated with phenothiazine overdose be treated?**

Lidocaine and phenytoin.

○   **What antibiotic may either increase or decrease lithium secretion?**

Tetracycline.

○   **How is lithium overdose treated?**

Lavage, saline diuresis, furosemide, and hemodialysis. Alkalinization may be appropriate.

○   **Is phenobarbital more quickly metabolized by children or by adults?**

Adults. Neonates are especially slow at metabolizing phenobarbital.

○   **How should barbiturate poisoning be treated?**

Support, charcoal, alkalinization of the urine, charcoal hemoperfusion, or hemodialy-sis.

○   **What drugs increase the half-life of phenytoin?**

Sulfonamides, isoniazid, dicumarol, and chloramphenicol.

○   **What hypersensitivity skin rashes are noted with phenytoin use?**

Lupus-like and Stevens-Johnson syndrome.

○   **What are the cardiac effects of phenytoin?**

It inhibits sodium channels, decreases the effective refractory period and automaticity in the Purkinje fibers. It has little effect on QRS width or action potential duration.

○   **What is the lethal dose of phenytoin?**

20 mg/kg.

○   **What symptoms are expected with a phenytoin level of > 20, > 30, and > 40 μg/mL?**

> 20: Lateral gaze nystagmus.
> 30: Lateral gaze nystagmus plus increased vertical nystagmus with upward gaze.
> 40: Lethargy, confusion, dysarthrias, and psychosis.

○   **What is the most common causative bacterium associated with right-sided endo-carditis in IV drug abusers?**

Staphylococcus aureus. Left-sided endocarditis in IV drug abusers is usually due to *E. coli*, *Streptococcus*, *Klebsiella*, *Pseudomonas*, or *Candida*.

○   **A heroin addict presents with pulmonary edema. What is the best treatment?**
Naloxone, O_2, and ventilatory support (not diuretics).

○   **What is the most common neurologic complication of IV drug abuse?**

Nontraumatic mononeuritis (i.e., painless weakness 2 to 3 hours after injection).

○   **Name two frequently observed organisms causing septic arthritis in drug ad-dicts.**

Serratia and *Pseudomonas*. These are rare causes in non-addicts.

○   **An alcoholic patient presents with complaints of abdominal pain and blurred vision. The patient is very photophobic, and blood gases reveal a metabolic acidosis. Diagnosis?**

Methanol poisoning. Patients may describe seeing something resembling a snow-storm.

○   **What is the lethal dose of methanol?**

30 mL. Formate levels in methanol poisoning are greatest in vitreous humor.

○   **What is clonidine's mechanism of action?**

Clonidine is a central acting a-agonist. It leads to decreased sympathetic outflow and lowers catecholamine levels.

○   **What alcohol poisoning is suggested by a plasma bicarbonate level of zero (cipher, null, empty set, zip, Ø)?**

Methanol. It also produces a large osmolar gap and a large anion gap. Methanol poisoning is treated with IV ethanol and hemodialysis.

○   **Positive birefringent calcium oxalate crystals in the urine are pathognomonic for poisoning with what substance?**

Ethylene glycol. The lethal dose of ethylene glycol is 100 mL.

○   **What are the signs and symptoms of ethylene glycol poisoning?**

Hallucinations, nystagmus, ataxia, papilledema, and a large anion gap.

○   **How should ethylene glycol poisoning be treated?**

This should be treated with gastric lavage, sodium bicarbonate, thiamine and pyridoxine, IV ethanol, and hemodialysis.

○   **A patient presents with ataxia, altered mental status, and sixth nerve palsy. What is your diagnosis?**

Wernicke's encephalopathy.

○   **What are the signs and symptoms of isopropanol poisoning?**

Sweet breath odor (acetone), hypotension, hemorrhagic gastritis, and CNS depression from isopropanol and from its metabolite, acetone.

○   **What is the treatment of cocaine toxicity?**

Sedate with benzodiazepine. Treat unresponsive hypertension with nitroprusside or phentolamine.

○   **What is the x-ray finding in a patient with salicylate toxicity?**

Noncardiogenic pulmonary edema.

○   **Describe the effects of salicylate poisoning on the central nervous system.**

Lethargy, confusion, seizures, and respiratory arrest.

○   **Salicylate levels should ideally be checked how long after an inges-tion?**

6 hours.

○   **What is the minimum toxic dose of salicylates?**

150 mg/kg.

○   **What salicylate level, measured 6 hours after ingestion, is as-soci-ated with toxicity?**

45 mg/dL.

○   **What Acetaminophen level, measured 4 hours after ingestion, is associated with toxicity?**

150 μg/mL.

○   **Alkalinization of urine will increase the excretion of which drugs?**

Cyclic antidepressants, salicylates, and long-acting barbiturates.

○   **What are the signs of salicylate poisoning?**

Hyperventilation, hyperthermia, mental status change, nausea, vomiting, abdominal pain, dehydration, diaphoresis, ketonuria, metabolic acidosis, and respiratory alkalosis.

○   **A child presents with lethargy, seizures, and hypoglycemia. He has had viral syndrome symptoms for several days. Mom states she has only been giving him aspirin. Name two disorders that should be considered.**

Reye's syndrome and salicylate intoxication.

○   **What laboratory test can aid in the evaluation of a possible toxic iron ingestion?**

Total iron binding capacity measured 3 to 5 hours after ingestion. If serum iron level is significantly less than the total iron binding capacity, a toxic iron ingestion is less likely.

○   **What is the antidote for a toxic ingestion of iron?**

Deferoxamine chelates only free iron. It should be given if the iron level is greater than 350 μg/dL.

O   **Which type of hydrocarbons are most toxic?**

Substances with low viscosities (measured in Saybolt Seconds Universal (SSU)) are more toxic than compounds with high viscosities. Gasoline, kerosene, and paint thinner (all aliphatic hydrocarbons with SSUs < 60) are all more toxic than motor oil, tar, and petroleum jelly, which all have SSUs > 100. Of the compounds with SSUs < 60, the most toxic are those that are not aliphatic, including benzene, toluene, xylene, and tetrachloroethylene.

O   **Where is the most reliable site for detecting central cyanosis?**

The tongue.

O   **You are taking boards and are presented with a patient who has a history of abdominal aortic aneurysm. The patient has been vomiting coffee grind emesis. What infrequent entity needs to be con-sidered?**

The dreaded aortoenteric fistula. Patients may present with a limited herald bleed before massive bleeding develops. A CT showing air in the periaortic area indicates the need for immediate surgery. An aortoenteric fistula may also follow aortic graft surgery.

O   **What is a common complication of pancuronium?**

Tachycardia from its vagolytic action.

O   **What is the most common cause of hypermagnesemia in a patient with renal failure?**

Patient use of compounds high in magnesium, such as antacids. This can result in neuromuscular paralysis. Consider IV calcium. Saline and furosemide assisted diuresis may not help a patient with renal failure, so consider dialysis as well.

O   **How much energy should be used to cardiovert an unstable infant with a wide complex tachycardia?**

0.5 to 1.0 J/kg.

O   **How much energy should be used to cardiovert unstable VF in an infant?**

2 J/kg.

O   **What is the most common malposition of the nasotracheal tube?**

The piriform sinus. The second most common malposition is the esophagus.

O   **What is the most common physical sign of a PE?**

Tachypnea.

O   **What are the three most common presenting signs of aortic stenosis?**

Syncope, angina, and heart failure.

O   **In an MI, when do CK levels begin to rise, and when do they peak?**

CK levels begin to rise at 6 to 8 hours; they peak at 24 to 30; and they stabilize at 48.

○   **In an MI, when does LDH begin to rise, and when does it peak?**

LDH-I (from heart) begins to rise at 12 to 24 hours; it peaks at 48 to 96.

○   **What is the effect of nitrates on preload and afterload?**

Nitrates mostly dilate veins and venules to decrease preload.

○   **Inferior wall MIs commonly lead to what two types of heart block (via mechanism of damage to autonomic fibers in the atrial septum giving increased vagal tone impairing AV node conduction)?**

First degree AV block and Mobitz Type I (Wenckebach) second degree AV block. Sinus bradycardia can also occur. Progression to complete AV block is not common.

○   **Anterior wall MIs may directly damage intracardiac conduction. This may lead to which type of arrhythmias?**

The dangerous type! A Mobitz II second degree AV block can suddenly progress to complete AV block.

○   **What are the potential, often rare, complications of Mycoplasma pneumonia?**

Non-pulmonary: Hemolytic anemia, aseptic meningitis, encephalitis, Guillain-Barré syndrome, pericarditis, and myocarditis

Pulmonary: ARDS, atelectasis, mediastinal adenopathy, pneumothorax, pleural effusion, and abscess

○   **Under what conditions should staphylococcal pneumonia be considered as a possible diagnosis?**

Although it only accounts for 1% of bacterial pneumonias, it should be considered in patients with sudden chills, hectic fever, pleurisy, and cough—especially following a viral illness, such as measles or influenza.

○   **Of the following anesthetics, which has the shortest duration of action—lidocaine, procaine, bupivacaine, or mepivacaine?**

Procaine.

○   **What is the differential diagnosis of a ring lesion on CT scan?**

Toxoplasmosis, lymphoma, fungal infection, TB, CMV, Kaposi's sarcoma, and hemorrhage.

○   **Does erythema multiforme itch?**

Not typically. It may be tender.

○   **A patient presents with granuloma inguinale. What does it look like?**

Papular, nodular, or vesicular painless lesions. These can result in extensive destruc-tion of local tissues. Cause is *Calymmatobacterium granulomatis.*

○   **What causes chancroid?**

Haemophilus ducreyi.

○   **Describe lesions associated with chlamydia.**

Painless, shallow ulcerations, papular or nodular lesions, and herpetiform vesicles that wax and wane.

○   **Which type of diarrhea-causing disease may be transmitted by pets?**

Yersinia.

○   **What state is associated with akinetic mutism?**

Abulic state, which is like a coma vigil. Patients seem awake and may have their eyes open. They respond to questions very slowly. The cause is typically due to depressed frontal lobe function.

○   **What is normal systolic blood pressure in a newborn?**

60 mm Hg.

○   **What is the initial drug of choice to treat SVT in a pediatric patient?**

Adenosine 0.1 mg/kg is drug of choice. Digoxin 0.02 mg/kg may take ~ 4 hours for conversion. Verapamil may be used in children > 2 years of age; however, it is has caused several deaths in children younger than 2. Synchronized cardioversion at 0.5 to 1.0 J/kg.

○   **After the first month of life, what is the cause of meningitis and the number one cause of pneumonia in children?**

Meningitis: *H. influenzae.*
Pneumonia: *Streptococcus pneumoniae. H. influenzae* is the second most common cause.

○   **Discuss infantile spasms.**

Onset is by 3 to 9 months of age. It typically lasts seconds, and may occur in single episodes or bursts. The EEG is often abnormal. 85% of these patients will be mentally handicapped.

○   **Hepatic failure is commonly associated with what anticonvulsant?**

Valproic acid.

○   **Does H. influenzae typically cause abscesses?**

No.

○   **What drugs, activities, and cooking habits are associated with an increased clearance of theophylline (decreasing the theophylline level)?**

Phenytoin, phenobarbital, cigarette smoking, and charcoal barbecuing.

○   **Anaphylaxis is a common cause of which type of renal failure?**

Prerenal.

○   **What are the end products of methanol, ethylene glycol, and isopropyl alcohol metabolism?**

Methanol: Formate.
Ethylene glycol: Oxalate and formate.
Isopropyl alcohol: Acetone.

○   **Which type of alcohol ingestion is associated with hypocalcemia?**

Ethylene glycol.

○   **Which type of alcohol ingestion is associated with hemorrhagic pancreatitis?**

Methanol.

○   **For what disorder is vigorous digital massage of the orbit indicated?**

Central retinal artery occlusion. Do not do this in central vein occlusion!

○   **What pathogen is suggested by a pneumonia with a single rigor?**

Pneumococcus.

○   **What pathogen does a strawberry cervix suggest?**

Trichomonas.

○   **What are the key features of Ellis Type I, II, and III dental fractures?**

Type I: Enamel, dentin, and pulp.
Type II: Enamel, dentin, and pulp.
Type III: Pulp bleeds.

○   **What is the vector and causative organism of Lyme's disease?**

The vector is *Ixodes dammini*, and the organism is *Borrelia burgdorferi*. It is the most frequently transmitted tick-borne disease.

○   **What causes Q fever?**

Coxiella burnetii, also known as *Rickettsia burnetii*. It is found in the *Dermacentor andersoni* tick.

○   **What is a hordeolum?**

A Meibomian gland infection, usually of the upper lid.

○   **Where are the three most common locations of malignant melanomas?**

(1) The skin, (2) eye, and (3) anal canal.

○   **What is the initial dose of blood given to children?**

10 mL/kg of packed RBCs.

○   **What is achalasia?**

Disorder of esophageal motility and incomplete relaxation of the lower esophagus.

❍   **Other than laparotomy, what invasive examination will confirm suspected mesenteric ischemia?**

Angiography.

❍   **Name four enterotoxin-producing organisms that can cause food poisoning.**

(1) *Clostridium*, (2) *Staphylococcus aureus*, (3) *Vibrio cholerae*, and (4) *E. coli*.

❍   **Antibiotics should be avoided with what infectious diarrhea?**

Salmonella. Clear exceptions are severe cases of diarrhea in immunocompromised patients and in children less than 6 months old.

❍   **Name three disorders associated with decreased DTRs.**

(1) Guillain-Barré, (2) tick paralysis due to *Dermacentor andersoni* (wood tick) bite, and (3) diphtheria exotoxin.

❍   **What is the most likely cause of CHF in a premature infant?**

PDA.

❍   **What is the most likely cause of CHF in the first 3 days of life?**

Transposition of the great vessels which leads to cyanosis and failure.

❍   **In the first week of life?**

Hypoplastic left ventricle.

❍   **In the second week of life?**

Coarctation.

❍   **Do you treat *Shigella* with antibiotics?**

In general, yes.

❍   **What is a pinguecula?**

It is a yellowish nodule, particularly on the nasal aspect of the eye, but it may be lateral. It is often caused by wind and dust.

❍   **What is a pterygium?**

It is a chronic growth over the medial or lateral aspect of the cornea approaching the pupil. It is much thicker than pingueculae.

❍   **What is the most common cause of painless upper GI bleeding in an infant or child?**

Varices from portal hypertension.

❍   **What is the most common cause of major painless lower GI bleeding in an infant or child?**

Meckel's diverticulum.

❍   **What is the most common cause of orbital cellulitis?**

Staphylococcus aureus.

❍   **Who should receive prophylaxis after exposure to *Neisseria meningitidis*?**

People living or having close contact with the patient.

❍   **Name some hydrocarbons that are considered to be the most toxic and have SSUs under 60.**

Aromatic hydrocarbons, halogenated hydrocarbons, mineral seal oil, kerosene, naphtha, turpentine, gasoline and lighter fluid. Those considered less toxic (with SSUs over 100) include grease, diesel oil, mineral oil, petroleum jelly, paraffin wax, and tar.

❍   **What drug is absolutely contraindicated when treating hydrocarbon poisoning?**

Epinephrine, as it sensitizes the myocardium and potentially leads to arrest.

❍   **What drug is contraindicated in a glue sniffing patient?**

Epinephrine. Like solvent abusers, these patients may be scared to death.

❍   **What is a delayed complication of acid ingestion?**

Pyloric stricture.

❍   **What is the difference between carbamates and organophosphates?**

Carbamates produce similar symptoms as organophosphates, however, the bonds in car-bamate toxicity are reversible.

❍   **A patient presents with miotic pupils, muscle fasciculations, diaphore-sis, and diffuse oral and bronchial secretions. The patient has a garlic odor on his breath. What is your diagnosis?**

Organophosphate poisoning.

❍   **What ECG changes may be associated with organophosphate poisoning?**

Prolongation of the QT interval, and ST and T wave abnormalities.

❍   **What is the key laboratory finding in the diagnosis of organophosphate poison-ing?**

Decreased RBC cholinesterase activity. The serum cholinesterase level (pseudocholinesterase) is more sensitive but less specific. RBC cholinesterase is regenerated slowly and can take months to approach normal levels.

❍   **What is the treatment for organophosphate poisoning?**

Decontaminate, charcoal, atropine, and pralidoxime prn.

❍   **What are the key features in the diagnosis of trench foot?**

Trench foot represents a superficial partial burn with no deep tissue damage. It results from exposure to wet and cold (above freezing) for 1 to 2 days.

○   **What is chilblain?**

Chilblain is prolonged exposure to dry cold.

○   **What is the sequence of arrhythmia development in a patient with hypothermia?**

Bradycardia, atrial fibrillation, ventricular fibrillation and asystole.

○   **What is the common pathogen in a cat bite?**

Pasteurella multocida.

○   **What would you expect to find in the hippocampus of a patient with rabies?**

Negri bodies. Incubation for rabies is 30 to 60 days. Treatment includes cleaning of the wound, rabies immune globulin, and human diploid cell vaccine. Remember, half the rabies immune globulin goes around the wound; the other half goes IM.

○   **How do you treat the bite of a Megalopyge opercularis caterpillar?**

Calcium gluconate, 10 mL of a 10% solution IV. Stings cause immediate rhythmic pain.

○   **What kind of tick transmits Rocky Mountain spotted fever (RMSF)?**

The female andersoni tick. It transmits *Rickettsia rickettsii.*

○   **What is the most common symptom in RMSF?**

Headache. This occurs in 90% of patients.

○   **Describe the skin lesion seen in Lyme disease.**

A large distinct circular skin lesion called erythema chronicum migrans. It is an annular erythematous lesion with central clearing.

○   **Describe a patient with tick paralysis.**

Bulbar paralysis, ascending flaccid paralysis, paresthesias of hands and feet, symmetric loss of deep tendon reflexes, and respiratory paralysis.

○   **What drug is contraindicated in a Gila monster bite?**

Meperidine (Demerol), as it may be synergistic with venom.

○   **What is the most common causative organism of otitis externa?**

Pseudomonas sp.

○   **What are the signs and symptoms of Lyme disease, stages I through III?**

Stage I: Erythema chronicum migrans, malaise, fatigue, headache, arthralgias, fever, and chills.

Stage II: Neurologic and cardiac symptoms that include headache, meningoencephalitis, facial nerve palsy, radiculoneuropathy, ophthalmitis, and first, second, and third degree AV blocks.

Stage III: Arthritis (knee > shoulder > elbow > TMJ > ankle > wrist > hip > hands > feet).

○   **A diver levels off at 33 feet. How many atmospheres of pressure is she experiencing?**

2 atm. Starting with 1 atm at sea level, atmospheric pressure doubles every 33 ft (10 meters).

○   **A person working in a plant making chemical deodorizers was exposed to phenol. What is a possible field treatment?**

Clean him or her with olive oil and water.

○   **What are the most common complaints in a patient with carbon monoxide poisoning?**

A headache is most common, followed by dizziness, weakness, and nausea.

○   **What signs and symptoms are expected after radiation exposures of 100 REM, 300 REM, 400 REM, and 2000 REM, less than 2 hours after exposure?**

100 REM: Nausea and vomiting.
300 REM: Erythema.
400 REM: Diarrhea.
2000 REM: Seizures.

○   **What drug blocks the uptake of radioactive iodine?**

Potassium iodine.

○   **Psilocybin mushroom is associated with:**

Hallucinations.

○   **With brain stem herniation, is decorticate or decerebrate posturing expected?**

Decerebrate posturing (hyperextension). Decorticate posturing is flexion of the upper extremities and extension of the lower extremities.

○   **A patient presents after experiencing trauma to the head. He has an elevated systolic blood pressure and bradycardia. What is this reflex?**

Cushing reflex.

○   **What are the three components to the Glasgow coma scale, and how many points is each worth?**

Eye opening: 4 points.
Verbal response: 5 points.
Motor response: 6 points.

○   **What is the name for a flexion mechanism fracture through the anterior aspect of a vertebral body that is associated with ligamentous damage and an ante-rior cord syndrome?**

A teardrop fracture.

○   **What nerves control the corneal reflex?**

The ophthalmic branch of the fifth nerve and the afferent branch of the facial (seventh) nerve.

❍ **Name the most unstable C-spine injuries.**

Rupture of transverse atlantal ligament > dens fracture > burst fracture (flexion teardrop) > bilateral facet dislocation.

❍ **What is the eponym for a C1 burst fracture from vertical compression?**

Jefferson fracture.

❍ **A patient in a motor vehicle accident sustains a hyperextension injury to the neck. Plain films reveal a C2 bilateral facet fracture through the pedicles. You describe this fracture in consultation with the neurosurgeon. Which type of fracture have you de-scribed?**

A hangman's fracture.

❍ **A patient has an avulsion fracture of the spinous process of C7 with a history of a hyperflexion mechanism. Diagnosis?**

Clay shoveler's fracture—a fracture involving the spinous process of C6, C7, or T1. The mechanism is usually flexion or a direct blow.

❍ **A patient suffers a bilateral interfacetal dislocation. What is your concern?**

Injury occurs as a result of flexion, and the C-spine is very unstable with ligament disruption.

❍ **Stable or unstable: Clay shoveler's fracture?**

Stable.

❍ **Stable or unstable: fracture of the posterior arch of C1?**

Stable.

❍ **Name the four stable C-spine fractures.**

(1) Simple wedge, (2) clay shoveler's, (3) pillar, and (4) C1 posterior neural arch. All other C-spine fractures are unstable or potentially unstable.

❍ **A patient presents after receiving a blow to the forehead. Her neck is hyperextended, and she complains of weakness in her arms and minimal weakness in her lower extremities. Diagnosis?**

Central cord syndrome.

❍ **You see a patient with an obvious traumatic spinal cord lesion. On physical examination, he has motor paralysis, loss of gross proprioception, loss of vibratory sensation on one side, and loss of pain and temperature sensation on the opposite side. Diagnosis?**

Brown-Séquard's syndrome.

❍ **What is the most common cause of shock in patients with blunt chest trauma?**

Pelvic (or extremity) fracture concomitant with massive bleeding.

❍ **What is a frequent complication of ethmoid sinusitis?**

Orbital cellulitis.

O   **Where is the most common site of aspiration pneumonitis?**

Right lower lobe.

O   **What are the most common ECG findings associated with a myocardial contusion?**

ST and T wave abnormalities.

O   **What is the most common valvular injury associated with blunt cardiac injury?**

A ruptured aortic valve.

O   **Where is the most common site of a traumatic aortic laceration?**

The vast majority of these lacerations occur just distal to the left subclavian artery.

O   **A patient presents with high speed traumatic injury to the chest. A systolic murmur over the precordium is auscultated. The patient has a slightly hoarse voice, and her pulse is stronger in the upper extremities. Diagnosis?**

Traumatic rupture of the aorta.

O   **What is the most common x-ray finding in traumatic rupture of the aorta?**

Widening of the superior mediastinum.

O   **What is the most accurate x-ray finding in traumatic rupture of the aorta?**

Rightward deviation of the esophagus greater than 1 to 2 cm.

O   **A patient presents with a history of chest trauma, a systolic murmur, and an infarct pattern on ECG. Diagnosis?**

Traumatic ventricular septal defect. X-rays would show widening of the superior mediastinum and rightward deviation of the esophagus greater than 1 to 2 cm.

O   **A patient who has been involved in a motor vehicle accident has x-ray findings of retroperitoneal air seen on a flat plate of the abdomen. What is a likely diagnosis?**

Duodenal injury. Tentative test is a contrast study with gastrograffin. Extravasation confirms a duodenal injury.

O   **On an x-ray of the hand, the AP view shows a triangular shaped lunate. Diagnosis?**

Lunate dislocation. Lateral films will reveal what resembles a cup spilling water.

O   **What x-ray view is required to diagnose a perilunate dislocation?**

Lateral view.

O   **A patient presents with a snapping sensation in the wrist and a click. The x-ray of a patient's hand reveals a 3 mm space between the scaphoid and the lunate. What is your diagnosis**

Scaphoid dislocation.

○   **In a boxer's fracture, how much angulation of the fifth metacarpal neck is acceptable.**

50 degrees.

○   **What ligament in the hand is commonly injured in a fall while skiing?**

Thumb MCP joint ulnar collateral ligament rupture (Gamekeeper's thumb).

○   **Posterior dislocation of the shoulder is often missed with a standard ra-diographic shoulder series. What x-ray view aids in this diagnosis?**

The scapular Y view.

○   **Name the four muscles of the rotator cuff.**

(1) Supraspinatus, (2) infraspinatus, (3) teres minor, and (4) the subscapularis. Patients with a rotator cuff tear will not be able to fully abduct or internally or externally rotate the arm.

○   **What is the usual mechanism of injury in a supracondylar fracture?**

A fall on the outstretched arm.

○   **What artery is commonly injured with a supracondylar fracture?**

Brachial artery.

○   **What nerve is commonly injured with a supracondylar fracture?**

Injury to the anterior interosseous nerve, which is a branch of the median nerve.

○   **On x-ray of the elbow, you find a posterior fat pad sign. Diagnosis?**

Occult fracture, such as a supracondylar fracture of the humerus. Posterior fat pad seen on a lateral radiograph of the flexed elbow is usually due to hemarthrosis caused by a fracture.

○   **What nerve injury is associated with a medial epicondyle fracture?**

Ulnar nerve.

○   **About how many liters of blood can a patient lose in the retroperitoneal space?**

6 L.

○   **Which type of pelvic fracture has the greatest amount of bleeding?**

Vertical sheer.

○   **What nerve may be injured with a knee dislocation?**

The peroneal nerve.

○   **Where are the most common sites of stress fractures in the foot?**

Second and third metatarsals.

○ **What is the most common cause of superior vena cava obstruction?**

Bronchogenic carcinoma.

Thoracic.

○ **Where is the most common site of bursitis?**

Olecranon.

○ **What is the most common cause of subarachnoid hemorrhage in teenagers?**

AV malformations.

○ **A patient presents with a painful, red eye and a decrease in visual acuity. What is the differential?**

Central corneal lesions, glaucoma, and iritis.

○ **What are the most common findings of osteomyelitis on x-ray?**

Periosteal elevation and demineralization.

○ **What is the most common cause of acute aortic regurgitation?**

Infectious endocarditis.

○ **What is the most common congenital valvular disease?**

Bicuspid aortic valve.

○ **What infarct is most commonly associated with acute mitral regurgitation?**

Inferior wall.

○ **What metabolic abnormality is commonly associated with hypercalcemia?**

Up to one-third will have hypokalemia.

○ **What form of hepatitis is most commonly transmitted through blood transfusions?**

Hepatitis C.

○ **On funduscopic examination, microaneurysms and soft exudates are typical of:**

Hypertension.

○ **On funduscopic examination, macular microaneurysms and hard exudates are typical of:**

Diabetes.

○ **What is the most common cause of retrobulbar optic neuritis?**